New Perspective in Atrial Fibrillation

New Perspective in Atrial Fibrillation

Editor

Charles Guenancia

MDPI • Basel • Beijing • Wuhan • Barcelona • Belgrade • Manchester • Tokyo • Cluj • Tianjin

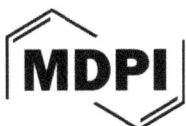

Editor
Charles Guenancia
Cardiology, Dijon University Hospital
Université de Bourgogne-Franche-Comté
Dijon
France

Editorial Office
MDPI
St. Alban-Anlage 66
4052 Basel, Switzerland

This is a reprint of articles from the Special Issue published online in the open access journal *Journal of Clinical Medicine* (ISSN 2077-0383) (available at: www.mdpi.com/journal/jcm/special_issues/atrial_fibrillation_research).

For citation purposes, cite each article independently as indicated on the article page online and as indicated below:

LastName, A.A.; LastName, B.B.; LastName, C.C. Article Title. *Journal Name* **Year**, *Volume Number*, Page Range.

ISBN 978-3-0365-1822-0 (Hbk)
ISBN 978-3-0365-1821-3 (PDF)

© 2021 by the authors. Articles in this book are Open Access and distributed under the Creative Commons Attribution (CC BY) license, which allows users to download, copy and build upon published articles, as long as the author and publisher are properly credited, which ensures maximum dissemination and a wider impact of our publications.

The book as a whole is distributed by MDPI under the terms and conditions of the Creative Commons license CC BY-NC-ND.

Contents

About the Editor vii

Preface to "New Perspective in Atrial Fibrillation" ix

Audrey Sagnard, Nefissa Hammache, Jean-Marc Sellal and Charles Guenancia
New Perspective in Atrial Fibrillation
Reprinted from: *Journal of Clinical Medicine* **2020**, *9*, 3713, doi:10.3390/jcm9113713 1

Néfissa Hammache, Hugo Pegorer-Sfes, Karim Benali, Isabelle Magnin Poull, Arnaud Olivier, Mathieu Echivard, Nathalie Pace, Damien Minois, Nicolas Sadoul, Damien Mandry, Jean Marc Sellal and Christian de Chillou
Is There an Association between Epicardial Adipose Tissue and Outcomes after Paroxysmal Atrial Fibrillation Catheter Ablation?
Reprinted from: *Journal of Clinical Medicine* **2021**, *10*, 3037, doi:10.3390/jcm10143037 5

Edouard Gitenay, Clément Bars, Michel Bremondy, Anis Ayari, Nicolas Maillot, Florian Baptiste, Antonio Taormina, Aicha Fofana, Sabrina Siame, Jérôme Kalifa and Julien Seitz
Localized Atrial Tachycardia and Dispersion Regions in Atrial Fibrillation: Evidence of Spatial Concordance
Reprinted from: *Journal of Clinical Medicine* **2021**, *10*, 3170, doi:10.3390/jcm10143170 19

Shauna McBride, Sahar Avazzadeh, Antony M. Wheatley, Barry O'Brien, Ken Coffey, Adnan Elahi, Martin O'Halloran and Leo R. Quinlan
Ablation Modalities for Therapeutic Intervention in Arrhythmia-Related Cardiovascular Disease: Focus on Electroporation
Reprinted from: *Journal of Clinical Medicine* **2021**, *10*, 2657, doi:10.3390/jcm10122657 31

Riyaz A. Kaba, Aziz Momin and John Camm
Persistent Atrial Fibrillation: The Role of Left Atrial Posterior Wall Isolation and Ablation Strategies
Reprinted from: *Journal of Clinical Medicine* **2021**, *10*, 3129, doi:10.3390/jcm10143129 51

Sahar Avazzadeh, Shauna McBride, Barry O'Brien, Ken Coffey, Adnan Elahi, Martin O'Halloran, Alan Soo and Leo. R Quinlan
Ganglionated Plexi Ablation for the Treatment of Atrial Fibrillation
Reprinted from: *Journal of Clinical Medicine* **2020**, *9*, 3081, doi:10.3390/jcm9103081 65

Paweł Wańkowicz, Jacek Staszewski, Aleksander Debiec, Marta Nowakowska-Kotas, Aleksandra Szylińska, Agnieszka Turoń-Skrzypińska and Iwona Rotter
Pre-Stroke Statin Therapy Improves In-Hospital Prognosis Following Acute Ischemic Stroke Associated with Well-Controlled Nonvalvular Atrial Fibrillation
Reprinted from: *Journal of Clinical Medicine* **2021**, *10*, 3036, doi:10.3390/jcm10143036 87

Yoon Jung Park, Pil-Sung Yang, Hee Tae Yu, Tae-Hoon Kim, Eunsun Jang, Jae-Sun Uhm, Hui-Nam Pak, Moon-Hyoung Lee, Gregory Y.H. Lip and Boyoung Joung
What Is the Ideal Blood Pressure Threshold for the Prevention of Atrial Fibrillation in Elderly General Population?
Reprinted from: *Journal of Clinical Medicine* **2020**, *9*, 2988, doi:10.3390/jcm9092988 97

Paweł Wańkowicz, Jacek Staszewski, Aleksander Debiec, Marta Nowakowska-Kotas, Aleksandra Szylińska and Iwona Rotter
Ischemic Stroke Risk Factors in Patients with Atrial Fibrillation Treated with New Oral Anticoagulants
Reprinted from: *Journal of Clinical Medicine* **2021**, *10*, 1223, doi:10.3390/jcm10061223 113

Dongmin Kim, Pil-Sung Yang, Gregory Y.H. Lip and Boyoung Joung
Atrial Fibrillation Increases the Risk of Early-Onset Dementia in the General Population: Data from a Population-Based Cohort
Reprinted from: *Journal of Clinical Medicine* **2020**, *9*, 3665, doi:10.3390/jcm9113665 121

Audrey Sagnard, Charles Guenancia, Basile Mouhat, Maud Maza, Marie Fichot, Daniel Moreau, Fabien Garnier, Luc Lorgis, Yves Cottin and Marianne Zeller
Involvement of Autonomic Nervous System in New-Onset Atrial Fibrillation during Acute Myocardial Infarction
Reprinted from: *Journal of Clinical Medicine* **2020**, *9*, 1481, doi:10.3390/jcm9051481 133

Sandro Ninni, Gilles Lemesle, Thibaud Meurice, Olivier Tricot, Nicolas Lamblin and Christophe Bauters
Real-Life Incident Atrial Fibrillation in Outpatients with Coronary Artery Disease
Reprinted from: *Journal of Clinical Medicine* **2020**, *9*, 2367, doi:10.3390/jcm9082367 145

Paweł Muszyński and Tomasz A. Bonda
Mitochondrial Dysfunction in Atrial Fibrillation—Mechanisms and Pharmacological Interventions
Reprinted from: *Journal of Clinical Medicine* **2021**, *10*, 2385, doi:10.3390/jcm10112385 157

Muhammad Shuja Khan, Kennosuke Yamashita, Vikas Sharma, Ravi Ranjan and Derek James Dosdall
RNAs and Gene Expression Predicting Postoperative Atrial Fibrillation in Cardiac Surgery Patients Undergoing Coronary Artery Bypass Grafting
Reprinted from: *Journal of Clinical Medicine* **2020**, *9*, 1139, doi:10.3390/jcm9041139 175

Thibaut Pommier, Thibault Leclercq, Charles Guenancia, Carole Richard, Guillaume Porot, Gabriel Laurent and Luc Lorgis
Left Atrial Remodeling and Brain Natriuretic Peptide Levels Variation after Left Atrial Appendage Occlusion
Reprinted from: *Journal of Clinical Medicine* **2021**, *10*, 3443, doi:10.3390/jcm10153443 191

José Ramón López-Mínguez, Juan Manuel Nogales-Asensio, Eduardo Infante De Oliveira, Lino Santos, Rafael Ruiz-Salmerón, Dabit Arzamendi-Aizpurua, Marco Costa, Hipólito Gutiérrez-García, Jose Antonio Fernández-Díaz, Xavier Freixa, Ignacio Cruz-González, Raúl Moreno, Andrés Íñiguez-Romo and Fernando Alfonso-Manterola
Major Bleeding Predictors in Patients with Left Atrial Appendage Closure: The Iberian Registry II
Reprinted from: *Journal of Clinical Medicine* **2020**, *9*, 2295, doi:10.3390/jcm9072295 201

About the Editor

Charles Guenancia

Charles Guenancia, MD, PhD, is an associate professor of physiology and a cardiac electrophysiologist. His research focuses on atrial fibrillation pathophysiology and heart–brain interactions in the PEC2 Laboratory, D, France.

Preface to "New Perspective in Atrial Fibrillation"

In spite of the large volume of associated research, the pathophysiological mechanisms involved in atrial fibrillation (AF) onset and recurrence remain uncertain. This may explain why the performances of thromboembolic and bleeding prediction scores in AF patients are limited. In the past few years, the concept of atrial cardiopathy has emerged as a promising lead to connect AF to stroke, heart failure, and inflammatory processes: indeed, all of the mechanisms associated with atrial remodeling and the development of atrial cardiopathy are also likely to promote the development of AF. This recent concept of atrial cardiopathy suggests that the real trigger of stroke may be an abnormal atrial substrate rather than atrial rhythm itself. In this setting, AF could be seen as a symptom of atrial cardiopathy rather than a risk factor for stroke. In the absence of validated clinical markers of atrial cardiopathy, the search for the mechanism of AF remains the cornerstone of cardioembolic stroke prevention for now.

The aim of this Special Issue is to gather basic research as well as pathophysiological and epidemiological papers focused on the relationship between atrial substrates and atrial fibrillation onset, recurrence, and outcomes.

Charles Guenancia
Editor

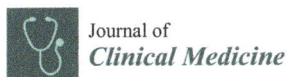

Editorial

New Perspective in Atrial Fibrillation

Audrey Sagnard [1], Nefissa Hammache [2], Jean-Marc Sellal [2,3] and Charles Guenancia [1,3,4,*,†]

1. Cardiology Department, University Hospital, 21079 Dijon, France; audrey.sagnard@chu-dijon.fr
2. Département de Cardiologie, Centre Hospitalier Universitaire (CHU de Nancy), 54500 Vandœuvre lès-Nancy, France; n.hammache@chru-nancy.fr (N.H.); jm.sellal@chru-nancy.fr (J.-M.S.)
3. INSERM-IADI U1254, 54500 Vandœuvre lès-Nancy, France
4. PEC 2 EA 7460, University of Burgundy and Franche-Comté, 21000 Dijon, France
* Correspondence: charles.guenancia@chu-dijon.fr; Tel.: +3-338-029-3536; Fax: +3-338-029-3536
† This author takes responsibility for all aspects of the reliability and freedom from bias of the data presented and their discussed interpretation.

Received: 13 November 2020; Accepted: 18 November 2020; Published: 19 November 2020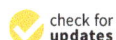

Despite a large number of publications on this subject, the pathophysiological mechanisms involved in atrial fibrillation (AF) onset and recurrence are uncertain. Moreover, though several thrombo-embolic and bleeding prediction [1] scores for AF patients have been developed, their performance is still limited [2]. Taken together, these facts suggest that we are still missing a global theory of atrial fibrillation pathophysiology (or at least some parts of it).

A better understanding of AF pathophysiology could come from the integration of all the cardiac environment modulators, including "Coumel triangle" components [3]. Indeed, apart from the pulmonary vein triggers that have been extensively studied [4], the relationship between other triggers (inflammation as in acute AF [5–7], stable coronary artery disease [8], or post-operative AF [9]), the modulator (mainly autonomic nervous system dysregulation [10]) and substrate alterations (fibrosis but also changes in the conduction properties of the atrial cells even in the absence of a quantifiable "scar" [11]) have been recently brought to light by several papers [12,13]. The interplay between cardiovascular risk factors, mainly high blood pressure [14] and obesity [6], atrial epicardial fat, and atrial ganglionated plexi [15], is complex and critical for the understanding of AF, but also in the search for new treatments. In this regard, a particular focus should be placed on the new anti-diabetic therapies (SGLT-2 inhibitors [16] and GLP-1 receptor agonists [17]) that have not only proven a benefit for major cardiovascular events (MACE) occurrence but also a decrease in AF burden. These treatments do not act so much as glycemia regulators, as Hb1Ac is usually only slightly decreased, but on the complex metabolic pathways involved in diabetic cardiomyopathy and possibly also in metabolic syndrome patients without diabetes. Thus, a fascinating field of research is open for the characterization of the metabolism's role in AF onset and persistence and perhaps also as a therapeutic target, as suggested by the major results obtained through weight loss in obese patients suffering from AF [18].

In the past few years, the concept of atrial cardiopathy has emerged as a promising lead to connect AF to stroke, heart failure, and inflammatory processes; indeed, all of the mechanisms associated with atrial remodeling and the development of atrial cardiopathy are also likely to promote the development of AF [19]. An international expert consensus defined atrial cardiopathy as "any complex of structural, architectural, contractile, or electrophysiological changes affecting the atria with the potential to produce clinically-relevant manifestations" [20]. This recent concept suggests that the real trigger of stroke may be an abnormal atrial substrate rather than the atrial rhythm itself. Indeed, evidence from studies analyzing the data obtained from implantable cardiac devices has recently demonstrated that there is no temporal correlation between AF and stroke [21]. This finding is in line with current thinking on the pathophysiology of the relationship between AF and cardioembolic stroke [22]: AF seems to be more of a risk marker than the cardioembolic risk vector itself. It is, therefore, only a symptom of underlying atrial cardiomyopathy, which, even in sinus rhythm, increases thromboembolic risk. For now, however, the lack of a clinically validated definition of atrial cardiopathy limits its clinical applications and the reproducibility of the results obtained using these various definitions. Indeed, several clinical, electrocardiographic, biological, and imaging markers [23] have been suggested [24], but few of them have been correlated to atrial tissue abnormalities as defined by the international expert consensus [20].

The aim of this Special Issue is to gather basic research, as well as pathophysiological and epidemiological papers, focused on the relationship between atrial substrate and atrial fibrillation onset, recurrence, and outcomes.

Funding: This research received no external funding.

Acknowledgments: The authors thank Lindsey B. Gottschalk for English revision of the paper.

Conflicts of Interest: The authors declare no conflict of interest.

References

1. Lopez-Minguez, J.R.; Nogales-Asensio, J.M.; De Oliveira, E.I.; Santos, L.; Ruiz-Salmeron, R.; Arzamendi-Aizpurua, D.; Costa, M.; Gutierrez-Garcia, H.; Fernandez-Diaz, J.A.; Freixa, X.; et al. Major Bleeding Predictors in Patients with Left Atrial Appendage Closure: The Iberian Registry II. *J. Clin. Med.* **2020**, *9*, 2295. [CrossRef]
2. Hirsh, B.J.; Copeland-Halperin, R.S.; Halperin, J.L. Fibrotic atrial cardiomyopathy, atrial fibrillation, and thromboembolism: Mechanistic links and clinical inferences. *J. Am. Coll. Cardiol.* **2015**, *65*, 2239–2251. [CrossRef] [PubMed]
3. Coumel, P. Cardiac arrhythmias and the autonomic nervous system. *J. Cardiovasc. Electrophysiol.* **1993**, *4*, 338–355. [CrossRef]
4. Haissaguerre, M.; Jais, P.; Shah, D.C.; Takahashi, A.; Hocini, M.; Quiniou, G.; Garrigue, S.; Le Mouroux, A.; Le Metayer, P.; Clementy, J. Spontaneous initiation of atrial fibrillation by ectopic beats originating in the pulmonary veins. *N. Engl. J. Med.* **1998**, *339*, 659–666. [CrossRef] [PubMed]
5. Guenancia, C.; Binquet, C.; Laurent, G.; Vinault, S.; Bruyère, R.; Prin, S.; Pavon, A.; Charles, P.E.; Quenot, J.P. Incidence and Predictors of New-Onset Atrial Fibrillation in Septic Shock Patients in a Medical ICU: Data from 7-Day Holter ECG Monitoring. *PLoS ONE* **2015**, *10*, e0127168. [CrossRef] [PubMed]
6. Guenancia, C.; Stamboul, K.; Garnier, F.; Beer, J.C.; Touzery, C.; Lorgis, L.; Cottin, Y.; Zeller, M. Obesity and new-onset atrial fibrillation in acute myocardial infarction: A gender specific risk factor. *Int. J. Cardiol.* **2014**, *176*, 1039–1041. [CrossRef]
7. Guenancia, C.; Toucas, C.; Fauchier, L.; Stamboul, K.; Garnier, F.; Mouhat, B.; Sagnard, A.; Lorgis, L.; Zeller, M.; Cottin, Y. High rate of recurrence at long-term follow-up after new-onset atrial fibrillation during acute myocardial infarction. *Europace* **2018**, *20*, e179–e188. [CrossRef]
8. Ninni, S.; Lemesle, G.; Meurice, T.; Tricot, O.; Lamblin, N.; Bauters, C. Real-Life Incident Atrial Fibrillation in Outpatients with Coronary Artery Disease. *J. Clin. Med.* **2020**, *9*, 2367. [CrossRef]
9. Khan, M.S.; Yamashita, K.; Sharma, V.; Ranjan, R.; Dosdall, D.J. RNAs and Gene Expression Predicting Postoperative Atrial Fibrillation in Cardiac Surgery Patients Undergoing Coronary Artery Bypass Grafting. *J. Clin. Med.* **2020**, *9*, 1139. [CrossRef]
10. Sagnard, A.; Guenancia, C.; Mouhat, B.; Maza, M.; Fichot, M.; Moreau, D.; Garnier, F.; Lorgis, L.; Cottin, Y.; Zeller, M. Involvement of Autonomic Nervous System in New-Onset Atrial Fibrillation during Acute Myocardial Infarction. *J. Clin. Med.* **2020**, *9*, 1481. [CrossRef]
11. Guichard, J.B.; Nattel, S. Atrial Cardiomyopathy: A Useful Notion in Cardiac Disease Management or a Passing Fad? *J. Am. Coll. Cardiol.* **2017**, *70*, 756–765. [CrossRef] [PubMed]
12. Gaeta, M.; Bandera, F.; Tassinari, F.; Capasso, L.; Cargnelutti, M.; Pelissero, G.; Malavazos, A.E.; Ricci, C. Is epicardial fat depot associated with atrial fibrillation? A systematic review and meta-analysis. *Europace* **2017**, *19*, 747–752. [CrossRef] [PubMed]

13. Nalliah, C.J.; Bell, J.R.; Raaijmakers, A.J.A.; Waddell, H.M.; Wells, S.P.; Bernasochi, G.B.; Montgomery, M.K.; Binny, S.; Watts, T.; Joshi, S.B.; et al. Epicardial Adipose Tissue Accumulation Confers Atrial Conduction Abnormality. *J. Am. Coll. Cardiol.* **2020**, *76*, 1197–1211. [CrossRef] [PubMed]
14. Park, Y.J.; Yang, P.S.; Yu, H.T.; Kim, T.H.; Jang, E.; Uhm, J.S.; Pak, H.N.; Lee, M.H.; Lip, G.Y.H.; Joung, B. What Is the Ideal Blood Pressure Threshold for the Prevention of Atrial Fibrillation in Elderly General Population? *J. Clin. Med.* **2020**, *9*, 2988. [CrossRef] [PubMed]
15. Avazzadeh, S.; McBride, S.; O'Brien, B.; Coffey, K.; Elahi, A.; O'Halloran, M.; Soo, A.; Quinlan, L.R. Ganglionated Plexi Ablation for the Treatment of Atrial Fibrillation. *J. Clin. Med.* **2020**, *9*, 3081. [CrossRef]
16. Li, W.J.; Chen, X.Q.; Xu, L.L.; Li, Y.Q.; Luo, B.H. SGLT2 inhibitors and atrial fibrillation in type 2 diabetes: A systematic review with meta-analysis of 16 randomized controlled trials. *Cardiovasc. Diabetol.* **2020**, *19*, 130. [CrossRef]
17. Nreu, B.; Dicembrini, I.; Tinti, F.; Sesti, G.; Mannucci, E.; Monami, M. Major cardiovascular events, heart failure, and atrial fibrillation in patients treated with glucagon-like peptide-1 receptor agonists: An updated meta-analysis of randomized controlled trials. *Nutr. Metab. Cardiovasc. Dis.* **2020**, *30*, 1106–1114. [CrossRef]
18. Pathak, R.K.; Middeldorp, M.E.; Meredith, M.; Mehta, A.B.; Mahajan, R.; Wong, C.X.; Twomey, D.; Elliott, A.D.; Kalman, J.M.; Abhayaratna, W.P.; et al. Long-Term Effect of Goal-Directed Weight Management in an Atrial Fibrillation Cohort: A Long-Term Follow-Up Study (LEGACY). *J. Am. Coll. Cardiol.* **2015**, *65*, 2159–2169. [CrossRef]
19. Guenancia, C.; Garnier, F.; Fichot, M.; Sagnard, A.; Laurent, G.; Lorgis, L. Silent atrial fibrillation: Clinical management and perspectives. *Future Cardiol.* **2020**, *16*, 133–142. [CrossRef]
20. Goette, A.; Kalman, J.M.; Aguinaga, L.; Akar, J.; Cabrera, J.A.; Chen, S.A.; Chugh, S.S.; Corradi, D.; D'Avila, A.; Dobrev, D.; et al. EHRA/HRS/APHRS/SOLAECE expert consensus on atrial cardiomyopathies: Definition, characterization, and clinical implication. *Europace* **2016**, *18*, 1455–1490. [CrossRef]
21. Brambatti, M.; Connolly, S.J.; Gold, M.R.; Morillo, C.A.; Capucci, A.; Muto, C.; Lau, C.P.; Van Gelder, I.C.; Hohnloser, S.H.; Carlson, M.; et al. Temporal relationship between subclinical atrial fibrillation and embolic events. *Circulation* **2014**, *129*, 2094–2099. [CrossRef] [PubMed]
22. Calenda, B.W.; Fuster, V.; Halperin, J.L.; Granger, C.B. Stroke risk assessment in atrial fibrillation: Risk factors and markers of atrial myopathy. *Nat. Rev. Cardiol.* **2016**, *13*, 549–559. [CrossRef] [PubMed]
23. Bernard, A.; Leclercq, T.; Comby, P.-O.; Duloquin, G.; Ricolfi, F.; Béjot, Y.; Guenancia, C. High rate of cardiac thrombus diagnosed by adding cardiac imaging in acute stroke computed tomography protocol. *Int. J. Stroke* **2020**. [CrossRef] [PubMed]
24. Kamel, H.; Okin, P.M.; Longstreth, W.T., Jr.; Elkind, M.S.; Soliman, E.Z. Atrial cardiopathy: A broadened concept of left atrial thromboembolism beyond atrial fibrillation. *Future Cardiol.* **2015**, *11*, 323–331. [CrossRef]

Publisher's Note: MDPI stays neutral with regard to jurisdictional claims in published maps and institutional affiliations.

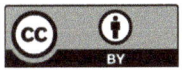

© 2020 by the authors. Licensee MDPI, Basel, Switzerland. This article is an open access article distributed under the terms and conditions of the Creative Commons Attribution (CC BY) license (http://creativecommons.org/licenses/by/4.0/).

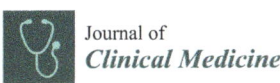

Article

Is There an Association between Epicardial Adipose Tissue and Outcomes after Paroxystic Atrial Fibrillation Catheter Ablation?

Néfissa Hammache [1,2,*,†], Hugo Pegorer-Sfes [1,†], Karim Benali [1,2,3], Isabelle Magnin Poull [1,2], Arnaud Olivier [1], Mathieu Echivard [1], Nathalie Pace [1], Damien Minois [1,2,4], Nicolas Sadoul [1,2], Damien Mandry [2,5], Jean Marc Sellal [1,2] and Christian de Chillou [1,2]

1. Département de Cardiologie, CHRU de Nancy, F-54500 Vandœuvre-lès-Nancy, France; h.pegorersfes@chru-nancy.fr (H.P.-S.); k.benali@chru-nancy.fr (K.B.); i.magnin-poull@chru-nancy.fr (I.M.P.); a.olivier@chru-nancy.fr (A.O.); m.echivard@chru-nancy.fr (M.E.); n.pace@chru-nancy.fr (N.P.); damien.minois@gmail.com (D.M.); n.sadoul@chru-nancy.fr (N.S.); jm.sellal@chru-nancy.fr (J.M.S.); c.dechillou@chru-nancy.fr (C.d.C.)
2. INSERM-IADI, U1254, F-54500 Vandœuvre-lès-Nancy, France; d.mandry@chru-nancy.fr
3. Département de Cardiologie, CHU de Saint-Etienne, 42270 Saint-Priest-en-Jarez, France
4. Département de Cardiologie, CHU de Nantes, 44000 Nantes, France
5. Département de Radiologie, CHRU de Nancy, F-54500 Vandœuvre-lès-Nancy, France
* Correspondence: n.hammache@chru-nancy.fr; Tel.: +33-3-83-15-74-43; Fax: +33-3-83-15-49-17
† These authors equally contributed.

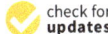

Abstract: Background: In patients undergoing paroxysmal atrial fibrillation (PAF) ablation, pulmonary vein isolation (PVI) alone fails in maintaining sinus rhythm in up to one third of patients after a first catheter ablation. Epicardial adipose tissue (EAT), as an endocrine-active organ, could play a role in the recurrence of AF after catheter ablation. Objective: To evaluate the predictive value of clinical, echocardiographic, biological parameters and epicardial fat density measured by computed tomography scan (CT-scan) on AF recurrence in PAF patients who underwent a first pulmonary vein isolation procedure using radiofrequency (RF). Methods: This monocentric retrospective study included all patients undergoing first-time RF PAF ablation at the Nancy University Hospital between March 2015 and December 2018 with one-year follow-up. Results: 389 patients were included, of whom 128 (32.9%) had AF recurrence at one-year follow-up. Neither total-EAT volume (88.6 ± 37.2 cm^3 vs. 91.4 ± 40.5 cm^3, $p = 0.519$), nor total-EAT radiodensity (-98.8 ± 4.1 HU vs. -98.8 ± 3.8 HU, $p = 0.892$) and left atrium-EAT radiodensity (-93.7 ± 4.3 HU vs. -93.4 ± 6.0 HU, $p = 0.556$) were significantly associated with AF recurrence after PAF ablation. In multivariate analysis, previous cavo-tricuspid isthmus (CTI) ablation, ablation procedure duration, BNP and triglyceride levels remained independently associated with AF recurrence after catheter ablation at 12-months follow-up. Conclusion: Contrary to persistent AF, EAT parameters are not associated with AF recurrence after paroxysmal AF ablation. Thus, the role of the metabolic atrial substrate in PAF pathophysiology appears less obvious than in persistent AF.

Keywords: paroxysmal atrial fibrillation; catheter ablation; epicardial adipose tissue

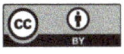

1. Introduction

Atrial fibrillation (AF) is the most common cardiac arrhythmia affecting approximatively 33.5 million persons worldwide [1]. Current guidelines recommend catheter ablation (CA) in order to maintain sinus rhythm and improve quality of life in symptomatic patients in whom drugs have already failed [2]. Currently, pulmonary vein isolation (PVI) is the cornerstone of the ablation strategy in patients with paroxystic atrial fibrillation (PAF). This is a well-established treatment for the prevention of PAF recurrence. The 12-month success rate is approximately 65% after a first procedure and 80% after multiple procedures [3–6]. Recently, it has been shown that first-line PAF ablation is superior to antiarrhythmic therapy in terms of recurrence, but also in terms of symptom improvement, physical capacity, and quality of life, reinforcing the place of catheter ablation [7–9]. Thus, determining the factors contributing to recurrence after a catheter ablation becomes essential. Prognostic models, which combine several predictors (such as left atrium volume, sex, age, coronary artery disease) to generate an individualized risk estimate, have been developed for prediction of AF recurrence after catheter ablation [10]. None of them has proven to be effective, especially in PAF, where only PV reconnections have proven to be a significant predictive factor for AF recurrences.

Epicardial adipose tissue (EAT) serves as a biologically active organ with important endocrine and inflammatory function [11,12]. An accumulating body of evidence suggests that EAT is associated with the initiation, perpetuation, and recurrence of AF, especially in case of persistent AF (PersAF) [13–15]. Quantitative and qualitative evaluation of EAT, aided by the development of imaging techniques, is of growing interest [16]. The role of EAT in recurrence after PAF catheter ablation has not been clearly elucidated.

The aim of this study was to evaluate the predictive value of clinical, echocardiographic, biological parameters and EAT characteristics measured by computed tomography scan (CT-scan) on AF recurrence in PAF patients after a first radiofrequency (RF) PVI.

2. Materials and Methods

2.1. Study Population

Consecutive adult patients with symptomatic drug-refractory PAF referred for a first RF catheter ablation between April 2015 and December 2018 in Nancy University Hospital were included. Preprocedural CT-scan was routinely performed before AF catheter ablation. AF was considered to be paroxysmal if it terminated spontaneously or with intervention within 7 days of onset.

Inclusion criteria were: first procedure of catheter ablation for PAF with CT scan, transthoracic echocardiography and transesophageal echocardiography before the procedure and >12-month follow-up. Exclusion criteria were: prior AF catheter ablation and cryo-balloon ablation, LA linear lesions, LA defragmentation and intervention aborted due to a procedural complication. All patients were adults and provided written informed consent for the CA and all procedures were in line with current guidelines (see Figure 1).

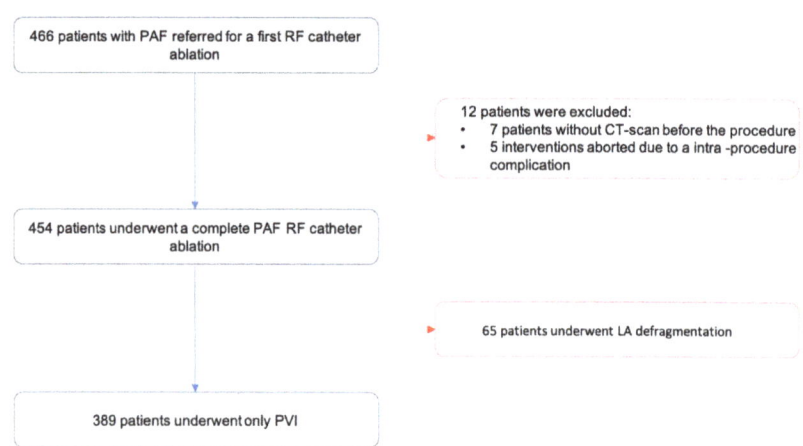

Figure 1. Flowchart for inclusion of patients in the study.

2.2. Echocardiography

Transthoracic and transesophageal echocardiography were performed within 24 h before intervention using a Vivid S6 cardiovascular ultrasound system (General Electric, Horten, Norway). The following data were collected: left ventricular ejection fraction (biplane Simpson's method), left atrial (LA) surface area (apical four-chamber view at end-systole), indexed LA volume (biplane area-length method at end-systole), LA diameter (parasternal long axis view), diastolic function according to the 2016 ASE recommendations (E/A, lateral e' velocity, average E/e', TR velocity), measurement of the interventricular septum at end-diastole.

2.3. Cardiac Computed Tomography

A 256-slice multidetector cardiac scanner (Revolution CT, General Electric) with iodinated contrast product injection was performed before the procedure to assess PVs and LA anatomy, and to check the absence of thrombus in the left atrial appendage. Cardiac CT angiography, with electrocardiographic gating, was acquired using a scanner allowing up to 16 cm of detector coverage, so that the whole heart could be captured in a single heartbeat. ECG-gated acquisitions were obtained during end-systole (approximately 40% of R–R interval). The injection protocol included an initial contrast injection of 50 mL (iodine concentration of 350 mg/mL) at the rate of 5 mL/s followed by 40 mL of saline at the rate of 4 mL/s. The acquisitions settings were 100 kV tube potential, 500 mA tube charge, 0.28 s rotation. Images were reconstructed with a slice thickness of 0.625 mm. Total EAT volume and density were assessed using a semi-automatic procedure with the CardIQ Xpress 2.0 v post-processing software on an Advantage workstation 4.7 v (General Electric) (see Figure 2).

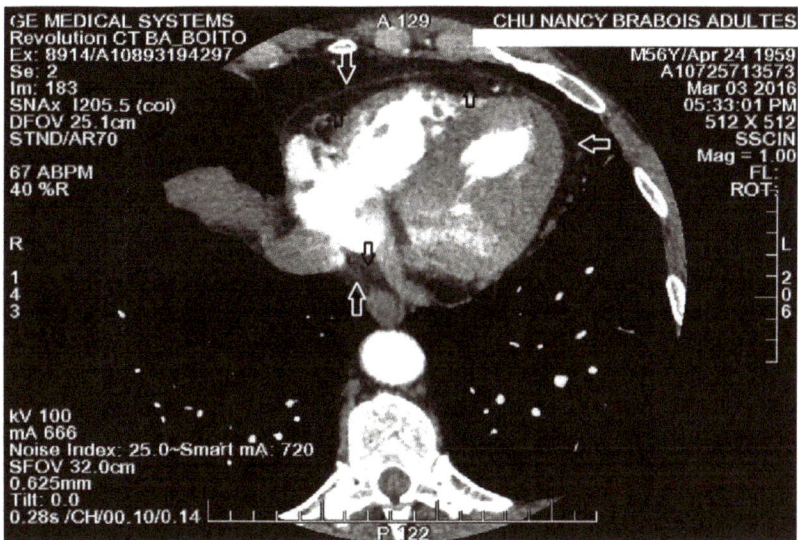

Figure 2. EAT measurement on a multiplanar reformatted CT image of the heart. Fibrous pericardium (white arrows) and epicardial fat (black arrows).

2.4. Cardiac CT Image Analysis

Manual contouring of the fibrous pericardium was performed on axial planes, for every 10 mm, from the pulmonary artery bifurcation to the diaphragm (see Figure 3). EAT was detected by assigning an attenuation threshold from −50 to −250 Hounsfield units (HU) to fat [17]. After three-dimensional reconstruction, volume (in cm^3), mean density (in HU) ± standard deviation (SD) were automatically calculated by the software. In order to assess left atrial (LA)-EAT density, three areas were identified: superior left region (SL), inferior left region (IL) and inferior right region (IR), near the pulmonary vein ostia. A circular region of interest (ROI) of 20 mm^2, or the largest possible size < 20 mm^2, was manually drawn and placed in each region (see Figure 4). LA density was calculated as the average of all regional densities. Data were evaluated by one operator, blinded to clinical outcomes.

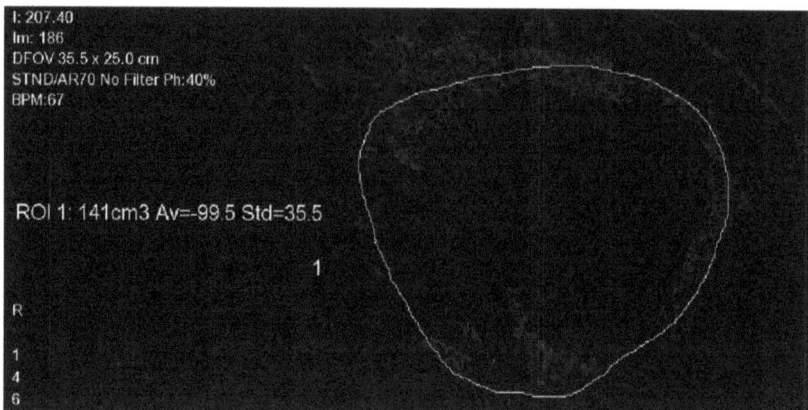

Figure 3. EAT measurement: contouring of the fibrous pericardium.

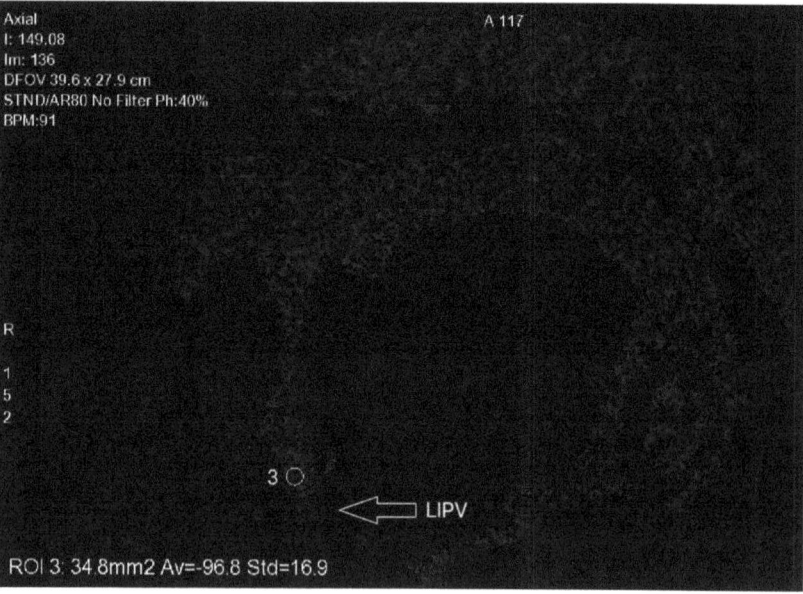

Figure 4. EAT measurement: Inferior left region (IL) near the LIPV (left inferior pulmonary vein) ostium.

Fibrous pericardium was manually traced, on axial planes, for every 10 mm, from the pulmonary artery bifurcation to the diaphragm. EAT was detected by assigning an attenuation threshold from -50 to -250 Hounsfield units (HU) to fat.

In order to assess LA-EAT density, three areas were identified: superior left region (SL), inferior right region (IL) and inferior left region (IR), near the PV ostia. A circular ROI of 20 mm^2, failing the largest possible size, was manually drawn and placed in each region. LA density was calculated as the average of all regional densities.

2.5. Atrial Fibrillation Ablation

AF ablation procedures were performed under local anesthesia and conscious sedation. Two catheters were advanced from the right femoral vein to the LA through transseptal puncture, under fluoroscopic guidance, a 10-pole circular mapping catheter (Lasso, Biosense Webster, Diamond Bar, CA, USA) and a 3.5-mm externally irrigated-tip ablation catheter (3.5-mm tip, ThermoCool, Biosense Webster, Diamond Bar, CA, USA/ 3.5-mm tip, Flexability, St. Jude Medical, St. Paul, MN, USA). A steerable quadripolar catheter (Xtrem, SORIN Group, Clamart, France) was placed into the coronary sinus and used as an electro anatomical mapping reference.

A 3-dimensional navigation system (CARTO®, Biosense Webster, Inc, Irvine, CA, USA or EnSite NavX system St. Jude Medical, St Paul, MN, USA) was used to create a 3-dimensional electro-anatomical map of the LA, which was integrated with computed tomography of the LA. PVI was performed with radiofrequency energy in a point-by-point wide area circumferential ablation (two by two PVI) pattern using a Thermocool SmartTouch irrigated tip CF-sensing ablation catheter (Biosense Webster, Inc., Irvine, CA, USA) or a FlexAbility™ Ablation Catheter (St. Jude Medical, St. Paul, MN, USA) introduced via a non-steerable sheath. The point-by-point circumferential lesion sets were created while navigating the catheter under the guidance of a 3-D electro-anatomical mapping system. During ablation, computerized LA reconstruction and mapping was conducted using the CARTO® mapping system (Biosense Webster, Inc. Irvine, CA, USA) or the EnSite NavX system (St. Jude Medical, St Paul, MN, USA). Contiguous lesions were performed. Each lesion was respectively guided by ablation index (AI) targets using 450 at the roof and anterior walls and 350 at the posterior and inferior walls or lesion size index (LSI) targets using 5.5 at the roof and anterior walls and 4.5 at the posterior and inferior wall. RF pulses were delivered by using a 550-kHz RF Stockert-Cordis generator and the ablation catheter, in a power-controlled mode, with RF energy up to 30 Watts at the anterior part of the veins and 25 Watts at their posterior part.

2.6. Endpoints and Data Collection

The objective was to assess the association between clinical, biological, echocardiographic and EAT characteristics and PAF recurrence after radiofrequency catheter ablation. The medical software DxCare® was used to collect all patients' data needed for the study. We evaluated: demographic and physical features, comorbidities, treatments, AF history, laboratory analysis, electrocardiogram features at the beginning of the procedure and at hospital discharge, and ablation procedure modalities.

2.7. Follow-Up and AF Recurrence Assessment

AF recurrences were assessed after a 3-month blanking period, and defined as ≥ 1 AF episode recorded during a 12 lead ECG or ≥ 1 AF episode lasting ≥ 30 s documented by Holter monitoring. All patients underwent an electrocardiographic evaluation before discharge from hospital. Arrhythmia monitoring included clinical evaluation, 12-lead electrocardiogram in case of symptom recurrence, and systematic 24-h Holter monitor recording by the referring cardiologist at months 3, 6 and 12. Our investigative team was unaware of the follow-up assessment outcomes.

The continuation or initiation of anti-arrhythmic drug therapy post-procedure and at 3 months was left to the referring physician preference. Successful ablation was defined as the absence of a documented episode of AF with or without anti-arrhythmic at one year after the procedure.

2.8. Statistical Analysis

Statistical analyzes were performed using IBM SPSS® version 26 software. Continuous variables were reported as mean ± standard deviation if normally distributed or median with interquartile range (IQR) if not. Categorical variables were expressed as frequencies with percentages. The Student's *t*-test or Mann-Whitney U-test (depending on whether the values were normally distributed) allowed comparison of continuous variables while comparison of percentages was performed using the Pearson's chi-squared test.

Simple logistic regression analysis was conducted to identify the relationship between baseline characteristics and recurrence. Variables with $p < 0.100$ were included in multivariate regression analysis. Because our study was focused on EAT, we planned to include EAT parameters in the multivariate analysis whatever the result in univariate analysis. A p-value < 0.05 was considered statistically significant.

3. Results

3.1. Baseline Characteristics

Between March 2015 and December 2018, 466 patients underwent their first CA for PAF. 77 patients were excluded (seven patients without CT scan; five aborted interventions due to intra-procedural tamponade [3], stroke [1], and intolerable pain [1], as well as 65 patients that underwent LA defragmentation). The population was divided into two groups, AF recurrence and successful CA, after 12-months follow-up. Patients' characteristics are summarized in Table 1.

Table 1. Baseline data of the overall study cohort and 1-year-follow-up (divided into patients with and without AF recurrence during 1-year-follow-up).

Variable	Total Population (n = 389)	AF Recurrence (n = 128)	Successful Procedure (n = 261)	p Value
Demographics				
Age—years	58.1 ± 11.1	57.1 ± 12	58.6 ± 10.7	0.343
Male sex—no. (%)	256 (65.8)	83 (64.8)	173 (67.6)	0.778
Co-morbidities				
HFrEF—no. (%)	25 (6.5)	5 (3.9)	20 (7.7)	0.125
Hypertension—no. (%)	156 (40.1)	47 (36.7)	109 (41.8)	0.340
Diabetes—no. (%)	28 (7.2)	8 (6.3)	20 (7.7)	0.612
Dyslipidemia—no (%)	104 (26.4)	27 (21.1)	77 (29.5)	0.078
CHA2DS2-VASc Score	1.3 ± 1.3	1.2 ± 1.2	1.4 ± 1.3	0.274
Active or previous smoking—no. (%)	85 (21.9)	29 (22.7)	56 (21.5)	0.788
Obstructive sleep apnea—no. (%)	38 (9.8)	9 (7.0)	29 (11.1)	0.403
COBP—no (%)	8 (2.1)	5 (3.9)	3 (1.1)	0.072
Obesity—no (%)	82 (22.1)	30 (23.4)	52 (19.9)	0.436
Stroke —no (%)	20 (5.1)	5 (3.9)	15 (5.7)	0.476
Previous CTI ablation—no (%)	53 (13.6)	25 (19.5)	28 (10.7)	0.017
AF history and management				
Time between diagnosis and ablation—months	30.1 ± 24.2	27.6 ± 23.0	31.1 ± 24.6	0.263
Number of AF episode $\geq$ 1/24 h—(%)	93 (23.9)	30 (23.5)	63 (23.9)	0.308
AF at the beginning of procedure—no (%)	22 (5.7)	8 (6,5)	14 (5.6)	0.722
AF during procedure—no (%)	149 (36.1)	54 (42.2)	86 (32.9)	0.079
AF at the end of procedure no (%)	21 (5.4)	9 (7.0)	12 (4.6)	0.318
RF time (minutes)	34.4 ± 15.6	36.8 ± 15.9	33.2 ± 15.1	0.033
AF recurrence (first year)	153 (33.7)			
Medication				
B-blocker—no (%)	211 (54.2)	69 (53.9)	142 (54.4)	0.926
ACEI—no (%)	57 (14.7)	15 (11.7)	42 (16.1)	0.252
ARB—no (%)	71 (18.3)	23 (18.0)	48 (18.4)	0.919
MRA—no (%)	17 (4.4)	3 (2.3)	14 (5.4)	0.171
Statines—no (%)	78 (23.6)	20 (15.6)	58 (22.2)	0.088
Physical features				
Body Mass Index—kg/m^2	27.1 ± 4.7	27.7 ± 5.2	26.9 ± 4.8	0.255
NYHA functional class—no. (%)				
II/III/IV	89 (22.8)	30 (23.4)	59 (22.6)	0.089

Table 1. Cont.

Variable	Total Population (n = 389)	AF Recurrence (n = 128)	Successful Procedure (n = 261)	p Value
Laboratory analysis				
Total cholesterol level—g/L	2.36 ± 0.78	1.89 ± 0.39	2.59 ± 0.39	0.509
Triglycerides level—g/L	1.10 ± 0.73	1.17± 0.92	1.10 ± 0.62	0.168
LDL level—g/dl	1.15 ± 0.32	1.16 ± 0.33	1.14 ± 0.32	0.693
HDL level—g/dl	0.50 ± 0.13	0.51 ± 0.13	0.50 ± 0.13	0.738
Creatinine—umol/L	84.7 ± 38.2	82.7 ± 22.8	85.7 ± 34.1	0.632
CRP—mg/L	3.8 ± 8.8	3.8 ± 7.0	3.8 ± 9.7	0.962
Fibrinogen—g/L	3.2 ± 0.8	3.2 ± 0.8	3.1 ± 0.8	0.372
BNP—pg/mL	83.9 ± 107.3	99.9± 133	77.7± 88.8	0.028
Echocardiography features				
LVEF—%	59.7 ± 7.4	59.4 ± 7.2	59.9 ± 7.6	0.524
Left atrial enlargement—no (%)	168 (46.2)	58 (45.3)	110 (42.1)	0.638
Left atrial surface area—cm^2	20.2 ± 5.1	20.5 ± 5.3	20.0 ± 5.0	0.516
Left atrial volume—ml/m^2	34.2 ± 11.2	34.7 ± 11.6	34.0 ± 10.9	0.527
Left ventricular hypertrophy—no (%)	34 (9)	13 (10.2)	21 (8)	0.480
Left ventricular diastolic dysfunction—no (%)	66 (17.0)	23 (17.6)	43 (16.4)	0.830
CT features				
Total EAT Volume—cm^3	90.5 ± 39.4	88.6 ± 37.2	91.4 ± 40.5	0.519
Total-EAT Density—HU	−98.9 ± 3.9	−98.8 ± 4.1	−98.8 ± 3.8	0.892
LA-EAT Density—HU	−93.5 ± 5.5	−93.7 ± 4.3	−93.4 ± 6.0	0.556
LA EAT (LS GP) Density—HU	−93.8 ± 12.1	−94.1 ± 6.9	−93.7± 14.0	0.784
LA EAT (RI GP) Density—HU	−93.4 ± 7.6	−92.7 ± 7.4	−93.7 ± 7.7	0.198
LA EAT (LI GP) Density—HU	−93.3 ± 7.6	94.4 ± 7.3	−92.8 ± 7.7	0.175

COBP: chronic obstructive broncho-pneumopathy; MRA: mineralocorticoid receptor antagonist.

Cardiac Computed Tomography Features

Total EAT volume and density were 90.5 ± 39.4 cm^3 and −98.9 ± 3.9 HU, respectively. LA-EAT density was −93.5 ± 5.5 HU. EAT density of the LS region, LI region and RI region were respectively −93.8 ± 12.1, −93.4 ± 7.6 and −93.3 ± 7.6 HU.

3.2. Ablation Results

During the 12 months' follow-up, 128 patients (32.9%) presented recurrence of AF.

Independent Predictors of AF Recurrence

Among the variables, only dyslipidemia, CHADsVASc score, previous CTI ablation, AF during procedure, RF time, presence of dyspnea, triglycerides level and BNP were significantly associated with AF recurrences after univariate analysis (Table 2).

The associations with AF recurrence at 12 months after CA remained significant following multivariate analysis (Table 3) for previous CTI ablation (p = 0.013, OR 2.43, 95% CI 1.22–4.85), RF time per ten minutes (p = 0.033, OR 1.20, 95% CI 1.12–1.30), BNP per 100 pg/mL (p = 0.019, OR 1.35, 95% CI 1.22–1.49) and triglycerides level (p = 0.047, OR 1.54, 95% CI 1.02–2.26). No association was found between AF recurrence and EAT, either total volume, total density or LA density with, respectively, p = 0.968, OR 1.00, 95% CI 0.99–1.01, p = 0.432, OR 1.02 95% CI (0.96–1.1) and p = 0.771, OR 1.06 95% CI (0.96–1.16).

Table 2. Univariate analysis of AF recurrence after CA after 12-months Follow-Up.

Variables	Odds Ratio (95% CI)	p Value
Demographics		
Age—years	0.99 (0.97~1.01)	0.232
Male sex	0.93 (0.60~1.46)	0.779
Co-morbidities		
HFrEF	0.49 (0.2~1.24)	0.133
Hypertension	0.81 (0.52~1.25)	0.341
Diabete	0.80 (0.34~1.88)	0.613
Dyslipidemia	0.64 (0.39~1.05)	0.080
CHA2DS2-VASc Score	0.85 (0.72~1.0)	0.056
Active or previous smoking	1.07 (0.65~1.78)	0.788
Obstructive sleep apnea	0.71 (0.32~1.58)	0.405
Stroke	0.52 (0.18~1.54)	0.24
Previous CTI ablation	2.02 (1.19~3.68)	0.019
AF history and management		
Time between diagnosis and ablation—months	0.99 (0.98~1.00)	0.223
Number of AF episodes $\geq 1/24$ h	1.03 (0.78~1.36)	0.847
AF at the beginning of procedure	1.2 (0.48~2.88)	0.722
AF during procedure	1.48 (1.0~2.3)	0.08
AF at hospital discharge	1.57 (0.64~3.83)	0.322
RF time—minutes	1.01 (1.00~1.02)	0.035
Medication		
Beta-blocker	0.98 (0.64~1.5)	0.926
ACEI	0.69 (0.37~1.3)	0.254
ARB	0.97 (0.56~1.68)	0.919
MRA	0.42 (0.12~1.5)	0.183
Statine	0.99 (0.69~1.42)	0.957
Physical features		
Body Mass Index—kg/m^2	1.03 (0.98~1.03)	0.256
NYHA functional class		
NYHA > I	1.8 (1.01~3.0)	0.085
Laboratory analysis		
Total cholesterol level—g/L	0.99 (0.92~1.05)	0.983
Triglycerides level—g/L	1.32 (1.02~1.71)	0.036
LDL level—g/L	1.12 (0.57~2.18)	0.741
HDL level—g/dl	1.33 (0.25~6.9)	0.737
CRP—mg/L	1.00 (0.98~1.02)	0.941
Creatinine—umol/L	1.00 (0.99~1.01)	0.64
Fibrinogen—g/L	1.15 (0.89~1.49)	0.292
BNP—pg/mL	1.00 (1.00~1.00)	0.017
Echocardiography features		
Left ventricular ejection fraction	1.00 (0.97~1.02)	0.523
Left atrial surface area—cm^2	1.02 (0.98~1.07)	0.321
Left atrial volume—mL/m^2	1.01 (0.99~1.03)	0.526
Left atrial dilatation	1.19 (0.80~1.78)	0.408
Left ventricular diastolic dysfunction	1.04 (0.96~1.12)	0.392
Left ventricular hypertrophy	1.07 (0.55~2.06)	0.912
CT features		
Total EAT Volume—cm^3	1.00 (0.99~1.00)	0.518
Total EAT Density—HU	1.00 (0.95~1.06)	0.892
Total LA-EAT Density—HU	0.99 (0.94~1.03)	0.556
LA EAT (LS GP) Density—HU	1.01 (0.99~1.02)	0.784
LA EAT (RI GP) Density—HU	1.02 (0.99~1.05)	0.198
LA EAT (LI GP) Density—HU	0.97 (0.95~1.00)	0.108

Table 3. Multivariate analysis of AF recurrence after CA after 12-months Follow-Up.

Variables	Odds Ratio (95% CI)	p Value
NYHA > I	1.77 (1.04~3)	0.058
Dyslipidemia	0.58 (0.33~1.11)	0.106
CHADs VASc	0.5 (0.14~1.71)	0.268
Previous CTI ablation	2.43 (1.22~4.85)	0.013
AF during procedure	1.35 (0.8~2.29)	0.264
RF time—10 min	1.2 (1.11~1.3)	0.033
Triglycerides level—g/L	1.54 (1.02~2.26)	0.047
BNP—100 pg/mL	1.35 (1.22~1.49)	0.019
Total EAT Volume—cm^3	1.0 (0.99~1.01)	0.968
Total EAT Density—HU	1.02 (0.96~1.10)	0.432
Total LA-EAT Density—HU	1.06 (0.96~1.16)	0.771
LA EAT (LS GP) Density—HU	0.98 (0.94~1.02)	0.249
LA EAT (RI GP) Density—HU	1.02 (0.99~1.04)	0.780
LA EAT (LI GP) Density—HU	0.97 (0.94~1.00)	0.067

4. Discussion

4.1. Main Results

The main finding of our study is that EAT parameters are not associated with the recurrence of PAF at one-year follow-up after a first CA. On the other hand, previous CTI ablation, longer RF time, high BNP and triglyceride levels appear to be factors associated with AF recurrence after the first CA procedure in patients treated for PAF.

4.2. EAT and PAF Recurrence after CA

To our knowledge, this is the first study designed to examine the association between EAT, assessed by cardiac CT, solely in a PAF population and not in a mixed population of PersAF and PAF. Numerous studies have demonstrated a relationship between EAT and the risk of AF recurrence after ablation [18]. These studies included mostly PersAF. However, in subgroup analyses according to the type of AF, the results differed between paroxysmal and persistent AF [19]. In these studies, EAT appeared to have a prognostic value for AF recurrences only in the persistent AF subgroup, without significant association in the PAF subgroup. Our results are consistent with these previous findings, suggesting the existence of different pathophysiological mechanisms between paroxysmal and persistent AF regarding EAT involvement.

EAT volume has been shown to be bigger in persistent AF compared with PAF [20–22]. The volume and density of the EAT, reflecting its secretory activity, is a predictive factor of recurrence after ablation of PersAF. Studies on patients with AF undergoing cardiac CT and electroanatomic mapping showed that the presence of EAT was associated with lower bipolar voltage and more electrogram fractionation as electrophysiologic substrates for AF [23]. These changes underlie the pathophysiology of PersAF and are prime targets during CA. As the EAT is in contact with the atrial epicardium, the question of hybrid ablation is justified. A recent study by Vroomen et al. could not confirm that EAT-V was predictive of recurrence of atrial fibrillation in patients undergoing a hybrid AF ablation. It might be interesting to look at EAT density in order to target areas of interest during hybrid ablation.

In contrast, the majority of PAF patients can be treated by eliminating PV triggers, and PVI is enough, with only a minor role for the previously described substrate and thus of the associated EAT.

However, a recent study published by El Mahdiui et al. showed an association between the EAT density of the LA posterior wall and the risk of recurrence after ablation of any type of AF [24]. Batal et al. had previously reported that only posterior EAT thickness was associated with AF burden [21]. The importance of posterior EAT in PAF could be explained by the effect of direct local EAT secretion on the PVs. Our study focused on the fat density of the entire LA. It might be interesting to look specifically at the posterior EAT in our population.

Moreover, the recent study of Zaman et al. found that patients with PAF despite prior PVI show electrical substrates that resemble PersAF more closely than patients with PAF undergoing their first ablation [25]. In this study, the redo group had PVI only during the first CA. In the absence of LA defragmentation, a causal relationship between the first ablation and the presence of atrial substrate more similar to that of PersAF would be difficult to understand. Notably, these subgroups of PAF are indistinguishable by structural indices. It could be interesting to compare the EAT characteristics before the first and second CA procedures, looking for criteria that may indicate a heterogeneous population of PAF that may overlap with persistent AF.

4.3. Previous CTI Ablation and PAF Recurrence after CA

The association of AF and common-type atrial flutter has been previously described and is very frequent. In our study, we found that a previous CTI ablation is associated with a higher risk of recurrence of AF after a catheter ablation, with a two-fold relative risk of recurrence compared to patients without previous common-type atrial flutter.

Moreira et al. demonstrated that in patients with coexisting PAF/common-type atrial flutter, CTI ablation and PVI were used successfully to treat sustained common-type atrial flutter but appeared insufficient to prevent recurrences of AF. In this population, the very existence of a common-type atrial flutter can be a sign that non-PV substrates are involved [26].

4.4. RF Time and PAF Recurrence after CA

Increase of ten minutes of RF application was associated with a 1.2-fold increase in risk of recurrence of AF after a catheter ablation. This can suggest that PVI was not easy to achieve in the case of longer RF time. Since PVI is a cornerstone of AF management, difficulties in achieving this outcome may be linked to an increased risk of recurrence. An increased RF time can also be caused by larger pulmonary veins ostia. Unfortunately, we did not collect this data. This criterion has never been specifically studied and is not included in the risk scores for AF recurrence after ablation.

4.5. BNP, Lipid Profile and Recurrence after CA

Studies suggested that elevated baseline BNP level is associated with AF recurrence after CA, suggesting that BNP could be a useful biomarker for predicting AF recurrence [27,28]. Our study is consistent with this result, describing that an increase of 100 pg/mL in the BNP was associated with a 1.2-fold increase in risk of recurrence of AF after a first PAF CA procedure.

AF is characterized by a loss of atrial contraction, leading to an increase of the LA volume and atrial stretch, promoting activation of the natriuretic system and the secretion of ANP and BNP, both of which are mainly produced in the atrium [28]. However, this effect seems to be more prominent in patients with persistent AF in whom BNP levels are significantly higher.

In our PAF population, other mechanisms are probably involved. On one hand, the increase of BNP level may reflect an electrophysiological disturbance, which could trigger AF by intracellular calcium overload, reduced conduction velocity and increased dispersion of the refractory period [28]. On the other hand, BNP may be arrhythmogenic by inhibiting sympathetic activity and potentiating vagal activity through the cGMP pathway [29].

Augmentation of 1 g/L of triglyceride level was associated with a 1.74-fold increase in risk of recurrence of AF after a catheter ablation. Metabolic syndrome, which includes high triglyceride levels, is associated with higher recurrence rates after CA, especially in case of PersAF. Metabolic syndrome is associated with PAF, but its role in recurrence is less clear [30,31]. Why metabolic syndrome markers failed to predict outcomes in patients with PAF is not known. We can speculate that their lower frequency in the PAF population may lead to a failure to show the association between recurrence after PAF catheter ablation and metabolic syndrome. Indeed, in our population the mean TG level was 1.11 g/L, which is well below the threshold value for metabolic syndrome. Under these conditions, it might be interesting to compare the characteristics of the EAT in our population according to the presence or absence of a metabolic syndrome.

4.6. Study Limitations

The present study has several limitations that must be considered. First, it is a retrospective monocentric study, therefore there is a non-negligible risk of selection bias. In order to assess left atrial (LA)-EAT density, three areas were identified: superior left region (SL), inferior left region (IL) and inferior right region (IR), near the pulmonary vein ostia. Other authors have decided to focus on the posterior wall of the LA. We decided to make another choice because we were interested only in the PAF where the pulmonary veins are at the center of the physiopathology. Finally, the current study evaluated the outcomes 12 months after ablation. Further studies will be necessary to evaluate the impact of EAT on late recurrence beyond 12 months.

5. Conclusions

Contrary to persistent AF, EAT parameters are not associated with AF recurrence after paroxysmal AF ablation. Thus, the role of the metabolic atrial substrate in PAF pathophysiology appears less obvious than in persistent AF.

Author Contributions: Conceptualization: N.H. and H.P.-S.; Methodology: N.H.; Supervision: N.H.; C.d.C., D.M. (Damien Mandry). and N.S.; formal analysis: N.H. and K.B.; investigation: H.P.-S.; resources, J.M.S., I.M.P., A.O., N.P., D.M. (Damien Minois) and M.E.; writing—original draft preparation: N.H. All authors have read and agreed to the published version of the manuscript.

Funding: This research received no external funding.

Informed Consent Statement: Informed consent was obtained from all subjects involved in the study.

Data Availability Statement: The data presented in this study are available on request from the corresponding author.

Conflicts of Interest: The authors declare no conflict of interest.

References

1. Chugh, S.S.; Havmoeller, R.; Narayanan, K.; Singh, D.; Rienstra, M.; Benjamin, E.J.; Gillum, R.F.; Kim, Y.H.; McAnulty, J.H., Jr.; Zheng, Z.J.; et al. Worldwide epidemiology of atrial fibrillation: A Global Burden of Disease 2010 Study. *Circulation* **2014**, *129*, 837–847. [CrossRef] [PubMed]
2. Hindricks, G.; Potpara, T.; Dagres, N.; Arbelo, E.; Bax, J.J.; Blomström-Lundqvist, C.; Boriani, G.; Castella, M.; Dan, G.A.; Dilaveris, P.E.; et al. 2020 ESC Guidelines for the diagnosis and management of atrial fibrillation developed in collaboration with the European Association for Cardio-Thoracic Surgery (EACTS): The Task Force for the diagnosis and management of atrial fibrillation of the European Society of Cardiology (ESC) Developed with the special contribution of the European Heart Rhythm Association (EHRA) of the ESC. *Eur. Heart J.* **2021**, *42*, 373–498.
3. Wilber, D.J.; Pappone, C.; Neuzil, P.; De Paola, A.; Marchlinski, F.; Natale, A.; Macle, L.; Daoud, E.G.; Calkins, H.; Hall, B.; et al. Comparison of antiarrhythmic drug therapy and radiofrequency catheter ablation in patients with paroxysmal atrial fibrillation: A randomized controlled trial. *JAMA* **2010**, *303*, 333–340. [CrossRef] [PubMed]
4. Ganesan, A.; Shipp, N.J.; Brooks, A.G.; Kuklik, P.; Lau, D.H.; Lim, H.S.; Sullivan, T.; Roberts-Thomson, K.C.; Sanders, P. Long-term outcomes of catheter ablation of atrial fibrillation: A systematic review and meta-analysis. *J. Am. Heart Assoc.* **2013**, *2*, e004549. [CrossRef] [PubMed]
5. Arbelo, E.; Brugada, J.; Lundqvist, C.B.; Laroche, C.; Kautzner, J.; Pokushalov, E.; Raatikainen, P.; Efremidis, M.; Hindricks, G.; Barrera, A.; et al. Contemporary management of patients undergoing atrial fibrillation ablation: In-hospital and 1-year follow-up findings from the ESC-EHRA atrial fibrillation ablation long-term registry. *Eur. Heart J.* **2017**, *38*, 1303–1316. [CrossRef] [PubMed]
6. Gaita, F.; Scaglione, M.; Battaglia, A.; Matta, M.; Gallo, C.; Galatà, M.; Caponi, D.; Di Donna, P.; Anselmino, M. Very long-term outcome following transcatheter ablation of atrial fibrillation. Are results maintained after 10 years of follow up? *Ep Eur.* **2018**, *20*, 443–450. [CrossRef] [PubMed]

7. Andrade, J.G.; Champagne, J.; Deyell, M.W.; Essebag, V.; Lauck, S.; Morillo, C.; Sapp, J.; Skanes, A.; Theoret-Patrick, P.; Wells, G.A.; et al. A randomized clinical trial of early invasive intervention for atrial fibrillation (EARLY-AF)—Methods and rationale. *Am. Heart J.* **2018**, *206*, 94–104. [CrossRef] [PubMed]
8. Kirchhof, P.; Camm, A.J.; Goette, A.; Brandes, A.; Eckardt, L.; Elvan, A.; Fetsch, T.; Van Gelder, I.C.; Haase, D.; Haegeli, L.M.; et al. Early Rhythm-Control Therapy in Patients with Atrial Fibrillation. *N. Engl. J. Med.* **2020**, *383*, 1305–1316. [CrossRef]
9. Wazni, O.M.; Dandamudi, G.; Sood, N.; Hoyt, R.; Tyler, J.; Durrani, S.; Niebauer, M.; Makati, K.; Halperin, B.; Gauri, A.; et al. Cryoballoon Ablation as Initial Therapy for Atrial Fibrillation. *N. Engl. J. Med.* **2021**, *384*, 316–324. [CrossRef] [PubMed]
10. Kornej, J.; Schumacher, K.; Dinov, B.; Kosich, F.; Sommer, P.; Arya, A.; Husser, D.; Bollmann, A.; Lip, G.Y.H.; Hindricks, G. Prediction of electro-anatomical substrate and arrhythmia recurrences using APPLE, DR-FLASH and MB-LATER scores in patients with atrial fibrillation undergoing catheter ablation. *Sci. Rep.* **2018**, *8*, 12686. [CrossRef]
11. Wong, C.X.; Ganesan, A.N.; Selvanayagam, J.B. Epicardial fat and atrial fibrillation: Current evidence, potential mechanisms, clinical implications, and future directions. *Eur. Heart J.* **2017**, *38*, 1294–1302. [CrossRef]
12. Goudis, C.A.; Vasileiadis, I.E.; Liu, T. Epicardial adipose tissue and atrial fibrillation: Pathophysiological mechanisms, clinical implications, and potential therapies. *Curr. Med. Res. Opin.* **2018**, *34*, 1933–1943. [CrossRef]
13. Al-Rawahi, M.; Proietti, R.; Thanassoulis, G. Pericardial fat and atrial fibrillation: Epidemiology, mechanisms and interventions. *Int. J. Cardiol.* **2015**, *195*, 98–103. [CrossRef]
14. van Rosendael, A.R.; Dimitriu-Leen, A.C.; van Rosendael, P.J.; Leung, M.; Smit, J.M.; Saraste, A.; Knuuti, J.; van der Geest, R.J.; van der Arend, B.W.; van Zwet, E.W.; et al. Association Between Posterior Left Atrial Adipose Tissue Mass and Atrial Fibrillation. *Circ. Arrhythm. Electrophysiol.* **2017**, *10*, e004614. [CrossRef] [PubMed]
15. Shamloo, A.S.; Dagres, N.; Dinov, B.; Sommer, P.; Husser-Bollmann, D.; Bollmann, A.; Hindricks, G.; Arya, A. Is epicardial fat tissue associated with atrial fibrillation recurrence after ablation? A systematic review and meta-analysis. *Int. J. Cardiol. Heart Vasc.* **2019**, *22*, 132–138.
16. Bonou, M.; Mavrogeni, S.; Kapelios, C.; Markousis-Mavrogenis, G.; Aggeli, C.; Cholongitas, E.; Protogerou, A.; Barbetseas, J. Cardiac Adiposity and Arrhythmias: The Role of Imaging. *Diagnostics* **2021**, *11*, 362. [CrossRef] [PubMed]
17. Pfannenberg, C.; Werner, M.K.; Ripkens, S.; Stef, I.; Deckert, A.; Schmadl, M.; Reimold, M.; Häring, H.-U.; Claussen, C.D.; Stefan, N. Impact of age on the relationships of brown adipose tissue with sex and adiposity in humans. *Diabetes* **2010**, *59*, 1789–1793. [CrossRef] [PubMed]
18. Wong, C.; Abed, H.S.; Molaee, P.; Nelson, A.; Brooks, A.G.; Sharma, G.; Leong, D.P.; Lau, D.H.; Middeldorp, M.; Roberts-Thomson, K.C.; et al. Pericardial fat is associated with atrial fibrillation severity and ablation outcome. *J. Am. Coll. Cardiol.* **2011**, *57*, 1745–1751. [CrossRef]
19. Kim, T.-H.; Park, J.; Park, J.-K.; Uhm, J.-S.; Joung, B.; Lee, M.-H.; Pak, H.-N. Pericardial fat volume is associated with clinical recurrence after catheter ablation for persistent atrial fibrillation, but not paroxysmal atrial fibrillation: An analysis of over 600-patients. *Int. J. Cardiol.* **2014**, *176*, 841–846. [CrossRef]
20. Al Chekakie, M.O.; Welles, C.C.; Metoyer, R.; Ibrahim, A.; Shapira, A.R.; Cytron, J.; Santucci, P.; Wilber, D.J.; Akar, J.G. Pericardial fat is independently associated with human atrial fibrillation. *J. Am. Coll. Cardiol.* **2010**, *56*, 784–788. [CrossRef]
21. Batal, O.; Schoenhagen, P.; Shao, M.; Ayyad, A.E.; Van Wagoner, D.R.; Halliburton, S.S.; Tchou, P.J.; Chung, M.K. Left atrial epicardial adiposity and atrial fibrillation. *Circ. Arrhythm. Electrophysiol.* **2010**, *3*, 230–236. [CrossRef]
22. Platonov, P.G.; Mitrofanova, L.B.; Orshanskaya, V.; Ho, S.Y. Structural abnormalities in atrial walls are associated with presence and persistency of atrial fibrillation but not with age. *J. Am. Coll. Cardiol.* **2011**, *58*, 2225–2232. [CrossRef] [PubMed]
23. Mahajan, R.; Nelson, A.; Pathak, R.K.; Middeldorp, M.E.; Wong, C.X.; Twomey, D.J.; Carbone, A.; Teo, K.; Agbaedeng, T.; Linz, D.; et al. Electroanatomical Remodeling of the Atria in Obesity: Impact of Adjacent Epicardial Fat. *JACC Clin. Electrophysiol.* **2018**, *4*, 1529–1540. [CrossRef] [PubMed]
24. El Mahdiui, M.; Simon, J.; Smit, J.M.; Kuneman, J.H.; van Rosendael, A.R.; Steyerberg, E.W.; van der Geest, R.J.; Száraz, L.; Herczeg, S.; Szegedi, N.; et al. Posterior Left Atrial Adipose Tissue Attenuation Assessed by Computed Tomography and Recurrence of Atrial Fibrillation After Catheter Ablation. *Circ. Arrhythm. Electrophysiol.* **2021**, *14*, e009135. [CrossRef]
25. Zaman, J.A.B.; Baykaner, T.; Clopton, P.; Swarup, V.; Kowal, R.C.; Daubert, J.P.; Day, J.D.; Hummel, J.; Schricker, A.A.; Krummen, D.E.; et al. Recurrent Post-Ablation Paroxysmal Atrial Fibrillation Shares Substrates With Persistent Atrial Fibrillation: An 11-Center Study. *JACC Clin. Electrophysiol.* **2017**, *3*, 393–402. [CrossRef] [PubMed]
26. Moreira, W.; Timmermans, C.; Wellens, H.J.J.; Mizusawa, Y.; Philippens, S.; Perez, D.; Rodriguez, L.-M. Can common-type atrial flutter be a sign of an arrhythmogenic substrate in paroxysmal atrial fibrillation? Clinical and ablative consequences in patients with coexistent paroxysmal atrial fibrillation/atrial flutter. *Circulation* **2007**, *116*, 2786–2792. [CrossRef] [PubMed]
27. Zhang, Y.; Chen, A.; Song, L.; Li, M.; Chen, Y.; He, B. Association Between Baseline Natriuretic Peptides and Atrial Fibrillation Recurrence After Catheter Ablation. *Int. Heart J.* **2016**, *57*, 183–189. [CrossRef]
28. Jiang, H.; Wang, W.; Wang, C.; Xie, X.; Hou, Y. Association of pre-ablation level of potential blood markers with atrial fibrillation recurrence after catheter ablation: A meta-analysis. *EP Eur.* **2017**, *19*, 392–400. [CrossRef]
29. Herring, N.; Zaman, J.A.; Paterson, D.J. Natriuretic peptides like NO facilitate cardiac vagal neurotransmission and bradycardia via a cGMP pathway. *Am. J. Physiol. Heart Circ. Physiol.* **2001**, *281*, H2318–H2327. [CrossRef]

30. Umetani, K.; Kodama, Y.; Nakamura, T.; Mende, A.; Kitta, Y.; Kawabata, K.; Obata, J.-E.; Takano, H.; Kugiyama, K. High prevalence of paroxysmal atrial fibrillation and/or atrial flutter in metabolic syndrome. *Circ. J. Off. J. Jpn. Circ. Soc.* **2007**, *71*, 252–255. [CrossRef]
31. Mohanty, S.; Mohanty, P.; Di Biase, L.; Bai, R.; Pump, A.; Santangeli, P.; Burkhardt, D.; Gallinghouse, J.G.; Horton, R.; Sanchez, J.E.; et al. Impact of metabolic syndrome on procedural outcomes in patients with atrial fibrillation undergoing catheter ablation. *J. Am. Coll. Cardiol.* **2012**, *59*, 1295–1301. [CrossRef] [PubMed]

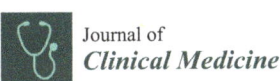

Article

Localized Atrial Tachycardia and Dispersion Regions in Atrial Fibrillation: Evidence of Spatial Concordance

Edouard Gitenay *, Clément Bars, Michel Bremondy, Anis Ayari, Nicolas Maillot, Florian Baptiste, Antonio Taormina, Aicha Fofana, Sabrina Siame, Jérôme Kalifa † and Julien Seitz †

Hôpital Saint Joseph, 26 bd de Louvain, 13008 Marseille, France; barsclement@yahoo.fr (C.B.); mbremondy@orange.fr (M.B.); anisayari84@yahoo.fr (A.A.); nicomaillot@yahoo.fr (N.M.); florian.baptiste@hotmail.fr (F.B.); antoniotaormina88@gmail.com (A.T.); aicha23@hotmail.fr (A.F.); ssiame@hopital-saint-joseph.fr (S.S.); jeromekalifa@gmail.com (J.K.); julienseitz13008@gmail.com (J.S.)
* Correspondence: egitenay@hopital-saint-joseph.fr
† Equal contribution.

Abstract: Introduction: During atrial fibrillation (AF) ablation, it is generally considered that atrial tachycardia (AT) episodes are a consequence of ablation. Objective: To investigate the spatial relationship between localized AT episodes and dispersion/ablation regions during persistent AF ablation procedures. Methods: We analyzed 72 consecutive patients who presented for an index persistent AF ablation procedure guided by the presence of spatiotemporal dispersion of multipolar electrograms. We characterized spontaneous or post-ablation ATs' mechanism and location in regard to dispersion regions and ablation lesions. Results: In 72 consecutive patients admitted for persistent AF ablation, 128 ATs occurred in 62 patients (1.9 ± 1.1/patient). Seventeen ATs were recorded before any ablation. In a total of 100 ATs with elucidated mechanism, there were 58 localized sources and 42 macro-reentries. A large number of localized ATs arose from regions exhibiting dispersion during AF ($n = 49$, 84%). Importantly, these ATs' locations were generally remote from the closest ablation lesion ($n = 42$, 72%). Conclusions: In patients undergoing a persistent AF ablation procedure guided by the presence of spatiotemporal dispersion of multipolar electrograms, localized ATs originate within dispersion regions but remotely from the closest ablation lesion. These results suggest that ATs represent a stabilized manifestation of co-existing AF drivers rather than ablation-induced arrhythmias.

Keywords: atrial tachycardia; ablation; persistent atrial fibrillation; mechanism; spatiotemporal dispersion

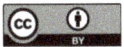

1. Introduction

Multiple groups have recently described patient-tailored, atrial fibrillation (AF) ablation approaches for patients in persistent AF [1–7]. Also named substrate-targeted approaches, these strategies differ in terms of the electrophysiological target that is selected for directing ablation, namely voltage, spatiotemporal dispersion, fractionation, or drivers. Regardless of the approach, most authors have reported the frequent occurrence of during or post-ablation atrial tachycardia (AT) episodes [3,8]. The etiology of these ATs, however, remains unclear. ATs during ablation have been viewed as a consequence of ablation [9,10] or, alternatively, as an arrhythmia relapse requiring reintervention [1–3,8]. Supporting the latter contention, a recent study suggested that post-ablation ATs most often originate from regions that were not previously ablated. In that study, the ECGi approach allowed for panoramic cutaneous phase mapping analysis of AF drivers and subsequent AF/AT ablation [11]. The authors suggested that post-ablation ATs exist prior to the ablation of AF drivers. When other substrate-based ablation approaches are implemented, however, the spatial relationship between AT locations and the substrate regions has been incompletely investigated. Here, we focused our attention on ATs occurring in patients undergoing ablation guided by the presence of spatiotemporal dispersion of electrograms, as described previously [3]. Specifically, we determined the location of localized ATs in regards of regions mapped as "dispersed" during AF.

2. Materials and Methods

We conducted a single center prospective observational study. All patients meeting the following criteria were included: (i) index dispersion-guided ablation for persistent AF between 1 November 2015 and 31 October 2016; (ii) 3D cartography performed with the CARTO 3 system.

2.1. Procedure

2.1.1. Peri-Procedural Aspects

Oral anticoagulation was maintained before intervention. Procedures were performed under general anesthesia. After the trans-esophageal echography-guided transseptal puncture, one or several 1 mg/kg heparin boluses were administered (goal: ACT > 350 ms).

2.1.2. Mapping Protocol

We used a single transseptal sheath. Mapping was performed in AF. For patients in sinus rhythm (SR), AF was induced by rapid atrial pacing using the coronary sinus (CS) catheter (from 500 to 180 ms). When AF was not inducible, isoproterenol (baseline dose: 2.4 mg/h, increased in 0.2 mg increments to reach a sinus rate > 100 beats/min) was infused. Baseline mapping in both atria was performed during AF with the PentaRay multispline catheter (Biosense Webster, Diamond Bar, CA, USA, 2-6-2 mm spacing) sequentially positioned in various regions of the RA and LA. At each location, the catheter was maintained in a stable position for a minimum of 2.5 s. As previously described [3], the operator conducted a mapping of dispersion regions. Briefly, dispersion corresponded to clusters of electrograms (EGMs), either fractionated or non-fractionated, that displayed interelectrode time and space dispersion at a minimum of three adjacent bipoles such that activation spread over all the AFCL. Dispersion regions were manually tagged on the 3D CARTO navigation system.

2.1.3. Ablation Protocol

Once the initial biatrial mapping with the PentaRay catheter was obtained, there was no further analysis/evaluation performed either visually or quantitatively on electrograms recorded with the ablation catheter, nor was there any voltage analysis. Previously mapped dispersion regions were targeted with ablation, while operators did not pursue pulmonary vein isolation or lines. Radiofrequency (RF) energy was delivered (15 to 45 W) at any atrial location including the PV antrum and the CS, using an open-tip irrigated 4 mm SmartTouch SF (Biosense Webster, Inc. Diamond Bar, CA, US). No ablation was performed inside the PVs. The power was adjusted to a range of 10 to 25 W when the ablation catheter was inside the CS or on the posterior LA wall. Irrigation flow rates were adjusted according to the power delivered: 15 mL/min for >30 W and 8 mL/min for $\leq$30 W.

A contact force of 7 g was considered a minimum to deliver RF energy at any location. The endpoint of ablation of areas of dispersion was AF termination defined as conversion to SR or a stable atrial tachycardia (AT).

Post-ablation ATs were mapped and ablated until conversion to SR. If AF did not terminate after ablation at dispersion regions, another sequential map was obtained. When two ablated areas were in close vicinity (<1 cm) or one ablation area was adjacent to an electrically neutral structure (PV, valve), additional RF applications were performed to connect regions or regions and structures. When AF did not terminate, direct current electrical cardioversion (DCCV) was conducted (see Figure 1 for the study flow chart).

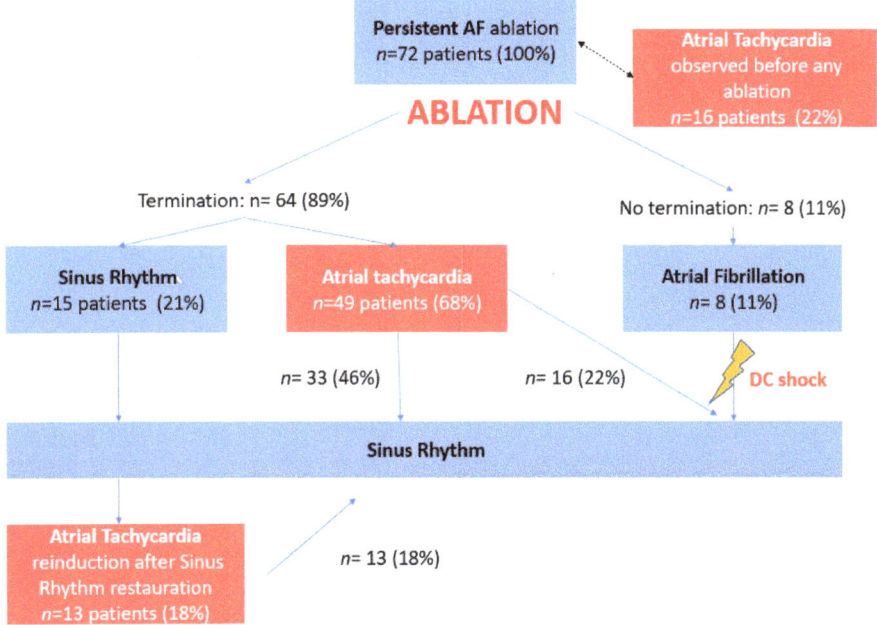

Figure 1. Study flow chart. AF, atrial fibrillation; AT, atrial tachycardia; SR, sinus rhythm.

When sinus rhythm was restored by ablation, reinduction (isoproterenol and/or burst pacing) was performed at the operator's discretion depending on the procedure duration until non-inducibility.

2.1.4. AT Mapping and Classification

AT was defined as a stable organized rhythm with consistent CS activation and monomorphic P-waves. We constructed an activation map for all ATs. Entrainment maneuvers were used when needed. ATs were classified into three categories:

(i) "Localized AT" includes focal AT pattern, i.e., centrifugal activation from a discrete location, and micro-reentry pattern, i.e., >75% of the cycle length represented in the activation map at a given location;

(ii) "Macro-reentries" includes cavotricuspid dependent flutters, peri-mitral flutter, roof flutter, and other more complex macro-reentries such as double loop ATs diagnosed with activation maps and/or entrainment pacing;

(iii) "Undetermined" indicates the above maps and maneuvers were not conclusive.

The spatial relationship between localized ATs and dispersion regions is shown in Figure 2.

Localized ATs were located according to the activation maps as well as the subsequent lesion which terminated the arrhythmia. We then assessed whether ATs were located within (AT-in, <1cm) or remotely (AT-out, ≥1 cm) from (i) a previously mapped dispersion region and (ii) the closest ablation lesion (Figures 2 and 3).

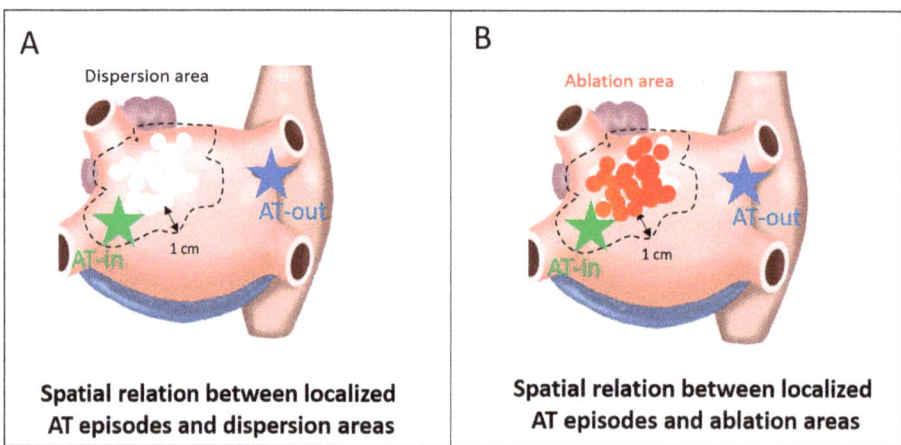

Figure 2. Binary classification of micro-reentrant AT localization. AT-in, localized AT located inside the boundary of the dispersion/ablation area (<1 cm); AT-out, localized AT located outside the boundary of the dispersion/ablation area (≥1 cm). (**A**) the blue star site is an example of localized AT considered distant (AT-out) from dispersion area, while the green star site is considered to be related (AT-in) to the dispersion region. (**B**) the blue star site is an example of localized AT considered distant (AT-out) from previously ablated area, while the green star localized AT site is considered to be related (AT-in) to the ablation region.

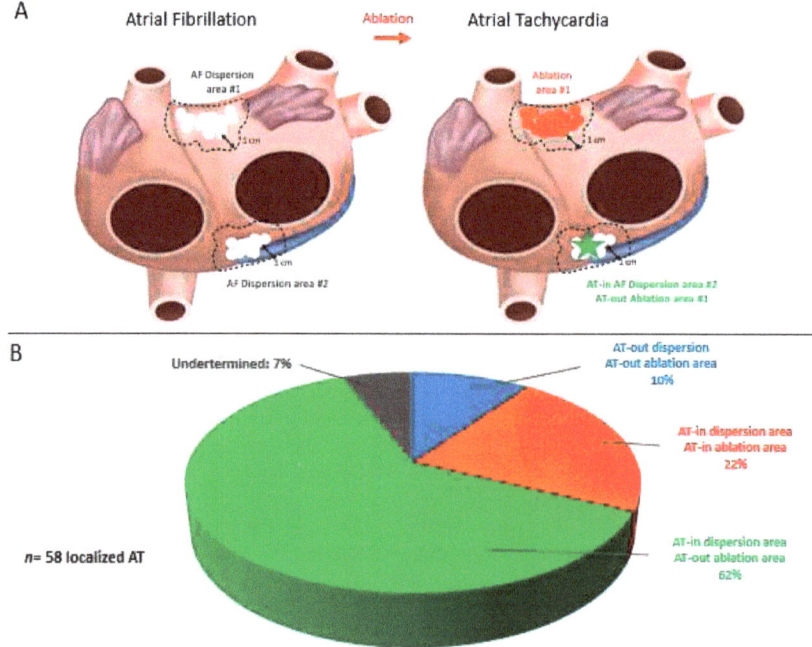

Figure 3. (**A**) Schematic of localized AT located in an AF dispersion unablated area. After bi-atrial dispersion mapping in AF (left picture), two regions of dispersion are highlighted. After ablation of the upper anterior dispersed site, AF turns into AT, found to be localized at the ostium of the coronary sinus (**B**). Spatial relationship between localized AT and dispersion and/or ablation areas. 62% of localized Ats were found to be in sites with dispersion pattern during AF, far from closest ablated region.

3. Statistical Analysis

Categorical variables are expressed as n (%) and numerical variables as mean $\pm$ SD.

4. Results

4.1. Population

From 1 November 2015 to 31 October 2016, we included 72 consecutive patients who underwent an index procedure of dispersion-guided persistent AF ablation with CARTO system. Patient characteristics are summarized in Table 1.

Table 1. Study population.

Study Population	n = 72
Age, years	67.2 $\pm$ 9
Female	19 (26%)
AF type	
Short-standing persistent *	38 (53%)
Long-standing persistent **	14 (19%)
Persistent/unknown duration	20 (28%)
Structural heart disease	25 (39%)
Systemic hypertension	26 (39%)
Diabetes mellitus	9 (12.5%)
Obesity (BMI > 30)	4 (5.5%)
LVEF (%)	46 $\pm$ 19
LA volume, mL	153 $\pm$ 41
RA volume, mL	135 $\pm$ 47
Spontaneous AF at the beginning of procedure	47 (65%)

Values are mean $\pm$ SD or n (%) unless otherwise indicated. AF, atrial fibrillation; BMI, body mass index; LA, left atrial/atrium; RA, right atrial/atrium; LVEF, left ventricular ejection fraction. * When arrhythmic episodes endure from 7 days to 12 months, AF is classified as short-standing persistent. ** Continuous incidences of AF extending greater than 12 months are classified as long-standing persistent.

4.2. Procedure, Mapping, and Analysis

Procedures were performed by four trained cardiac electrophysiologists in a single center: Hopital Saint Joseph, Marseille. The average procedure, fluoroscopy, and radiofrequency times were, respectively, 169 $\pm$ 37.8 $\pm$ 11 and 44 $\pm$ 25 min. The average radiation exposure was 3820c $\pm$ 4167c Gycm^2.

Forty-seven patients (65%) were in AF at the beginning of the procedure. In the other patients, AF was induced by burst pacing and/or isoproterenol infusion.

Before ablation, the CS, RA, and LA appendage reference CLs in AF were 212 $\pm$ 59, 208 $\pm$ 58, and 201 $\pm$ 60 ms, respectively. While all patients had an LA dispersion mapping, the dispersion mapping was biatrial in 57 patients (79%). The LA and RA average volumes were 153 $\pm$ 41 and 135 $\pm$ 47 mL, respectively.

AF terminated—i.e., conversion either to AT or SR—during ablation in 64 patients (89%).

The mean procedure time to terminate AF and the mean RF time to terminate AF were 53 $\pm$ 39 and 23 $\pm$ 21 min, respectively. When AF terminated, it converted directly to SR in 15 patients (21%) and to AT in the remaining 49 patients (68%). Site of AF termination, clearly identified in 49 patients are illustrated in Figure S1 (supplemental materials). There was a subsequent SR restauration by ablation in 33 patients, and DCCV was conducted in the 16 remaining patients. Overall, there was a SR restoration by ablation in 48 patients (67%). All patients underwent an LA ablation, while 57 patients (79%) underwent a biatrial ablation. Inducibility was tested in 29 patients and achieved in 20 patients.

4.3. Atrial Tachycardias

We observed 128 ATs in 62 patients (1.9 $\pm$ 1.1/patient) before any ablation in patients with clinically documented persistent AF, as a transitional rhythm after ablation, or as a re-induced arrhythmia (see Figure 1—study flow-chart). Overall, 58 ATs (45%) were characterized as localized ATs (see localization in Figure S2), while 42 (33%) were characterized as macro-reentries. Of 42 macro-reentries, we observed 16 peri-tricuspid flutters (38%), 15 peri-mitral flutters (36%), and 11 LA roof-dependent flutters (26%). In 22 ATs (17%), the AT mechanism was undetermined.

4.4. AT before Any Ablation

Among the 72 patients referred for documented persistent AF ablation, 17 ATs were seen before any ablation, including 9 peri-tricuspid flutters, 5 localized ATs, and 3 with an undetermined mechanism.

4.5. Spatial Relationship between Localized ATs and Dispersion Regions

A large number of localized ATs (48/58, 83%) arose from a previously mapped spatiotemporal dispersion region. In 41/58 ATs (71%), they also located remotely from the closest ablation lesion. A representative example of how localized ATs originated within a cluster of dispersion but remotely from the closest lesion is presented in Figure 4. In this patient, the initial biatrial map highlighted the presence of multiple dispersion regions in both the RA and LA. In the RA, one small-sized dispersion region was delineated on the superior aspect of the RA posterior wall. After ablation in the LA only, AF transitioned into a stable AT, which originated from the posterior-wall RA dispersion region. This example suggests that the progressive ablation of LA dispersion regions in AF was sufficient to alter the AF dynamics into the emergence of a localized AT from a non-ablated dispersion region.

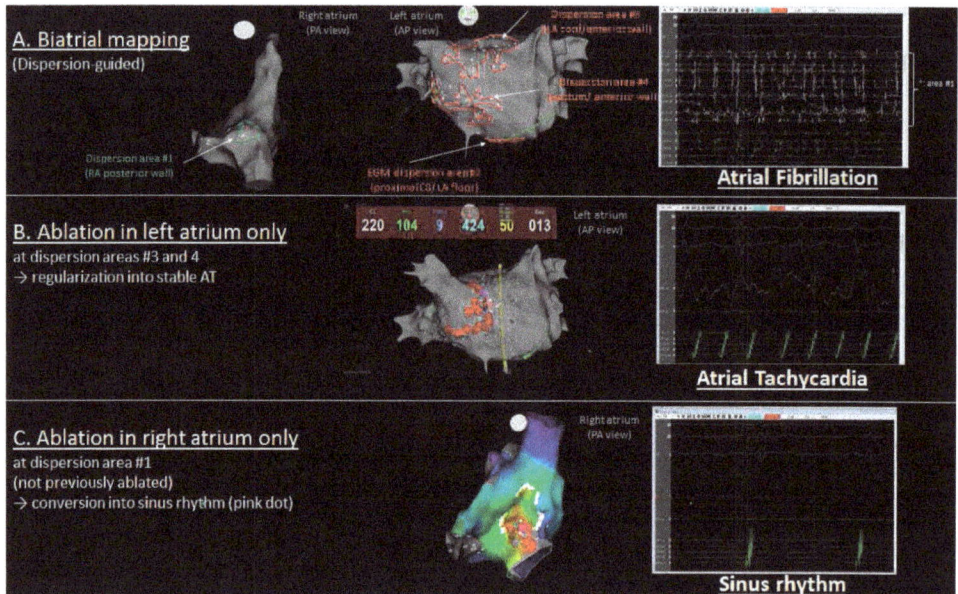

Figure 4. Representative example of the spatial concordance between spatiotemporal dispersion regions in persistent AF and a post-ablation localized AT emanating from the RA posterior wall, remotely from previously ablated regions. (**A**) Biatrial map showing spatiotemporal dispersion regions as encircled clusters of white dots, with the green and red lines indicating the RA and LA, respectively. (**B**) Ablation at dispersion regions in the LA led to AF regularization into a stable AT. (**C**) The localized AT presented in (**B**) terminated after ablation in the right atrium remotely from the closest ablation lesion. AF, atrial fibrillation; AT, atrial tachycardia.

Further, we observed that, in some patients, a pattern of spatiotemporal dispersion, which is typically seen in AF, may sequentially underlie AF or AT at the same location. An example is presented in Figure 5. In this patient, prior to any ablation, AF and AT sequentially occurred while dispersion was continually recorded with a PentaRay catheter stably positioned at the posterior LA (Figure 5).

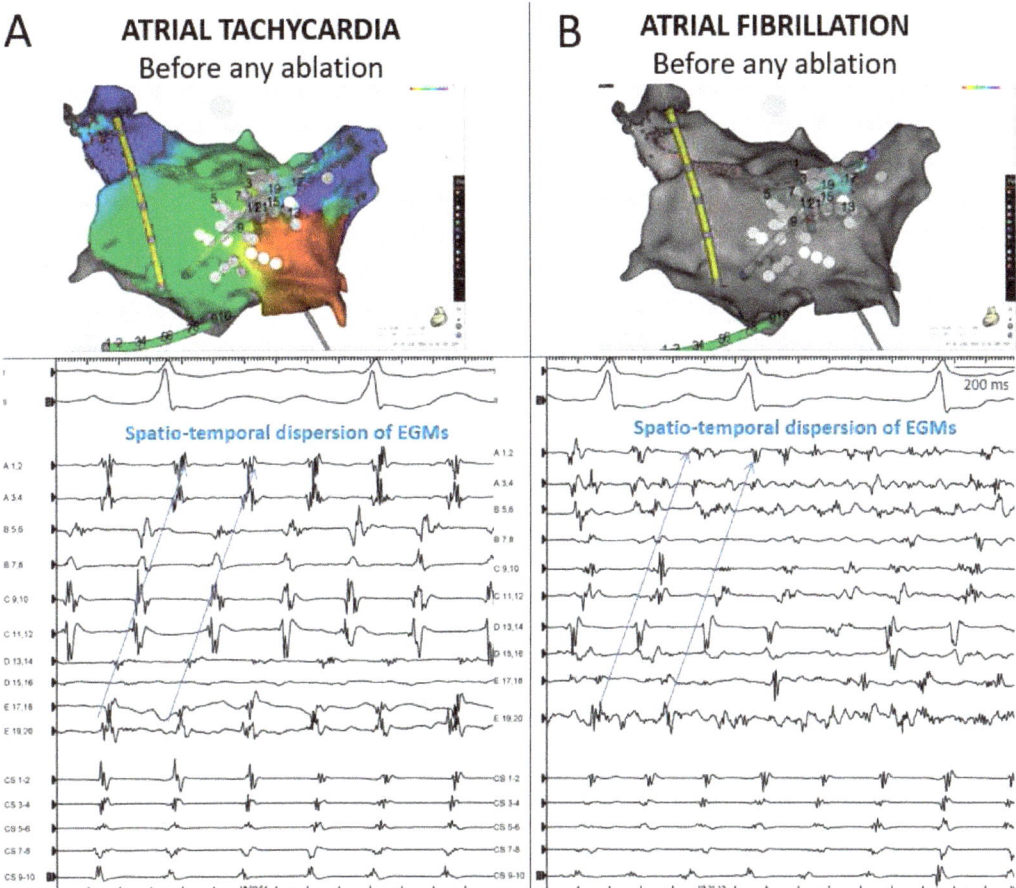

Figure 5. Posteroanterior 3D view of a left atrium alternatively in AT and AF prior to any ablation. The pattern of dispersion observed on a delineated posterior zone, during either AT ((**A**) the activation map on the right shows a micro-reentry at the same location) or AF ((**B**) the cluster of white tags indicates the area of dispersion beside the right pulmonary vein's posterior antrum). AF, atrial fibrillation; AT, atrial tachycardia; AT-in, AT located inside; AT-out, AT located outside.

4.6. Redo Ablation Procedures

In total, 55 redo ablation procedures in 35 patients were performed between 16 November 2016 and 20 January 2021 (67% for AT and 33% for AF). The arrhythmia type, mechanism, and termination sites are described in Supplementary Table S1.

5. Discussion

Our main findings are as follows: (i) Most localized ATs (84%) recorded during dispersion-guided persistent AF ablation originated from dispersion areas mapped in AF; (ii) of these localized ATs, 72% arose remotely from the closest ablation lesion; (iii) 13% (n = 17) of the ATs were observed prior to any ablation.

5.1. Spatial Concordance between Localized AT and AF Drivers

Here, we show that there is a spatial concordance between localized AT locations and dispersion regions. Using dispersion of multipolar electrograms as a beacon to localize AF drivers, we bring evidence that ATs mostly originate from the regions where AF drivers are found. Our findings corroborate previous investigations, which found that peri-ablation ATs tend to locate where previously mapped "active" AF sites had been delineated. For example, Ban et al. [12] examined patients who experienced AT episodes after pulmonary vein isolation and CFAE-guided ablation. They demonstrated that regions exhibiting CFAEs are frequently associated with the termination of AT occurring after AF ablation. In addition, Yamashita et al. [11] investigated patients referred for persistent AF ablation consisting of the targeting AF drivers mapped with body surface multi-electrode ECG (252-lead ECGi; Cardioinsight). Among the 26 focal and 52 micro-reentrant ATs observed, 82% located in the vicinity of an AF driver. Reminiscent of some of the criteria of spatiotemporal dispersion, the sites of ATs generally presented with low-voltage, fractionated, and long-duration electrograms in AF.

5.2. Mechanistic Significance of Organized AT in Patients with AF

Our findings support the contention that there is a common pathophysiological mechanism that underlies AT and AF drivers. Several experimental works showed that both AT and AF may be initiated and perpetuated by wavebreaks and micro-reentrant circuits [13,14]. Other works suggested that a discrete number of co-existing drivers may perpetuate AF [15,16]. Albeit indirectly, the present observation provides additional evidence that co-existing or interchangeable AF/AT drivers originate from a unique region, which may underlie both persistent AF and ATs. In addition, our results show that some ATs might exist before AF or could alternatively represent an organized manifestation of AF. In support of these contentions, our findings suggest that spatiotemporal dispersion may represent a common electrogram footprint of AF and AT drivers (Figure 5). We also provide insight into the commonly observed phenomenon of AF transitioning into AT—and vice versa—during an ablation procedure (Figure 6).

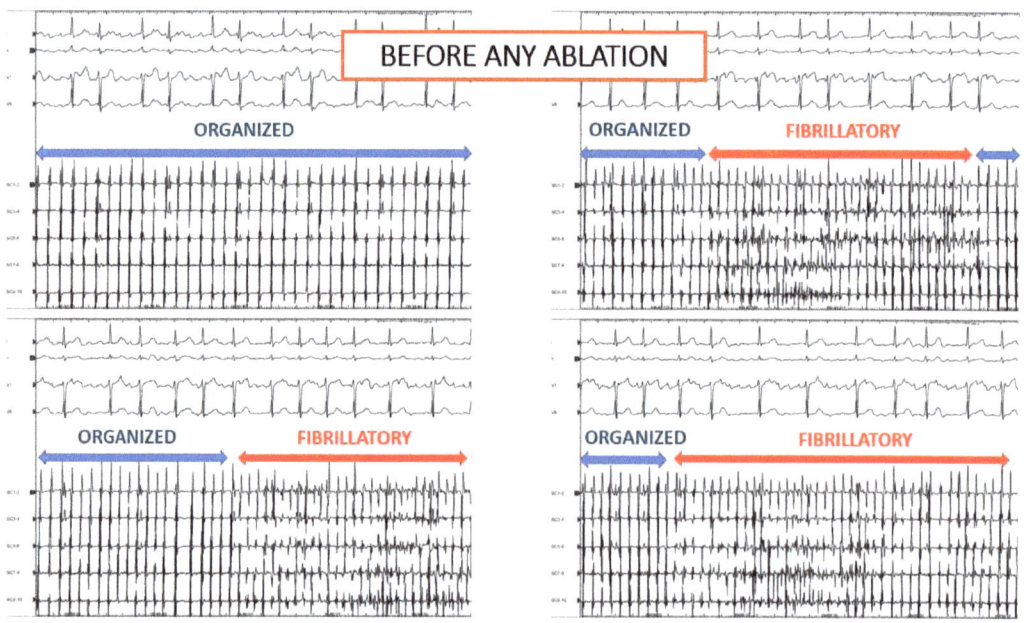

Figure 6. Coronary sinus EGMs showing subsequent AF and AT in a patient prior to any ablation.

5.3. Clinical Relevance in the Clinical Cardiac Electrophysiological Laboratory

ATs are highly prevalent in the population of patients with either paroxysmal [17] or persistent AF [18]. In a series of patients with AT, Israel et al. [19] concluded that most patients with a history of AF show both disorganized and highly organized AT episodes. In addition, the fact that regular ectopic beats can initiate AF episodes and play the role of a "trigger" has been abundantly demonstrated. Haissaguerre et al. [17] showed that such triggers are found in pulmonary vein regions. In addition, a focal, non-sustained monomorphic AT was seen in 40% of patients with persistent AF who underwent an electrical shock and a subsequent early AF recurrence [18]. Similarly, it is also well-known that anti-arrhythmic drugs may organize AF into a stable AT [20,21]. At the mechanistic level, Baykaner et al. [22] conducted a study in patients who underwent AF driver ablation after endocardial multi-electrode biatrial mapping using a 64-electrode catheter. The mapped AT spatially overlapped one AF source in 88% of patients, and three mechanisms were suggested: an ablation-related anchoring of AF rotor resulting in AT, a residual unablated AF source producing AT, or a spontaneous slowing of an AF rotor. In addition, Yoshida et al. [23] implemented a spectral analysis of the AF electrograms from the coronary sinus and lead V1 in patients referred for AF ablation with organization into AT during the procedure. In about half of the patients, a spectral component with a frequency that matched the frequency of subsequent AT was present in the baseline periodogram of AF. Finally, Rostock et al. [24] conducted a randomized investigation, which concluded that systematic mapping and ablation of ATs occurring during persistent AF ablation improves long-term outcomes.

Together with these studies, our work suggests that ATs could represent a so-called "simplified" manifestation of AF drivers. Thus, AF may be seen as a complex physiopathological phenomenon, whereby one or a small number of stable drivers initiate and/or perpetuate the arrhythmia. On the other hand, we acknowledge that an ablation lesion may represent an iatrogenic origin of ATs—in providing a substrate for a subsequent reentry. Our results, however, demonstrate that, during dispersion-guided ablation, RF lesions mostly cause AF driver termination, without which AT is initiated.

5.4. Ablation-Related ATs

Previously, ablation-related tissue injury has been shown to represent a substrate for reentry and focal discharges [25]. Karch et al. demonstrated that segmental pulmonary vein isolation leads to a higher number of post-ablation tachyarrhythmias than circumferential PVI [26]. In addition, Iwai et al. [27] showed that localized ATs during an index persistent AF ablation may differ from the ones seen in subsequent procedures and represent a poor prognosis. Such studies highlighted that ablation gaps may provide a substrate for the occurrence of localized atrial tachycardias, particularly around the PV region. In the present work, however, our observations suggest that only ~30% (17 AT episodes) of the localized ATs arose in the vicinity (within 1 cm) of the closest ablation lesion. Even if we were speculating that all these ATs were caused by prior ablative lesions, our results would still show that dispersion-guided ablation is mainly associated with non-iatrogenic localized ATs.

6. Study Limitations

Our work provides little information about the correlation between macro-reentrant ATs and dispersion. However, it should be mentioned that nine patients had spontaneous macro-reentries prior to any ablation. Furthermore, technical limitations prevented us from building voltage maps. In previous publications [11,22], however, localized ATs arising from AF driver sites have been associated with fragmented and low-voltage signals. Thus, future works are warranted to examine the relationship between post-ablation ATs and low-voltage regions. This study provides clinical observations and indirect evidence of a mechanistic commonality between AF and AT. Future works will need to further this investigation in examining the role of rotors and fibrotic scars in the development of AF and AT.

7. Conclusions

ATs are commonly observed during an index persistent AF ablation procedure guided by spatiotemporal dispersion. Our observations indicate that localized ATs mostly originate within dispersion regions but remotely from the closest ablation lesion. These results suggest a commonality of mechanism between AF and AT. Although incomplete ablation may be proarrhythmic, most ATs occurring during a dispersion-guided AF ablation procedure are unlikely to have been caused by ablation lesions.

Supplementary Materials: The following are available online at https://www.mdpi.com/article/10.3390/jcm10143170/s1, Figure S1: Bi-atrial cumulative schematic of atrial fibrillation termination sites clearly identified in 49 patients; Figure S2: Bi-atrial cumulative schematic of localized atrial tachycardia termination sites in 40 patients; Table S1: Arrhythmia type/mechanism/termination site for redo procedures performed between 16 November 2016 to 20 January 2021.

Author Contributions: E.G. and J.S., study design, data collection, data analysis, writing, and reviewing; J.K. and C.B., data collection, data analysis, and reviewing; S.S., database organization, administrative tasks, and reviewing; M.B., A.A., N.M., F.B., A.T. and A.F., reviewing. All authors have read and agreed to the published version of the manuscript.

Funding: This research received no external funding.

Institutional Review Board Statement: This study did not involve humans but only the reuse of already recorded data. This study falls within the scope of the French Reference Methodology MR-004 (according to 2016-41 law dated 26 January 2016 on the modernization of the French health system). As requested by the French regulation for such non-interventional study, after being informed about the study, the non-opposition of all included patients was collected and reported in their case report form by the investigators. The study was conducted in accordance with the ethical guidelines of the 1975 Declaration of Helsinki. The study was approved by the institutional and ethical review board of the Saint Joseph Hospital of Marseille (26 November 2020).

Informed Consent Statement: Informed consent was obtained from all subjects involved in the study.

Data Availability Statement: The data presented in this study are available on request from the corresponding author.

Conflicts of Interest: Gitenay received consulting fees from Abbott. Bars, Kalifa, and Seitz received Speaker Fees from Biosense Webster, Abbott, and Boston Scientific and are shareholders of VOLTA Medical.

Abbreviations

AAD	antiarrhythmic drug
AF	atrial fibrillation
AFCL	atrial fibrillation cycle length
AT	atrial tachycardia
CFAE	complex fractionated atrial electrogram
CL	cycle length
CS	coronary sinus
DCCV	direct current electrical cardioversion
LA	left atrial/atrium
PV	pulmonary vein
PVI	pulmonary vein isolation
RA	right atrial/atrium
RF	radiofrequency
SR	sinus rhythm

References

1. Nademanee, K.; McKenzie, J.; Kosar, E.; Schwab, M.; Sunsaneewitayakul, B.; Vasavakul, T.; Khunnawat, C.; Ngarmukos, T. A new approach for catheter ablation of atrial fibrillation: Mapping of the electrophysiologic substrate. *J. Am. Coll. Cardiol.* **2004**, *43*, 2044–2053. [CrossRef]
2. Jadidi, A.S.; Lehrmann, H.; Keyl, C.; Sorrel, J.; Markstein, V.; Minners, J.; Park, C.-I.; Denis, A.; Jaïs, P.; Hocini, M.; et al. Ablation of Persistent Atrial Fibrillation Targeting Low-Voltage Areas With Selective Activation Characteristics. *Circ. Arrhythmia Electrophysiol.* **2016**, *9*, e002962. [CrossRef] [PubMed]
3. Seitz, J.; Bars, C.; Théodore, G.; Beurtheret, S.; Lellouche, N.; Bremondy, M.; Ferracci, A.; Faure, J.; Penaranda, G.; Yamazaki, M.; et al. AF Ablation Guided by Spatiotemporal Electrogram Dispersion Without Pulmonary Vein Isolation. *J. Am. Coll. Cardiol.* **2017**, *69*, 303–321. [CrossRef]
4. Lin, R.; Zeng, C.; Xu, K.; Wu, S.; Qin, M.; Liu, X. Dispersion-guided ablation in conjunction with circumferential pulmonary vein isolation is superior to stepwise ablation approach for persistent atrial fibrillation. *Int. J. Cardiol.* **2019**, *278*, 97–103. [CrossRef] [PubMed]
5. Kottkamp, H.; Berg, J.; Bender, R.; Rieger, A.; Schreiber, D. Box Isolation of Fibrotic Areas (BIFA): A Patient-Tailored Substrate Modification Approach for Ablation of Atrial Fibrillation. *J. Cardiovasc. Electrophysiol.* **2016**, *27*, 22–30. [CrossRef]
6. Narayan, S.M.; Krummen, D.E.; Shivkumar, K.; Clopton, P.; Rappel, W.-J.; Miller, J.M. Treatment of Atrial Fibrillation by the Ablation of Localized Sources: CONFIRM (Conventional Ablation for Atrial Fibrillation With or Without Focal Impulse and Rotor Modulation) Trial. *J. Am. Coll. Cardiol.* **2012**, *60*, 628–636. [CrossRef]
7. Haissaguerre, M.; Hocini, M.; Denis, A.; Shah, A.J.; Komatsu, Y.; Yamashita, S.; Daly, M.; Amraoui, S.; Zellerhoff, S.; Picat, M.-Q.; et al. Driver Domains in Persistent Atrial Fibrillation. *Circulation* **2014**, *130*, 530–538. [CrossRef] [PubMed]
8. Scherr, D.; Khairy, P.; Miyazaki, S.; Aurillac-Lavignolle, V.; Pascale, P.; Wilton, S.B.; Ramoul, K.; Komatsu, Y.; Roten, L.; Jadidi, A.; et al. Five-Year Outcome of Catheter Ablation of Persistent Atrial Fibrillation Using Termination of Atrial Fibrillation as a Procedural Endpoint. *Circ. Arrhythmia Electrophysiol.* **2015**, *8*, 18–24. [CrossRef]
9. Tutuianu, C.; Szilagyi, J. Atrial Tachycardias Following Atrial Fibrillation Ablation. *Curr. Cardiol. Rev.* **2014**, *11*, 149–156. [CrossRef]
10. Kuck, K.-H.; Brugada, J.; Fürnkranz, A.; Metzner, A.; Ouyang, F.; Chun, K.J.; Elvan, A.; Arentz, T.; Bestehorn, K.; Pocock, S.J.; et al. Cryoballoon or Radiofrequency Ablation for Paroxysmal Atrial Fibrillation. *N. Engl. J. Med.* **2016**, *374*, 2235–2245. [CrossRef]
11. Yamashita, S.; Hooks, D.A.; Shah, A.; Relan, J.; Cheniti, G.; Kitamura, T.; Berte, B.; Mahida, S.; Sellal, J.-M.; Al Jefairi, N.; et al. Atrial tachycardias: Cause or effect with ablation of persistent atrial fibrillation? *J. Cardiovasc. Electrophysiol.* **2017**, *29*, 274–283. [CrossRef] [PubMed]
12. Ban, J.-E.; Chen, Y.-L.; Park, H.-C.; Lee, H.-S.; Lee, D.-I.; Choi, J.-I.; Lim, H.-E.; Park, S.-W.; Kim, Y.-H. Relationship Between Complex Fractionated Atrial Electrograms During Atrial Fibrillation and the Critical Site of Atrial Tachycardia That Develops After Catheter Ablation for Atrial Fibrillation. *J. Cardiovasc. Electrophysiol.* **2014**, *25*, 146–153. [CrossRef]
13. Mandapati, R.; Skanes, A.; Chen, J.; Berenfeld, O.; Jalife, J. Stable Microreentrant Sources as a Mechanism of Atrial Fibrillation in the Isolated Sheep Heart. *Circulation* **2000**, *101*, 194–199. [CrossRef]
14. Berenfeld, O.; Zaitsev, A.V.; Mironov, S.F.; Pertsov, A.M.; Jalife, J. Frequency-Dependent Breakdown of Wave Propagation Into Fibrillatory Conduction Across the Pectinate Muscle Network in the Isolated Sheep Right Atrium. *Circ. Res.* **2002**, *90*, 1173–1180. [CrossRef]
15. Berenfeld, O. Quantifying activation frequency in atrial fibrillation to establish underlying mechanisms and ablation guidance. *Heart Rhythm.* **2007**, *4*, 1225–1234. [CrossRef] [PubMed]
16. Atienza, F.; Almendral, J.; Jalife, J.; Zlochiver, S.; Ploutz-Snyder, R.; Torrecilla, E.G.; Arenal, Á.; Kalifa, J.; Fernández-Avilés, F.; Berenfeld, O. Real-time dominant frequency mapping and ablation of dominant frequency sites in atrial fibrillation with left-to-right frequency gradients predicts long-term maintenance of sinus rhythm. *Heart Rhythm.* **2009**, *6*, 33–40. [CrossRef]
17. Haïssaguerre, M.; Jaïs, P.; Shah, D.C.; Takahashi, A.; Hocini, M.; Quiniou, G.; Garrigue, S.; Le Mouroux, A.; Le Métayer, P.; Clémenty, J. Spontaneous Initiation of Atrial Fibrillation by Ectopic Beats Originating in the Pulmonary Veins. *N. Engl. J. Med.* **1998**, *339*, 659–666. [CrossRef] [PubMed]
18. Todd, D.M.; Fynn, S.P.; Hobbs, W.J.; Fitzpatrick, A.P.; Garratt, C.J. Prevalence and significance of focal sources of atrial arrhythmia in patients undergoing cardioversion of persistent atrial fibrillation. *J. Cardiovasc. Electrophysiol.* **2000**, *11*, 616–622. [CrossRef] [PubMed]
19. Israel, C.W.; Ehrlich, J.R.; Grönefeld, G.; Klesius, A.; Lawo, T.; Lemke, B.; Hohnloser, S.H. Prevalence, characteristics and clinical implications of regular atrial tachyarrhythmias in patients with atrial fibrillation: Insights from a study using a new implantable device. *J. Am. Coll. Cardiol.* **2001**, *38*, 355–363. [CrossRef]
20. Nabar, A. Class IC antiarrhythmic drug induced atrial flutter: Electrocardiographic and electrophysiological findings and their importance for long term outcome after right atrial isthmus ablation. *Heart Br. Card. Soc.* **2001**, *85*, 424–429. [CrossRef]
21. Bianconi, L.; Mennuni, M.; Lukic, V.; Castro, A.; Chieffi, M.; Santini, M. Effects of oral propafenone administration before electrical cardioversion of chronic atrial fibrillation: A placebo-controlled study. *J. Am. Coll. Cardiol.* **1996**, *28*, 700–706. [CrossRef]
22. Baykaner, T.; Zaman, J.A.; Rogers, A.J.; Navara, R.; Alhusseini, M.; Borne, R.T.; Park, S.; Wang, P.J.; Krummen, D.E.; Sauer, W.H.; et al. Spatial relationship of sites for atrial fibrillation drivers and atrial tachycardia in patients with both arrhythmias. *Int. J. Cardiol.* **2017**, *248*, 188–195. [CrossRef] [PubMed]

23. Yoshida, K.; Chugh, A.; Ulfarsson, M.; Good, E.; Kühne, M.; Crawford, T.; Sarrazin, J.F.; Chalfoun, N.; Wells, D.; Boonyapisit, W.; et al. Relationship between the spectral characteristics of atrial fibrillation and atrial tachycardias that occur after catheter ablation of atrial fibrillation. *Heart Rhythm.* **2009**, *6*, 11–17. [CrossRef]
24. Rostock, T.; Salukhe, T.V.; Hoffmann, B.A.; Steven, D.; Berner, I.; Müllerleile, K.; Theis, C.; Bock, K.; Servatius, H.; Sultan, A.; et al. Prognostic Role of Subsequent Atrial Tachycardias Occurring During Ablation of Persistent Atrial Fibrillation. *Circ. Arrhythmia Electrophysiol.* **2013**, *6*, 1059–1065. [CrossRef]
25. Gerstenfeld, E.P.; Dixit, S.; Bala, R.; Callans, D.J.; Lin, D.; Sauer, W.; Garcia, F.; Cooper, J.; Russo, A.M.; Marchlinski, F. Surface electrocardiogram characteristics of atrial tachycardias occurring after pulmonary vein isolation. *Heart Rhythm.* **2007**, *4*, 1136–1143. [CrossRef]
26. Karch, M.R.; Zrenner, B.; Deisenhofer, I.; Schreieck, J.; Ndrepepa, G.; Dong, J.; Lamprecht, K.; Barthel, P.; Luciani, E.; Schömig, A.; et al. Freedom From Atrial Tachyarrhythmias After Catheter Ablation of Atrial Fibrillation. *Circulation* **2005**, *111*, 2875–2880. [CrossRef] [PubMed]
27. Iwai, S.; Takahashi, Y.; Masumura, M.; Yamashita, S.; Doi, J.; Yamamoto, T.; Sakakibara, A.; Nomoto, H.; Yoshida, Y.; Sugiyama, T.; et al. Occurrence of Focal Atrial Tachycardia During the Ablation Procedure Is Associated with Arrhythmia Recurrence After Termination of Persistent Atrial Fibrillation. *J. Cardiovasc. Electrophysiol.* **2017**, *28*, 489–497. [CrossRef]

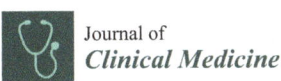

Review

Ablation Modalities for Therapeutic Intervention in Arrhythmia-Related Cardiovascular Disease: Focus on Electroporation

Shauna McBride [1], Sahar Avazzadeh [1], Antony M. Wheatley [1], Barry O'Brien [2], Ken Coffey [2], Adnan Elahi [3,4], Martin O'Halloran [3] and Leo R. Quinlan [1,5,*]

1. Physiology and Cellular Physiology Laboratory, CÚRAM SFI Centre for Research in Medical Devices, School of Medicine, Human Biology Building, National University of Ireland (NUI) Galway, H91 W5P7 Galway, Ireland; shauna.mcbride@nuigalway.ie (S.M.); sahar.avazzadeh@nuigalway.ie (S.A.); antony.wheatley@nuigalway.ie (A.M.W.)
2. AtriAN Medical Limited, Unit 204, NUIG Business Innovation Centre, Upper Newcastle, H91 R6W6 Galway, Ireland; barry.obrien@atrianmedical.com (B.O.); ken.coffey@atrianmedical.com (K.C.)
3. Translational Medical Device Lab (TMDL), Lamb Translational Research Facility, University College Hospital Galway, H91 V4AY Galway, Ireland; adnan.elahi@nuigalway.ie (A.E.); martin.ohalloran@nuigalway.ie (M.O.)
4. Electrical & Electronic Engineering, School of Engineering, National University of Ireland Galway, H91 HX31 Galway, Ireland
5. CÚRAM, SFI Research Centre for Medical Devices, National University of Ireland Galway, H92 W2TY Galway, Ireland
* Correspondence: leo.quinlan@nuigalway.ie

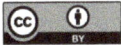

Citation: McBride, S.; Avazzadeh, S.; Wheatley, A.M.; O'Brien, B.; Coffey, K.; Elahi, A.; O'Halloran, M.; Quinlan, L.R. Ablation Modalities for Therapeutic Intervention in Arrhythmia-Related Cardiovascular Disease: Focus on Electroporation. *J. Clin. Med.* **2021**, *10*, 2657. https://doi.org/10.3390/jcm10122657

Academic Editor: Charles Guenancia

Received: 25 May 2021
Accepted: 14 June 2021
Published: 16 June 2021

Publisher's Note: MDPI stays neutral with regard to jurisdictional claims in published maps and institutional affiliations.

Copyright: © 2021 by the authors. Licensee MDPI, Basel, Switzerland. This article is an open access article distributed under the terms and conditions of the Creative Commons Attribution (CC BY) license (https://creativecommons.org/licenses/by/4.0/).

Abstract: Targeted cellular ablation is being increasingly used in the treatment of arrhythmias and structural heart disease. Catheter-based ablation for atrial fibrillation (AF) is considered a safe and effective approach for patients who are medication refractory. Electroporation (EPo) employs electrical energy to disrupt cell membranes which has a minimally thermal effect. The nanopores that arise from EPo can be temporary or permanent. Reversible electroporation is transitory in nature and cell viability is maintained, whereas irreversible electroporation causes permanent pore formation, leading to loss of cellular homeostasis and cell death. Several studies report that EPo displays a degree of specificity in terms of the lethal threshold required to induce cell death in different tissues. However, significantly more research is required to scope the profile of EPo thresholds for specific cell types within complex tissues. Irreversible electroporation (IRE) as an ablative approach appears to overcome the significant negative effects associated with thermal based techniques, particularly collateral damage to surrounding structures. With further fine-tuning of parameters and longer and larger clinical trials, EPo may lead the way of adapting a safer and efficient ablation modality for the treatment of persistent AF.

Keywords: electroporation; pulsed field ablation; cardiac; heart; arrhythmia; atrial fibrillation

1. Introduction

The Centers for Disease Control and Prevention in the USA reports that 1 in every 4 deaths in the United States is related to general cardiovascular disease, with an estimated 12.1 million people predicted to develop arrhythmias such as atrial fibrillation (AF) by 2030 [1]. In recent years there has been a rapid growth in the technology base and clinical appetite for targeted ablative procedures for arrhythmias, with some reports showing procedures to be effective, with quick procedural timelines, minimal associated risks and rapid recovery times [2,3]. Catheter-based ablation for AF is considered a safe and effective approach for patients who are refractory to medication. The cornerstone of catheter-based approaches to date is pulmonary vein isolation (PVI) but, increasingly, additional sites beyond the pulmonary veins are now being targeted [4]. In this review we report on the available data exploring energy-based ablative technologies, highlight the differing modalities that have been developed with a particular focus on anti-arrhythmic therapies. This review also considers the factors involved in achieving successful ablation of cardiac tissue and the evidence from in vitro and in vivo preclinical work which has informed clinical studies using EPo approaches.

2. Current Ablation Approaches for Treating Arrhythmia

Several relatively simple non-invasive ablative procedures have been developed to date, such as alcohol septal ablation, which involves the injection of ethanol into the septal coronary artery to target portions of the septal wall [5]. This minimally invasive ablation method has been extensively employed as a treatment for structural related heart defects such as hypertrophic cardiomyopathy, targeting the attenuation of outflow tract obstruction [2,6]. Alcohol septal ablation is often applied when previous lower intensity therapies have failed [5]. Stereotactic radioablation is another non-invasive modality under development. While not currently used in clinical practice to the best of our knowledge, a number of animal-based feasibility studies with stereotactic radioablation have been performed and reviewed elsewhere [7,8].

Typically, more invasive ablation techniques require entry into the body cavity to access targeted areas of the myocardium (Figure 1). These techniques up to more recently generally involved the use of thermal energy and either induced hyper- or hypo-thermal injury at the target site [9]. Hyperthermal approaches are most commonly based on the application of radiofrequency (RF) or laser energy. Hypothermal approaches, termed cryoablation, are commonly achieved by passing cooled, thermally conductive, fluids through hollow probes at the target site.

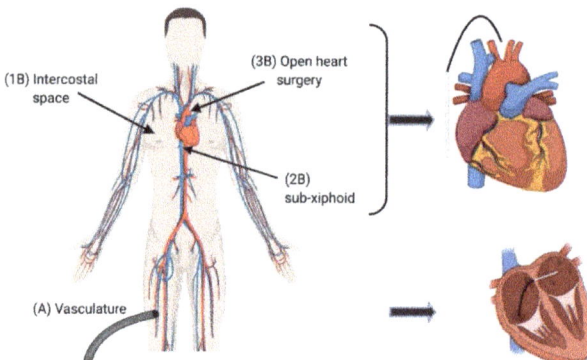

Figure 1. Access to the heart for invasive ablation purposes. This can be achieved via an internal endocardial approach (**A**) via the femoral vasculature (Table 2). Ablation catheter access can also be gained from an external epicardial (**B**) method. The extremities of the heart are reached by this technique. Access via an epicardial approach can be achieved through ports in the intercostal spaces (**1B**), a sub-xiphoid puncture (**2B**) or via open heart surgery (**3B**). The choice made between the two approaches is often made in relation to the target area and patient's disease substrate [10].

2.1. Hyperthermal Techniques

Hyperthermal approaches can use various energy sources including the use of ultrasound, lasers, radiofrequency technology applied via electrode catheter, or hot balloon ablation systems [11,12]. Focused ultrasound causes the destruction of a target area due to a thermal heating effect, while remaining minimally invasive [11,13,14]. Several studies have highlighted the challenges associated with using high-intensity ultrasound for cardiac ablation [15–17]. Due to the incidence of oesophageal fistula and subsequent fatalities, ultrasound as a modality needs considerably more development involving lower-intensity energy and better targeting if it is to be more widely adopted [15,18]. Similar techniques are employed using lasers and have often been applied to target tumours in a variety of locations in the body [11]. Laser-based approaches employ slow heating, with low-power lasers delivered through optical fibres to induce protein denaturation. However, areas targeted by hyperthermal techniques are often difficult to control, with blood circulation proving problematic, acting to dissipate the temperature field. Some of the initial negative associations with laser or ultrasound methods are being overcome as devices become smaller and more user friendly [11]. More recent developments in commercial laser ablation systems and low-intensity ultrasound systems are beginning to compete with RF technologies in PVI applications [19].

By far the most common hyperthermal approach is based on RF technology. This modality has been in use since the 1990s and has surpassed all other energy delivery methods in popularity for use in cardiac ablation [20]. Ablation with RF relies on thermal energy from high frequency sinusoidal waves (500–750 kHz), to induce controlled damage or region-specific necrosis of heart tissue [11,20–25]. Temperatures of ≥ 50 °C induce tissue necrosis; however, temperatures approaching 100 °C can cause a coagulum of denatured proteins and plasma to form on the catheter tip, impeding current delivery [20] (Figure 2). RF-induced lesions typically have well-defined borders and their shape can adopt a monopolar egg shape or a bipolar round-brick shape [25,26]. RF lesion shape is dependent on a number of factors including catheter tip diameter, inter-tip spacing, tissue contact, temperature and duration of energy pulse delivered [25–27]. RF is a clinically significant technique as an ablation treatment for atrial fibrillation (AF), with success rates generally ranging anywhere between 45% and 80% [4,28,29].

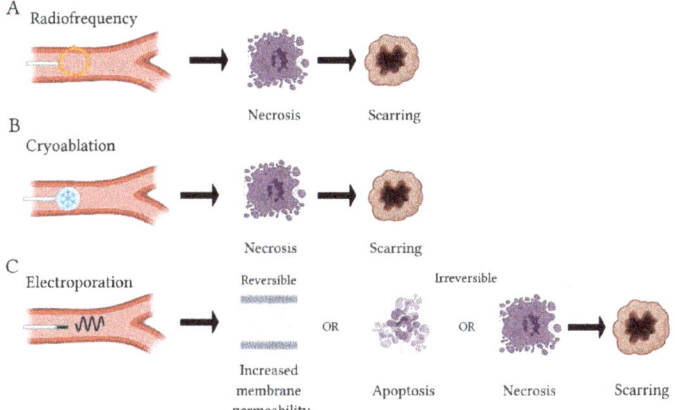

Figure 2. Effects of thermal and non-thermal energies. Diagram highlights the differing outcomes exhibited post-ablation between radiofrequency (**A**), cryoablation (**B**) and electroporation (EPo) (**C**) modalities. Radiofrequency and cryoablation can induce necrosis upon application which is followed by scarring with the intention to break arrhythmic circuits. Meanwhile, EPo increases membrane permeability which can lead to apoptotic or necrotic cell death, ultimately resulting in scarring.

2.2. Hypothermal or Cryoablation Techniques

Cryoablation has proven to be a clinically effective and a safe ablation method for use on cardiac tissue and has been studied since the early years of interventional cardiology [30]. Cryoablation uses hypothermal energy to induce ablation by freezing (≤ -40 °C) [21,31] (Figure 2). Lesion shape with cryoablation is sharper, more homogeneous and less thrombogenic than lesions resulting with RF [32]. Cryoablation has been employed as a treatment particularly for arrhythmias such as AF. A study by Bárta et al. yielded success rates of approximately 90% immediately post-ablation and 48.5% of patients were free from AF at 12-month follow-up [30,33,34]. A comparison study by Kim et al. showed atrial contractility recovery rates of 32.2% and 48.8% following RF or cryoablation treatment at 12-month follow-up, respectively [35]. Similar data were reported in the FIRE and ICE clinical trial with comparable numbers of patients requiring repeat ablation procedures to sufficiently isolate pulmonary veins (PVs) and terminate arrhythmias, highlighting the success, efficacy and challenges associated with both procedures [36].

2.3. Challenges with Current Ablative Approaches

While there have been many positive reports particularly for RF ablation and cryoablation, their efficacies rely on the precise positioning of catheters, adequate catheter-to-tissue contact and the energy level applied to the target area [37]. Collateral damage of surrounding areas is common during the application of thermal energy, including cardiac tamponade, thromboembolism, PV stenosis, phrenic nerve and oesophageal injury or fistula, and mitral valve trauma [21,38]. Overheating of the ablation site with RF energy has resulted in 'steam pop' and can cause myocardial perforation or cardiac tamponade [39–41]. Similarly, blood flow can cause a heat sink effect during RF and cryoablation procedures, preventing uniform tissue heating or lesion formation [42]. RF has also been shown to cause coagulation within coronary vessels, induce initial hyperplasia and instigate the shrinkage of collagen fibres within the coronary arterial walls [43].

Over the last decade, the interest and demand for a more controllable and safer alternative ablation technique has been growing. The advances in electroporation (EPo) and its refinement as pulsed electric field (PEF) technology, or pulsed-field ablation (PFA), has expanded to such a degree that it can now be considered a cutting-edge, nominally thermal ablation approach. The capacity to customise parameters for further enhanced application in humans may be a turning point in the treatment of specific targeted CVDs, improving procedure management and outcomes for both clinician and patient.

3. Electroporation as an Ablative Approach

Catheter-based electroporation (EPo) using monophasic pulses was first employed with cardiac tissue in the 1980s but it was found to be associated with negative side effects such as the induction of an electrically isolating "vapor globe" resulting in a spark (arcing), followed by an explosion and damaging pressure waves [44–46]. Serious complications such as barotrauma and a pro-arrhythmic effect saw voltage-based energy systems superseded by RF ablation [46,47]. However, Ahsan et al. demonstrated that the cautious use of electroporation at lower energies could successfully avoid arcing and produce sufficient therapeutic lesions [48]. Modern voltage-based systems typically employ pulsed electric fields (PEFs) [49,50]. Ablation based on EPo is growing in popularity as an alternative to thermal ablation and causes a biophysical phenomenon to arise following the application of PEF [2,51]. These electric fields induce irreparable pore formation in cell membranes [3]. As a result, so-called PFA is considered minimally thermal and creates more predictable and controllable lesions, with minimal interaction with blood flow.

Since 2005, both irreversible (IRE) and reversible (RE) EPo has received considerable attention as a method of disrupting cell membranes for drug delivery or inducing selective cell death, respectively [11]. Both IRE and RE have the potential to be tissue-specific in terms of lethal or effective thresholds, with extracellular and endothelial structures commonly remaining intact following exposure to electric fields [52,53]. The permanent opening of nanopores in cell membranes activates intracellular molecular pathways, increases ionic and molecular transport, resulting in an overall disruption of the cell membrane and intracellular homeostasis [11,21,54]. Exposure to sufficiently large field strength results in IRE, and permanent damage and cell death ensues due to localized rearrangement within membrane structures, while supporting structures remain unscathed [9,55–58]. RE, in contrast, only transiently opens membrane pores, maintaining cell viability, and is commonly employed in the targeted delivery of drugs and nucleotides [11].

The extent and targeting of ablation with IRE can be controlled at least to some degree by changing parameters such as pulse amplitude, frequency, duration of the application and pulse number [2,59]. The lethal thresholds for many cell types have been reported based on these parameters; however, many contradictory data exist as it is still an active area of ongoing research. On the face of it, short exposures and microsecond EPo impulses can be used for biomedical applications aimed at drug delivery and gene transfer, while more prolonged impulses are related to cellular injury and ablation by IRE [55,60,61]. The shape of the applied pulse is an under-explored, and in many cases a poorly documented, parameter that has not received the same degree of experimental testing as amplitude, frequency and others (Tables 1 and 2). Using a lung cell line, Kotnik et al. demonstrated that of the parameters used to describe pulse shape, the major factor determining electropermeabilization was the amount of time the pulse amplitude exceeded a certain threshold value [62]. They suggest that any differences observed between various pulse shapes may in fact be reflecting the difference in time the pulse is above the critical threshold for that cell type. Meanwhile, Stankevic et al. reported that it is the pulse shape and total energy input that contribute to the efficiency of IRE [63]. Sano et al. (2017) reported that asymmetric waveforms have significantly lower IRE thresholds compared to equivalent symmetrical waveforms, at least for neuroblastoma cells in vitro [64]. Both symmetrical and asymmetrical biphasic pulses have proven effective in IRE cardiac ablation procedures in both animals and a small number of pilot human trials [45,65–68]. Overall, asymmetric waveforms appear to produce more effective pore opening than symmetric pulses, possibly due to the different amplitudes of their phases. We recommend that all elements of pulse profile need to be reported, according to a set of recommended guidelines, as the extent that pulse shape contributes towards the safety and efficacy for AF treatment with IRE is unclear [69]. Overall, this is an area that requires substantial and more fundamental research before it can become part of standard clinical application [67].

More recently, the field has focused on pulse timing issues [70]. With nanosecond-PEFs in particular, this has been shown to improve the controllability of pore size. Short duration nsPEFs have been shown to minimise the electrophoretic effects associated with cell membrane transport [70,71]. When compared with longer pulse durations, shorter durations are reported to limit solute movement, overall reducing the osmotic imbalance and improving cell targeting with PEF exposure. nsPEF stimuli are too short to induce capacitive charging and instead aim to influence displacement currents over conduction currents [70]. Elementally, every cell behaves independently, deeming intercellular electric connections ineffective on membrane charging [72]. However, the mechanism by which such short stimuli can influence pore opening is still not fully understood and is the subject of ongoing research [70].

3.1. Pre-Clinical Evaluation of IRE, towards Optimization of Parameters for Clinical Use

Ex vivo studies were a milestone in the adaptation of IRE for in vivo applications as early work by Krassowska et al. emphasized the formation of pores in tissue exposed to EPo in a 2D model of cardiac tissue [73]. Selective pore formation can prevent excessively high transmembrane potentials, limiting damage in surrounding tissues. As work progressed, studies investigated the therapeutic thresholds and biophysical effects of EPo at a cellular level [3]. This was achieved by altering some therapeutic variables (pulse duration, pulse frequency, amplitude) and comparing the induction of injury on tissue through lactate dehydrogenase activity and the integrity of cell membranes.

Experiments involving the murine atrial cardiac cell line HL-1, cultured as adherent monolayers, showed that the damage was proportional to the number of IRE pulses and field strength applied [3] (Table 2). When compared to previous work from the same group looking at the human prostate cancer line LNCaP, data suggested that cardiac cells were more suspectable to IRE at higher field strengths greater than 1000 V/cm. Kaminska et al. showed that pulse intensities above 375 V/cm were destructive in the immature rat H9C2 myoblast cell line [74] (Table 2). A scan of the potential range of field strengths that might induce cell death is required and would be enhanced by the addition of threshold data on neuronal, cardiomyocyte and fat tissue found in the heart. Very recently, Hunter et al. showed that cardiac cells are more susceptible to electroporation damage than cortical neurons and oesophageal smooth muscle cells [75]. However, there are very few reports of this nature examining the different IRE thresholds of cardiac cells relative to other appropriate cardiac–neuronal model systems.

In animal studies, the application of IRE to cardiac tissue for the treatment of arrhythmias was found sufficient to block aberrant conductive pathways and reduce conduction and propagation of disruptive electrical signals [76]. In a study by Zager et al., it was shown that longer pulse durations (100 µs versus 70 µs) and increased pulse number (20 versus 10) were associated with a larger volume of damage in the ventricular myocardium in a rat model [2]. In a porcine model, the controlled delivery of electrical pulses both monophasic and biphasic, over a few microseconds or nanoseconds, has been shown to create tissue injury while avoiding negative effects [45].

In terms of pulse polarity, studies have found that biphasic pulses show better efficacy than monophasic stimuli in penetrating epicardial fat and overcomes the impedance by fatty cells during ablation of cardiac tissue [43,60]. Similarly, while both monophasic and biphasic pulses have proven efficient at producing feasible ablation outcomes, biphasic waveforms have been shown to create more durable lesions than monophasic applications [77]. This may be owing to biphasic pulses significantly altering electric field bias, reducing ion charging and prolonged post-ablation depolarizations [70]. Due to a "cancellation effect", higher amplitudes are often required to achieve ablation when using biphasic shocks at the nanosecond level [60]. Ablation success is seen to be influenced by the time between successive pulses. Nanosecond pulses can induce a uniform activation of the myocardium by forming a consistent electric field distribution [70]. This has been found to reduce the risk of new wave-fronts arising that could reinitiate arrhythmia and fibrillation [70]. Studies have also demonstrated that patients receiving monophasic pulses commonly require general anaesthesia and neuromuscular paralytics during procedures [78]. In comparison, patients that received biphasic pulses or high frequency energy were able to have the procedure under conscious sedation due to minimal resulting skeletal muscle activation [60,67,78] (Figure 3). It has been proposed that direct current (DC) monophasic energy be replaced by short alternating current (AC) biphasic energy to target larger areas, as it appears to reduce capture of nearby excitable tissues, thus reducing muscle spasms and acute pain during ablation [79].

3.2. Controlled Lesion Formation with IRE In Vivo

Human studies using comparably greater pulse durations and frequencies, ranging from microseconds to milliseconds (Table 2), show that the ablative effect and lesion area depends on the electric resistivity of the tissue, presence of cell membranes and the applied electric field [47]. Short electric field pulses cause rapid lesion formation, which is favorable to procedural work-flow [68]. However, the rapid nature of the delivery of IRE provides little, if any, opportunity for clinicians to change position of catheters or the profile of the energy delivered during the active phase of energy delivery.

While clinical outcome reports for IRE are limited, they are growing, and success has been noted in early clinical trials. Reddy et al. and Loh et al. have in a series of papers shown the safety and efficacy of IRE in the clinic [68,80,81]. Firstly, the authors highlighted the safety of the IRE procedure by successful acute pulmonary vein isolation (PVI) in 100% of patients [68,78,81]. This was a turning point in IRE ablation as it highlighted the potential of IRE and its capability to replace current thermal techniques in PVI procedures. Freedom from AF was later recorded in 94.4 ± 3.2% of patients by Reddy et al., in a recent trial using a either a combined RF/IRE (pulsed-field) approach or IRE as a standalone ablation procedure [80]. Similarly, 100% of PVs in patients with symptomatic paroxysmal or persistent AF were successfully isolated by Loh et al., using IRE alone [81].

Compared to thermal approaches, IRE appears to be less reliant on specific anatomical catheter positioning or catheter–tissue contact to produce adequate lesions, however this has not been examined systemically and requires more evidential data [51]. Successful ablations have been demonstrated even when delivering less precise, more widespread energy, suggesting that tissue vulnerability and lesion formation depends on tissue susceptibility and tissue type, facilitating cell-specific targeting with controlled parameter selection [51]. Studies have shown that IRE lesions occur locally in regions directly associated with electrodes [82,83]. Regions surrounding the electrodes are exposed to lower electric fields which induce RE, thus cells in this region recover and revert to normal function. Whether IRE lesions are transmural or not varies with the increasing thickness of the myocardium, requiring lesions to be wider to ensure adequate penetration [84]. IRE-induced lesions of the myocardium can be observed at a cellular level and are differentiated from unaffected tissue by a sharp border, similar to those induced by RF and cryoablation [9]. Appropriate transmural lesions are necessary to ensure the isolation of targeted regions to prevent disease relapse, thus avoiding the need for repeated procedures [9].

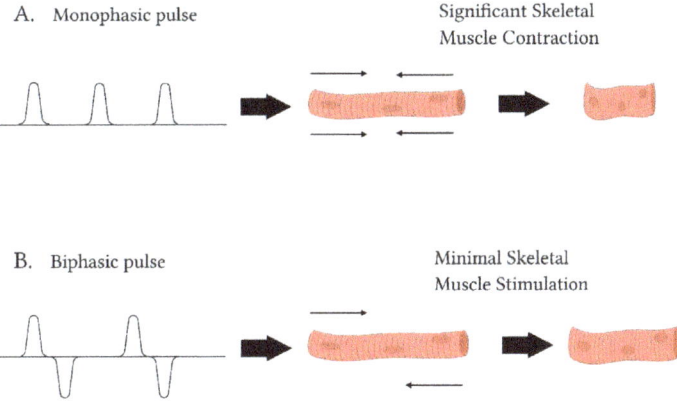

Figure 3. Structure of monophasic and biphasic pulses and their effect on muscle during ablation. (**A**) Monophasic pulses have been shown to induce excessive skeletal muscle spasm in patients thus requiring the use of general anaesthesia and paralytics. (**B**) Muscle activation induced by biphasic is minimal and therefore requires sedation.

It has been suggested that IRE parameters can be fine-tuned to achieve different lesion profiles [78]. The data to date, suggest that lesion geometry is significantly influenced by a number of pulse parameters and electrode spacing, with lesion size and depth corresponding mainly to the magnitude of field strength delivered [40,72,85] (Table 2). Early studies in which IRE was applied to porcine tissue noted that no charring or tissue disruption was visible upon gross inspection, and a clear demarcation line was evident around electroporated regions at the cellular level [9]. Further histological inspection demonstrated that while avoiding a significant local temperature change, successful electrical isolation was evident in the atria and was accompanied by transmural destruction. In addition, these studies demonstrated that lower field strengths can create sufficient lesions on PVs, while higher energies result in tissue shrinkage of the ventricle [53,86]. In porcine models, IRE-induced lesions were found to be similar to those formed with RF energy, however microscopic analysis revealed that IRE lesions have reduced epicardial fat-associated inflammation and fewer intralesional sequestered cardiomyocytes [45]. Furthermore, fibrotic regions formed during remodeling at the site of energy delivery were more homogenous in those areas exposed to IRE than to RF energy [45]. As expected, both modalities were linked to neointimal thickening on the undisrupted endocardium, fibrosis of intralesional nerves, and absence of endocardial thrombus formation. Similar histological results were recorded in canine studies upon the targeting of epicardial ganglia with IRE, highlighting preservation of cardiomyocyte architecture, minimal inflammatory response and fibrosis [76]. Studies have also shown that blood has a higher conductivity than tissues, which may affect IRE lesion depth of procedures done using an endocardial approach; however, unlike thermal techniques, this interaction with blood does not cause coagulation [87]. While substantial information has been collected from animal models, evidence of lesion geometry in humans cannot be assessed to such degrees. Instead, lesions are observed from a gross, clinical perspective and their electrical conduction is monitored during procedures. The inspection of the effect of IRE on vasculature is commonly achieved via imaging techniques.

3.3. Advantages and Disadvantages of EP

Preclinical and clinical data overall support the efficacy and safety of IRE with its capacity to limit injury to surrounding structures [51,68,73,74]. Due to the importance of protecting the coronary vasculature, several studies have investigated the short-term (3 weeks) and longer-term (3 months) effects of IRE on blood vessels (Table 2). Du Pre et al. investigated the effect of IRE when applied directly to the coronary vasculature in a porcine model. They observed that the coronary vessels remained free from clinically relevant damage, regardless of the lesion proximity to the vessel [43]. This further supports the targeting benefits of IRE which is not influenced by arterial blood flow, even when applied directly to vessels [43]. Long-term follow-up studies of porcine models by Neven et al. also highlighted the safety of IRE when targeted at the coronary vasculature [44]. They demonstrated that even deep lesions had no effect on luminal coronary artery diameter in their long-term study, proving IRE to be a safe ablation strategy for use on or in close approximation to the coronary vasculature.

The minimal damage IRE induces to vasculature makes it an attractive ablation modality for further development [77]. The major drawback with current thermal techniques is the induction of vessel stenosis, particularly of the PVs. The mechanism behind PV stenosis is believed to be a combination of intimal hyperplasia, medial thickening and smooth muscle activation, which is often followed by scar retraction and vein narrowing [88]. Comparative studies have drawn interesting comparisons between the use of RF energy and IRE for ablation of PVs. Early investigations were conducted on porcine models showing the effect of the given energies on inducing PV stenosis [89] (Table 2). A study revealed the significant damage caused by RF on PV tissue with observations of necrotic myocardium, large amounts of scar tissue surrounding the myocardial sleeve and intimal and elastic lamina proliferation. In contrast, only minor intimal proliferation was noted on tissue targeted with IRE. An initial decrease in PV diameter was noted in IRE experiments, however later studies revealed an overall increase in diameter [89]. It was evident that no PV stenosis arose due to IRE-exposed subjects at 3-month follow-up, while those who underwent RF ablation exhibited stenosis immediately that persisted for the follow-up survival period [89]. In recent years, the effects of IRE and RF were investigated in humans and research showed that the incidence of stenosis and narrowing of PV diameter following PFA was virtually eliminated (0%), while patients who received RF energy saw a 12.0% reduction in diameter and 32.5% incidence of stenosis at 3-month follow-up [90].

Some early preclinical work on porcine PVs by Wittkampf et al. reported that lower field strengths can create feasible and safe lesions on PV ostia, without evidence of collateral damage to surrounding structures [53,91] (Table 2). Preservation of nerve tissue was observed with no significant damage to the phrenic nerve post-IRE procedure [92]. With the oesophagus lying near the heart, the avoidance of trauma here is also a major concern of electrophysiologists. Similar findings were reported in a canine model, with subjects showing no signs of oesophageal injury [93]. In a porcine model, Neven et al. reported no disruption to oesophagus architecture, even with purposeful targeting of the adventitia [94]. This highlights the feasibility of IRE applications for cardiac tissue. In the first human trials IMPULSE and PEFCAT, incorporating the FARAPULSE endocardial ablation system, combined analysis by Reddy et al. showed the tissue-specific nature of IRE [78]. There were no reports of oesophageal or phrenic nerve injury in patients receiving the therapy, demonstrating that IRE possesses a major safety advantage over thermal techniques as an ablation modality for cardiac tissue [78].

Table 1. Comparison of clinical IRE studies on cardiac tissue.

Ref.	Follow-Up	Energy	Parameters	Monophasic/Biphasic Waveform	Monopolar/Bipolar Electrode Configuration	Reported Outcome Reported Outcome
[68]	N/A	900–2500 V	PF- 3.	Not specified	Bipolar	(1) PEF is a safe method for treating AF both endocardially and epicardially. (2) No incidences of atrial or ventricular arrythmia during procedure. (3) No collateral damage or PV stenosis recorded.
[78]	4 months	900–1000 V	Not specified	Monophasic	Bipolar	(1) Acute PVI achieved in 100% of patients using 6.4 ± 2.3 applications. (2) No injury to oesophagus or phrenic nerve.
[80]	12 months	0.011 ± 0.006 mV	PD- 3-5 s	Biphasic	Bipolar	(1) No adverse effects recorded related to PEF. (2) Freedom from AF was 94.4 ± 3.2%.
[81]	N/A	2154 ± 59 V	Not specified	Monophasic	Monopolar	(1) Acute bidirectional electrical PVI achieved in all 40 PVs. (2) No PV reconnections occurred during waiting period (30 min).
[90]	3 months	900–1000 V	Not specified	Monophasic	Monopolar and Bipolar	(1) No change (0%) in PV diameter and no stenosis in PFA patients, but reduction in diameter in 32.5% of patients who received RFA.

Another major difference between IRE and thermal catheter-based procedures is the time taken to perform the procedure. From a practical perspective, IRE procedures require significantly less time, energy and number of applications of energy in comparison to those of RF or cryoablation [3,59,72,78,93]. In the FIRE and ICE trial, studies by Reddy et al., on the isolation of PVs, highlighted a notable difference in mean total procedure time for IRE (92.2 min) compared to RF and cryoablation procedure times, which required 141 and 124 min, respectively [78]. Similarly, left atrial catheter-dwell time was much lower in IRE procedures (34 min) in contrast to RF and cryoablation (109 and 92 min, respectively) [78]. Similar results have been recorded in AF treatments with cryoablation yielding significantly shorter procedure times (ranging between 73.5 ± 16 min to 192.9 ± 44 min), in comparison to RF energy techniques (from 118.5 ± 15 min to 283.7 ± 78.0 min), with IRE procedures yielding even less time overall (from 22.6 ± 8.3 min to 92.2 ± 27.4 min) [78,80,95]. Shorter procedure times also incorporate less fluoroscopy duration, reducing a patient's radiation exposure [96]. While procedure time is not a crucial factor in ablation, shorter duration can enhance productivity by reducing healthcare costs overall. Therefore, IRE has a clear advantage over current procedures for efficacy, safety and reduced procedure times.

While IRE overcomes many complications associated with thermal ablation techniques, it does pose some similar risks such as thrombosis, haemorrhage and infection, however these are common to all procedures employing similar access techniques [50]. Specific to IRE there is an associated risk of electrolysis when untuned current is passed through body fluids with dissolved electrolytes, instigating gas formation [97,98]. One study reported that different current polarity may decrease gas bubble formation as a side-effect of IRE, highlighting that a reduced number of gas bubbles are released when using anodal IRE, compared to RF or cathodal IRE [98]. Gaseous microemboli could result in myocardial damage and in some instances with symptomatic cerebral ischemic events due to the obstruction of capillaries [98]. However, the risk of microemboli appears very low with preclinical canine reports by Neven et al. detailing that no treatment-related cerebral events occurred due to gas formation during IRE procedures [99]. In addition, MRI imaging and histopathology confirmed the absence of cerebral emboli, supporting the safety of this procedure [99].

The most immediate effects of electric field application to the myocardium are electrophysiological, leading to possible changes in ECG, such as in the ST segment and T-wave, or an overall decrease in resting cell membrane potential [50]. In some instances, the use of PEFs in non-cardiac applications has also been involved in the evolution of lethal and non-lethal cardiac arrhythmias in animal studies [51]. To minimise the risk of induced arrhythmia, it is presumed that ECG synchronisation integrated with pulse delivery is critical to ensure the energy is applied only during the absolute refractory period of the heart to avoid a critical increase in cell permeability [66,82,100]. A recent clinical trial by Loh et al. incorporated ECG synchronisation for the delivery of monophasic IRE pulses [81]. During this study, no peri-procedural complications were recorded. Likewise, in a study by Reddy et al. no adverse effects were reported when using biphasic pulses without synchronization to depolarization of the atria or ventricles [80]. Thus, the absolute requirement for synchronization is unclear. The use of IRE requires meticulous monitoring of blood pressure and electrolytes, as instances of induced mild hypertension and epileptic-like seizures have been reported with the use of high voltages and general anaesthesia during IRE procedures [81,90,101]. Cases of such intraoperative complications could jeopardize patient safety, therefore a clear understanding and rapid, appropriate management by the clinician is paramount. Nevertheless, it has been concluded that an application of irreversible PEFs directly to cardiac tissue both endocardially and epicardially in preclinical studies is safe when timed with the R-wave during sinus rhythm, and in early clinical studies regardless of timing [51,66,80–82,90,100,101]. However, as PEF is a novel technique, safety boundaries and significant safety data remain scarce for human application and further investigation is required.

Table 2. Comparison of preclinical IRE studies on cardiac tissue.

Ref.	Subject	Follow-Up	Energy	Parameters	Monophasic/Biphasic Waveform	Monopolar/Bipolar Electrode Configuration	Reported Outcome
				In Vitro			
[3]	HL-1 cell line	N/A	200 V; 1000 V/cm	PD- 50 µs, F- 10 Hz, PF- 10, 50, 99 pulses.	Not specified	Not specified	(1) IRE is effective for creating lesions on HL-1 cell line.
[73]	Cardiac strand-2D model	N/A	0.4–0.5 V; 25 V/cm	PD- 5 ms	Monophasic	Not specified	(1) Cardiac fibre exposed to a strong stimulus responds by developing pores in the first layer of cells immediately adjacent to the electrode. (2) IRE stops the growth of the macroscopic transmembrane potential, it does not affect intra- and extracellular potentials in the bulk of the tissue.
				In Vivo Animal			
[2]	Rat	1 month	50, 250, 500 V	PD- 70 vs. 100 µs, F- 1, 2, 3, 4 Hz, PF- 10 V's 20.	Not specified	Not specified	(1) Longer pulse duration (100 µs vs. 70 µs) is associated with larger volume reduction. (2) More pulses (20 vs. 10) are associated with larger volume reduction. (3) Pulse voltage (500 V vs. 250 V, 50 V) has an important effect on tissue damage. (4) Lower pulse frequency (10 Hz vs 20 Hz) is correlated with harsher tissue damage.
[9]	Porcine	24 h	1500–2000 V	PD- 100 µs, PF- 8, 16, 32.	Not specified	Not specified	(1) Lesions were mean 0.9 cm in depth. (2) Complete transmural destruction of atrial tissue at the site of the electrode application. (3) No local temperature change and with demonstration of electrical isolation.
[40]	Porcine	7 days	Not specified	F- 1 Hz, PF- 35	Not specified	Bipolar	(1) Unlike RF lesions, SW lesions showed only mild denaturation and little disruption of endocardium. (2) Lesion depth from SW correlated to amount of energy used. (3) SWCA lesions showed transient inflammatory responses followed by accelerated healing process with preserved myocardial blood flow.

Table 2. Cont.

Ref.	Subject	Follow-Up	Energy	Parameters	Monophasic/Biphasic Waveform	Monopolar/Bipolar Electrode Configuration	Reported Outcome
[43]	Porcine	3 weeks	Not specified	Not specified	Monophasic	Not specified	(1) Mean depths ranged from 2.9 + 1.2 mm–6.5 + 2.7 mm. (2) 32% of lesions were transmural. (3) Coronary arteries do not develop significant stenosis within 3 weeks after epicardial IRE.
[44]	Porcine	3 months	Not specified	PF- 3.	Monophasic	Not specified	(1) Mean value of the median lesion depths was 6.4 ± 2.6 mm. (2) 31% of lesions were transmural. (3) Apart from short-lasting (<30 min) coronary spasm, no long-term luminal narrowing was seen.
[45]	Porcine	2 weeks	500 V	PD- 90 µs, PF- 60.	Biphasic	Bipolar	(1) PFA lesions comparable to RFA lesions and had no collateral damage.
[51]	Canine	29 days	750 V	PD- 20 µs, F- 30–500 Hz, PF-10.	Not specified	Bipolar	(1) PEF can safely ablate Purkinje fibres. (2) Minimal collateral damage to myocardium.
[53]	Porcine	3 weeks	Not specified	PF- 4.	Monophasic	Bipolar	(1) Low energy IRE is safe and efficient in creating lesions on the PV ostia.
[57]	Rat	N/A	20 kV; 36 kV/cm	PD- 10 ns, F- 2 Hz, PF- 3.	Not specified	Not specified	(1) nsEP produces smaller pore size and reduced non-polar distribution of electro-pores over the cell body. (2) At near threshold intensities, both nsEPo and msEPo triggered Ca^{2+} transients.
[58]	Rabbit	N/A	50–500 V	F- 1–2 kHz, PF- 6–10.	Monophasic	Bipolar	(1) IRE thresholds were 229 ± 81 and 318 ± 84 V for the endocardium and the epicardium, respectively. (2) Selective transient impairment of electrical activity in endocardial bundles is caused by IRE. (3) IRE might transiently reduce myocardial vulnerability to arrhythmias.
[59]	Ovine	N/A	Not specified	PD- 100–400 µs, F- 1–5 Hz, PF- 10–40 pulses.	Not specified	Bipolar	(1) Lesions were well demarcated from the unaffected tissue. (2) The induced inflammatory reaction within these acute ablations was minimal.

Table 2. Cont.

Ref.	Subject	Follow-Up	Energy	Parameters	Monophasic/Biphasic Waveform	Monopolar/Bipolar Electrode Configuration	Reported Outcome
[67]	Porcine	3 weeks	600 V	PD- 2 ms, F- 10 kHz, PF- 10.	Biphasic	Not specified	(1) Demonstrated the feasibility of a novel asymmetrical high frequency (aHF) waveform for IRE. (2) The aHF waveform led to significantly deeper lesions than the symmetrical HF waveform. (3) Both methods showed lesions of more than 4 mm deep.
[70]	Murine, rat, porcine	N/A	100 V; 12.2 kV/cm	PD- 400 ns, PF- 20.	Not specified	Not specified	(1) Stimulation by 200 ns shocks can elicit Ca^{2+} transients. (2) Shortest shocks cause the least damage and their threshold energy is minimal. (3) Orientation of cardiomyocytes with respect for electric field does not affect threshold for ns shocks.
[71]	Murine	N/A	Not specified	PD- 200 μs	Not specified	Not specified	(1) 200 ns stimuli induced action potentials. (2) nsPEF caused Ca^{2+} entry, associated with a slow sustained depolarisation.
[72]	Rabbit	N/A	200 V	PD- 350 ns, F- 1, 3 Hz, PF- 20, 6.	Not specified	Monopolar	(1) Nonconducting lesions created in less than 2 s with nsPEF application per site and minimal heating (<0.2 °C) of the tissue. (2) Lesion was smoother and more uniform throughout the wall in comparison to RF lesions.
[76]	Canine	113 ± 7 days	1000 V	PD- 100 μs, PF- 10	Not specified	Bipolar	(1) Cardiac GP permanently damaged using DC for IRE. (2) Preservation of atrial myocardial architecture and absence of inflammatory reaction and fibrosis.
[77]	Porcine	63 ± 3.3 days	800–1800 V	Not specified	Monophasic	Bipolar	(1) Both waveforms created confluent myocardial lesions. (2) Biphasic PFA was more durable than monophasic PFA and radiofrequency ablation lesions.
[83]	Rabbit	4 weeks	300 V	Not specified	Monophasic	Bipolar	(1) Shock-induced IRE was spatially dependent on the location and dimension of the active region of the shock electrode. (2) The surviving anterior epicardial layers in the infarcted region were more susceptible to IRE.

Table 2. Cont.

Ref.	Subject	Follow-Up	Energy	Parameters	Monophasic/Biphasic Waveform	Monopolar/Bipolar Electrode Configuration	Reported Outcome
[84]	Rabbit	Not specified	200 V; 3 kV/cm	PD- 350 ns, F- 3 Hz, PF- 6.	Not specified	Not specified	(1) High anisotropy ratio substantially affects the ablation outcome, low anisotropy ratio does not.
[85]	Porcine	3 months	Not specified	Not specified	Monophasic	Not specified	(1) Lesion size, depth and width corresponds to magnitude of energy used. (2) Initial spasm of coronary vasculature was noted, but this did not persist and was not recorded at follow-up.
[86]	Porcine	3 months	Not specified	Not specified	Not specified	Not specified	(1) Mean depth of the 30 J, 100 J and 300 J lesions was 3.2 ± 0.7, 6.3 ± 1.8 and 8.0 ± 1.5 mm, respectively. (2) Mean width of the 30 J, 100 J, and 300 J lesions was 10.1 ± 0.8, 15.1 ± 1.5 and 17.1 ± 1.3 mm, respectively. (3) No luminal arterial narrowing was observed after 3 months.
[87]	Porcine	3 weeks	950–2150 V	PD- <10 ms, PF- 4.	Monophasic	Monopolar	(1) 200 J applications yielded median lesion depth of 5.2 ± 1.2 mm. (2) No signs of tissue heating. (3) Lesion would be sufficient for inducing PVI.
[88]	Canine	N/A	Not specified	PD- 60–300 s, F- 7 kHz.	Not specified	Not specified	(1) Device can successfully deliver both RF and IRE energy. (2) Addition of porous configuration on balloon can aid in enhancing drug delivery.
[89]	Porcine	3 months	Not specified	Not specified	Monophasic	Not specified	(1) IRE ablation: PV ostial diameter decreased $11 \pm 10\%$ directly after ablation but had increased $19 \pm 11\%$ after 3 months. (2) RF ablation: PV ostial diameter decreased $23 \pm 15\%$ directly after ablation and remained $7 \pm 17\%$ smaller after 3 months than pre-ablation diameter, despite a $21 \pm 7\%$ increase in heart size during aging from 6 to 9 months.
[91]	Canine	N/A	Not specified	F- 1 Hz.	Not specified	Bipolar	(1) No evidence of collateral damage to surrounding structures. (2) Ventricular arrhythmias can occur during DC application and are more likely with use of higher energy.

Table 2. *Cont.*

Ref.	Subject	Follow-Up	Energy	Parameters	Monophasic/Biphasic Waveform	Monopolar/Bipolar Electrode Configuration	Reported Outcome
[93]	Canine	27 days	2 kV/cm	PD- 100 µs, PF- 100.	Not specified	Bipolar	(1) No significant PV stenosis or oesophageal injury occurred.
[3]	Porcine	N/A	500 V; 1200 V/cm	PD- 50 µs, F- 10 Hz, PF- 50.	Not specified	Not specified	(1) IREis effective for creating lesions on PV tissue.
[102]	Porcine	35 days	2200 V	PD- <60 s	Biphasic	Bipolar	(1) Fibrous tissue homogeneously replaced myocytes. (2) When present, nerve fascicles and vasculature were preserved within surrounding fibrosis.
[103]	Canine ex vivo	N/A	750–2500 V; 250–833 V/cm	PD- 200 µs, F- 1 Hz, PF- 10	Biphasic	Not specified	(1) Delivery of IRE energy significantly reduced the window of vulnerability to ventricular arrhythmia. (2) No evidence of myocardial damage.

4. Conclusions

IRE has seen its stock rise substantially as a therapeutic intervention in recent decades and there has been much interest in its safety and feasibility for use on cardiac tissue. While significant advances have been made based on animal studies, particularly involving porcine and canine models, and preliminary parameters have been developed for use in humans (Table 1), much optimisation remains to be achieved. Further testing and fine-tuning are required to adapt and potentially individualise these parameters for specific patients or patient groups, while ensuring precise delivery of energy to achieve efficient EP ablation. There is significant room for the development of more complex representative in vitro model systems that incorporate both functional and histological outcomes, that are multi-cellular and more easily translatable. This will facilitate rapid development of pulse parameters and potentially catheter design by looking at the catheter not just to deliver energy, but to also provide feedback on target site and success of the ablation.

Similarly, while there are substantial preclinical data for IRE from animal models, the number of clinical trials is limited. Studies completed to date include small cohorts of approximately eighty patients with varying follow-up times of 3, 4 and 12 months [78,80,90]. Therefore, not only larger, multicentre trials are required to analyse the effects of IRE but also long-term evaluation of the permanence of the ablation.

Lesions are difficult to investigate in human studies, thus, most information is to be acquired regarding the true depth and volume of lesions is collected from animal studies. Follow-up times of preclinical trials generally exceed no longer than 3 or 4 months (Table 2). Similarly, long-term studies would challenge the durability of lesions in humans and examine any relapse to the electrical or structural induced CVD originally treated by IRE. Another limitation to current IRE trials is the lack of consistency between experiments. Some studies are limited to one energy magnitude, while others either use smaller or greater magnitudes on different sized animals (Table 2). While there are few published clinical trials related to the use of IRE on cardiac tissue, preclinical studies provide a promising baseline representation of its use. IRE bypasses many of the complications and drawbacks of the more commonly used thermal ablation modalities. With further improvements and refinement of parameter specifics, IRE may prove to be the gold standard for ablative CVD therapy.

Author Contributions: Conceptualization, S.M., S.A. and L.R.Q. Writing—Original draft preparation, S.M. and S.A.; Writing—review and editing, S.A., A.M.W., B.O., K.C., A.E., M.O. and L.R.Q. All authors have read and agreed to the published version of the manuscript.

Funding: This research was funded by Enterprise Ireland Disruptive technology (DTIF) grant number [DT20180123].

Institutional Review Board Statement: Not applicable.

Informed Consent Statement: Not applicable.

Data Availability Statement: Not applicable.

Conflicts of Interest: The authors declare no conflict of interest.

References

1. Heart Disease Facts | cdc.gov. Available online: https://www.cdc.gov/heartdisease/facts.htm (accessed on 9 June 2020).
2. Zager, Y.; Kain, D.; Landa, N.; Leor, J.; Maor, E. Optimization of irreversible electroporation protocols for in-vivo myocardial decellularization. *PLoS ONE* **2016**, *11*. [CrossRef] [PubMed]
3. Jiang, C.; Goff, R.; Patana-anake, P.; Iaizzo, P.A.; Bischof, J. Irreversible electroporation of cardiovascular cells and tissues. *J. Med. Devices Trans. ASME* **2013**, *7*. [CrossRef]
4. Avazzadeh, S.; McBride, S.; O'Brien, B.; Coffey, K.; Elahi, A.; O'Halloran, M.; Soo, A.; Quinlan, L.R. Ganglionated Plexi Ablation for the Treatment of Atrial Fibrillation. *J. Clin. Med.* **2020**, *9*, 3081. [CrossRef]
5. Holmes, D.R.; Valeti, U.S.; Nishimura, R.A. Alcohol septal ablation for hypertrophic cardiomyopathy: Indications and technique. *Catheter. Cardiovasc. Interv.* **2005**, *66*, 375–389. [CrossRef]

6. Nagueh, S.F.; Groves, B.M.; Schwartz, L.; Smith, K.M.; Wang, A.; Bach, R.G.; Nielsen, C.; Leya, F.; Buergler, J.M.; Rowe, S.K.; et al. Alcohol septal ablation for the treatment of hypertrophic obstructive cardiomyopathy: A multicenter north american registry. *J. Am. Coll. Cardiol.* **2011**, *58*, 2322–2328. [CrossRef]
7. Wei, C.; Qian, P.; Tedrow, U.; Mak, R.; Zei, P.C. Non-invasive stereotactic radioablation: A new option for the treatment of ventricular arrhythmias. *Arrhythmia Electrophysiol. Rev.* **2019**, *8*, 285–293. [CrossRef]
8. Chiu, M.H.; Mitchell, L.B.; Ploquin, N.; Faruqi, S.; Kuriachan, V.P.; Chiu, M. Review of Stereotactic Arrhythmia Radioablation Therapy for Cardiac Tachydysrhythmias. *CJC Open* **2020**, *3*, 236–247. [CrossRef] [PubMed]
9. Lavee, J.; Onik, G.; Rubinsky, B. A Novel Nonthermal Energy Source for Surgical Epicardial Atrial Ablation: Irreversible Electroporation Single cell manipulation and electroporation View project Isochoric Freezing: A new frontier for cryopreservation View project. *Heart Surg. Forum* **2007**, *10*, 96–101. [CrossRef]
10. Njeim, M.; Bogun, F. Selecting the appropriate ablation strategy: The role of endocardial and/or epicardial access. *Arrhythmia Electrophysiol. Rev.* **2015**, *4*, 184–188. [CrossRef] [PubMed]
11. Davalos, R.V.; Mir, L.M.; Rubinsky, B. Tissue ablation with irreversible electroporation. *Ann. Biomed. Eng.* **2005**, *33*, 223–231. [CrossRef] [PubMed]
12. Sohara, H.; Satake, S.; Takeda, H.; Yamaguchi, Y.; Toyama, H.; Kumagai, K.; Kuwahara, T.; Takahashi, A.; Ohe, T. Radiofrequency hot balloon catheter ablation for the treatment of atrial fibrillation: A 3-center study in Japan. *J. Arrhythmia* **2013**, *29*, 20–27. [CrossRef]
13. Okumura, Y.; Kolasa, M.W.; Johnson, S.B.; Bunch, T.J.; Henz, B.D.; O'brien, C.J.; Miller, D.V.; Packer, D.L. Mechanism of Tissue Heating During High Intensity Focused Ultrasound Pulmonary Vein Isolation: Implications for Atrial Fibrillation Ablation Efficacy and Phrenic Nerve Protection. *J. Cardiovasc. Electrophysiol.* **2008**, *19*, 945–951. [CrossRef]
14. Zhou, Y.-F. High intensity focused ultrasound in clinical tumor ablation. *World J. Clin. Oncol.* **2011**, *2*, 8. [CrossRef]
15. Borchert, B.; Lawrenz, T.; Hansky, B.; Stellbrink, C. Lethal atrioesophageal fistula after pulmonary vein isolation using high-intensity focused ultrasound (HIFU). *Heart Rhythm* **2008**, *5*, 145–148. [CrossRef]
16. Nakagawa, H.; Seres, K.A.; Jackman, W.M. Limitations of esophageal temperature-monitoring to prevent esophageal injury during atrial fibrillation ablation. *Circ. Arrhythm. Electrophysiol.* **2008**, *1*, 150–152. [CrossRef]
17. Prasertwitayakij, N.; Vodnala, D.; Pridjian, A.K.; Thakur, R.K. Esophageal injury after atrial fibrillation ablation with an epicardial high-intensity focused ultrasound device. *J. Interv. Card. Electrophysiol.* **2011**, *31*, 243–245. [CrossRef] [PubMed]
18. Bessiere, F.; N'djin, W.A.; Colas, E.C.; Chavrier, F.; Greillier, P.; Chapelon, J.Y.; Chevalier, P.; Lafon, C. Ultrasound-Guided Transesophageal High-Intensity Focused Ultrasound Cardiac Ablation in a Beating Heart: A Pilot Feasibility Study in Pigs. *Ultrasound Med. Biol.* **2016**, *42*, 1848–1861. [CrossRef]
19. Figueras i Ventura, R.M.; Mărgulescu, A.D.; Benito, E.M.; Alarcón, F.; Enomoto, N.; Prat-Gonzalez, S.; Perea, R.J.; Borràs, R.; Chipa, F.; Arbelo, E.; et al. Postprocedural LGE-CMR comparison of laser and radiofrequency ablation lesions after pulmonary vein isolation. *J. Cardiovasc. Electrophysiol.* **2018**, *29*, 1065–1072. [CrossRef]
20. Joseph, J.P.; Rajappan, K. Radiofrequency ablation of cardiac arrhythmias: Past, present and future. *An. Int. J. Med.* **2012**, *105*, 303–314. [CrossRef] [PubMed]
21. Wojtaszczyk, A.; Caluori, G.; Pešl, M.; Melajova, K.; Stárek, Z. Irreversible electroporation ablation for atrial fibrillation. *J. Cardiovasc. Electrophysiol.* **2018**, *29*, 643–651. [CrossRef] [PubMed]
22. Eisenberg Center at Oregon Health & Science University. Radiofrequency Ablation for Atrial Fibrillation: A Guide for Adults. In *Comparative Effectiveness Review Summary Guides for Consumers*; Agency for Healthcare Research and Quality: Rockville, MD, USA, 2005.
23. Wazni, O.M.; Marrouche, N.F.; Martin, D.O.; Verma, A.; Bhargava, M.; Saliba, W.; Bash, D.; Schweikert, R.; Brachmann, J.; Gunther, J.; et al. Radiofrequency ablation vs antiarrhythmic drugs as first-line treatment of symptomatic atrial fibrillation: A randomized trial. *J. Am. Med. Assoc.* **2005**, *293*, 2634–2640. [CrossRef] [PubMed]
24. Yokoyama, K.; Nakagawa, H.; Shah, D.C.; Lambert, H.; Leo, G.; Aeby, N.; Ikeda, A.; Pitha, J.V.; Sharma, T.; Lazzara, R.; et al. Novel contact force sensor incorporated in irrigated radiofrequency ablation catheter predicts lesion size and incidence of steam pop and thrombus. *Circ. Arrhythm. Electrophysiol.* **2008**, *1*, 354–362. [CrossRef] [PubMed]
25. Cosman, E.R.; Dolensky, J.R.; Hoffman, R.A. Factors that affect radiofrequency heat lesion size. *Pain Med.* **2014**, *15*, 2020–2036. [CrossRef]
26. Sweet, W.H.; Mark, V.H. Unipolar anodal electrolytic lesions in the brain of man and cat: Report of Five Human Cases with Electrically Produced Bulbar or Mesencephalic Tractotomies. *Arch. Neurol. Psychiatry* **1953**, *70*, 224–234. [CrossRef] [PubMed]
27. Wittkampf, F.H.M.; Nakagawa, H. RF catheter ablation: Lessons on lesions. *PACE-Pacing Clin. Electrophysiol.* **2006**, *29*, 1285–1297. [CrossRef]
28. Katritsis, D.G.; Giazitzoglou, E.; Zografos, T.; Pokushalov, E.; Po, S.S.; Camm, A.J. Rapid pulmonary vein isolation combined with autonomic ganglia modification: A randomized study. *Heart Rhythm* **2011**, *8*, 672–678. [CrossRef] [PubMed]
29. Budera, P.; Osmancik, P.; Herman, D.; Zdarska, J.; Talavera, D.; Mala, A.; Prochazkova, R.; Straka, Z. Midterm outcomes of two-staged hybrid ablation of persistent and long-standing persistent atrial fibrillation using the versapolar epicardial surgical device and subsequent catheter ablation. *J. Interv. Card. Electrophysiol.* **2017**, *50*, 187–194. [CrossRef]
30. Friedman, P.L. Catheter Cryoablation of Cardiac Arrhythmias. *Curr. Opin. Cardiol.* **2005**, *20*, 48–54. [PubMed]

31. Hunter, R.J.; Baker, V.; Finlay, M.C.; Duncan, E.R.; Lovell, M.J.; Tayebjee, M.H.; Ullah, W.; Siddiqui, M.S.; Mclean, A.; Richmond, L.; et al. Point-by-Point Radiofrequency Ablation Versus the Cryoballoon or a Novel Combined Approach: A Randomized Trial Comparing 3 Methods of Pulmonary Vein Isolation for Paroxysmal Atrial Fibrillation (The Cryo Versus RF Trial). *J. Cardiovasc. Electrophysiol.* **2015**, *26*, 1307–1314. [CrossRef]
32. Wasserlauf, J.; Pelchovitz, D.J.; Rhyner, J.; Verma, N.; Bohn, M.; Li, Z.; Arora, R.; Chicos, A.B.; Goldberger, J.J.; Kim, S.S.; et al. Cryoballoon versus Radiofrequency Catheter Ablation for Paroxysmal Atrial Fibrillation. *Pacing Clin. Electrophysiol.* **2015**, *38*, 483–489. [CrossRef]
33. Bárta, J.; Brát, R. Assessment of the effect of left atrial cryoablation enhanced by ganglionated plexi ablation in the treatment of atrial fibrillation in patients undergoing open heart surgery. *J. Cardiothorac. Surg.* **2017**, *12*, 69. [CrossRef] [PubMed]
34. Boveda, S. Cryoablation for Atrial Fibrillation: A Useful Technique beyond Paroxysmal Forms of Arrhythmia? *Rev. Española Cardiol.* **2017**, *70*, 236–238. [CrossRef]
35. Kim, K.M.; Chung, S.; Kim, S.Y.; Kim, D.J.; Kim, J.S.; Lim, C.; Park, K.H. Comparison of radiofrequency ablation and cryoablation for the recovery of atrial contractility and survival. *Korean J. Thorac. Cardiovasc. Surg.* **2018**, *51*, 266–272. [CrossRef] [PubMed]
36. Kuck, K.-H.; Albenque, J.-P.; Chun, K.R.J.; Fürnkranz, A.; Busch, M.; Elvan, A.; Schlüter, M.; Braegelmann, K.M.; Kueffer, F.J.; Hemingway, L.; et al. Repeat Ablation for Atrial Fibrillation Recurrence Post Cryoballoon or Radiofrequency Ablation in the FIRE AND ICE Trial. *Circ. Arrhythmia Electrophysiol.* **2019**, *12*. [CrossRef]
37. Strickberger, S.A.; Hummel, J.; Gallagher, M.; Hasse, C.; Man, K.C.; Williamson, B.; Vorperian, V.R.; Kalbfleisch, S.J.; Morady, F.; Langberg, J.J. Effect of accessory pathway location on the efficiency of heating during radiofrequency catheter ablation. *Am. Heart J.* **1995**, *129*, 54–58. [CrossRef]
38. Safaei, N.; Montazerghaem, H.; Azarfarin, R.; Alizadehasl, A.; Alikhah, H. Radiofrequency ablation for treatment of atrial fibrillation. *BioImpacts* **2011**, *1*, 171–177. [CrossRef]
39. Koruth, J.S.; Dukkipati, S.; Gangireddy, S.; McCarthy, J.; Spencer, D.; Weinberg, A.D.; Miller, M.A.; D'Avila, A.; Reddy, V.Y. Occurrence of steam pops during irrigated RF ablation: Novel insights from Microwave Radiometry. *J. Cardiovasc. Electrophysiol.* **2013**, *24*, 1271–1277. [CrossRef] [PubMed]
40. Hirano, M.; Yamamoto, H.; Hasebe, Y.; Fukuda, K.; Morosawa, S.; Amamizu, H.; Ohyama, K.; Uzuka, H.; Takayama, K.; Shimokawa, H. Development of a Novel Shock Wave Catheter Ablation system—A Validation Study in Pigs in Vivo. *EP Eur.* **2018**, *20*, 1856–1865. [CrossRef]
41. Tokuda, M.; Kojodjojo, P.; Epstein, L.M.; Koplan, B.A.; Michaud, G.F.; Tedrow, U.B.; Stevenson, W.G.; John, R.M. Outcomes of Cardiac Perforation Complicating Catheter Ablation of Ventricular Arrhythmias. *Circ. Arrhythmia Electrophysiol.* **2011**, *4*, 660–666. [CrossRef] [PubMed]
42. Kaszala, K.; Ellenbogen, K.A. Biophysics of the second-generation cryoballoon: Cryobiology of the big freeze. *Circ. Arrhythmia Electrophysiol.* **2015**, *8*, 15–17. [CrossRef]
43. Du Pre, B.C.; van Driel, V.J.; van Wessel, H.; Loh, P.; Doevendans, P.A.; Goldschmeding, R.; Wittkampf, F.H.; Vink, A. Minimal Coronary Artery Damage by Myocardial Electroporation Ablation. *EP Eur.* **2013**, *15*, 144–149. [CrossRef]
44. Neven, K.; van Driel, V.; van Wessel, H.; van Es, R.; du Pré, B.; Doevendans, P.A.; Wittkampf, F. Safety and feasibility of closed chest epicardial catheter ablation using electroporation. *Circ. Arrhythm. Electrophysiol.* **2014**, *7*, 913–919. [CrossRef]
45. Stewart, M.T.; Haines, D.E.; Verma, A.; Kirchhof, N.; Barka, N.; Grassl, E.; Howard, B. Intracardiac pulsed field ablation: Proof of feasibility in a chronic porcine model. *Heart Rhythm* **2019**, *16*, 754–764. [CrossRef] [PubMed]
46. Coltorti, F.; Bardy, G.H.; Reichenbach, D.; Greene, H.L.; Thomas, R.; Breazeale, D.G.; Alferness, C.; Ivey, T.D. Catheter-mediated electrical ablation of the posterior septum via the coronary sinus: Electrophysiologic and histologic observations in dogs. *Circulation* **1985**, *72*, 612–622. [CrossRef] [PubMed]
47. Nakagawa, H.; Jackman, M. Electroporation (revival of direct current ablation) new approach for increasing epicardial ablation safety in close proximity to a coronary artery. *Circ. Arrhythmia Electrophysiol.* **2014**, *7*, 779–780. [CrossRef]
48. Ahsan, A.J.; Cunningham, D.; Rowland, E.; Rickards, A.F. Catheter Ablation without Fulguration: Design and Performance of a New System. *Pacing Clin. Electrophysiol.* **1989**, *12*, 1557–1561. [CrossRef]
49. Wittkampf, F.H.M.; van Es, R.; Neven, K. Electroporation and its Relevance for Cardiac Catheter Ablation. *JACC Clin. Electrophysiol.* **2018**, *4*, 977–986. [CrossRef]
50. Tung, L.; Tovar, O.; Neunlist, M.; Jain, S.K.; O'neill, R.J. Effects of Strong Electrical Shock on Cardiac Muscle Tissue. *Ann. N. Y. Acad. Sci.* **1994**, *720*, 160–175. [CrossRef] [PubMed]
51. Sugrue, A.; Vaidya, V.R.; Livia, C.; Padmanabhan, D.; Abudan, A.; Isath, A.; Witt, T.; DeSimone, C.V.; Stalboerger, P.; Kapa, S.; et al. Feasibility of selective cardiac ventricular electroporation. *PLoS ONE* **2020**, *15*. [CrossRef]
52. Maor, E.; Ivorra, A.; Mitchell, J.J.; Rubinsky, B. Vascular smooth muscle cells ablation with endovascular nonthermal irreversible electroporation. *J. Vasc. Interv. Radiol.* **2010**, *21*, 1708–1715. [CrossRef]
53. Wittkampf, F.H.; Van Driel, V.J.; Van Wessel, H.; Vink, A.; Hof, I.E.; GrÜndeman, P.F.; Hauer, R.N.; Loh, P. Feasibility of electroporation for the creation of pulmonary vein ostial lesions. *J. Cardiovasc. Electrophysiol.* **2011**, *22*, 302–309. [CrossRef]
54. Frandsen, S.K.; Gissel, H.; Hojman, P.; Tramm, T.; Eriksen, J.; Gehl, J. Direct therapeutic applications of calcium electroporation to effectively induce tumor necrosis. *Cancer Res.* **2012**, *72*, 1336–1341. [CrossRef] [PubMed]
55. Weaver, J.C. Electroporation of cells and tissues. *IEEE Trans. Plasma Sci.* **2000**, *28*, 24–33. [CrossRef]

56. Neumann, E.; Rosenheck, K. Permeability changes induced by electric impulses in vesicular membranes. *J. Membr. Biol.* **1972**, *10*, 279–290. [CrossRef]
57. Semenov, I.; Zemlin, C.; Pakhomova, O.N.; Xiao, S.; Pakhomov, A.G. Diffuse, non-polar electropermeabilization and reduced propidium uptake distinguish the effect of nanosecond electric pulses. *Biochim. Biophys. Acta Biomembr.* **2015**, *1848*, 2118–2125. [CrossRef]
58. Al-Khadra, A.; Nikolski, V.; Efimov, I.R. The role of electroporation in defibrillation. *Circ. Res.* **2000**, *87*, 797–804. [CrossRef] [PubMed]
59. Hong, J.; Stewart, M.T.; Cheek, D.S.; Francischelli, D.E.; Kirchhof, N. Cardiac ablation via electroporation. In Proceedings of the 31st Annual International Conference of the IEEE Engineering in Medicine and Biology Society: Engineering the Future of Biomedicine, EMBC 2009, Minneapolis, MN, USA, 3–6 September 2009; Volume 2009, pp. 3381–3384.
60. Vižintin, A.; Vidmar, J.; Ščančar, J.; Miklavčič, D. Effect of interphase and interpulse delay in high-frequency irreversible electroporation pulses on cell survival, membrane permeabilization and electrode material release. *Bioelectrochemistry* **2020**, *134*, 107523. [CrossRef]
61. Andrei, G.; Pakhomov, D.; Miklavcic, M.S.M. Advanced Electroporation Techniques in Biology and Medicine. Available online: https://books.google.ie/books?id=sTHNBQAAQBAJ&pg=PA160&lpg=PA160&dq=U.+Zimmermann,+Ed.,+The+Effects+of+High+Intensity+Electric+Field+Pulses+on+Eukaryotic+Cell+Membranes:+Fundamentals+and+Applications.+Boca+Raton,+FL:+CRC,+1996&source=bl&ots=WvQ3rRMyfg&sig (accessed on 27 March 2020).
62. Kotnik, T.; Pucihar, G.; Rebersek, M.; Miklavčič, D.; Mir, L.M. Role of pulse shape in cell membrane electropermeabilization. *Biochim. Biophys. Acta Biomembr.* **2003**, *1614*, 193–200. [CrossRef]
63. Stankevic, V.; Simonis, P.; Zurauskiene, N.; Stirke, A.; Dervinis, A.; Bleizgys, V.; Kersulis, S.; Balevicius, S. Compact square-wave pulse electroporator with controlled electroporation efficiency and cell viability. *Symmetry* **2020**, *12*, 412. [CrossRef]
64. Sano, M.B.; Fan, R.E.; Xing, L. Asymmetric Waveforms Decrease Lethal Thresholds in High Frequency Irreversible Electroporation Therapies. *Sci. Rep.* **2017**, *7*, 1–13. [CrossRef]
65. Polajžer, T.; Dermol-Cerne, J.; Erne, J.; Reberšek, M.; O'connor, R.; Miklavčič, D. Cancellation effect is present in high-frequency reversible and irreversible electroporation. *Bioelectrochemistry* **2019**. [CrossRef]
66. Caluori, G.; Odehnalova, E.; Jadczyk, T.; Pesl, M.; Pavlova, I.; Valikova, L.; Holzinger, S.; Novotna, V.; Rotrekl, V.; Hampl, A.; et al. AC Pulsed Field Ablation Is Feasible and Safe in Atrial and Ventricular Settings: A Proof-of-Concept Chronic Animal Study. *Front. Bioeng. Biotechnol.* **2020**, *8*, 1374. [CrossRef]
67. Van Es, R.; Konings, M.K.; Du Pré, B.C.; Neven, K.; Van Wessel, H.; Van Driel, V.J.H.M.; Westra, A.H.; Doevendans, P.A.F.; Wittkampf, F.H.M. High-frequency irreversible electroporation for cardiac ablation using an asymmetrical waveform. *Biomed. Eng. Online* **2019**, *18*. [CrossRef] [PubMed]
68. Reddy, V.Y.; Koruth, J.; Jais, P.; Petru, J.; Timko, F.; Skalsky, I.; Hebeler, R.; Labrousse, L.; Barandon, L.; Kralovec, S.; et al. Ablation of Atrial Fibrillation With Pulsed Electric Fields: An Ultra-Rapid, Tissue-Selective Modality for Cardiac Ablation. *JACC Clin. Electrophysiol.* **2018**, *4*, 987–995. [CrossRef] [PubMed]
69. Cemazar, M.; Sersa, G.; Frey, W.; Miklavcic, D.; Teissié, J. Recommendations and requirements for reporting on applications of electric pulse delivery for electroporation of biological samples. *Bioelectrochemistry* **2018**, *122*, 69–76. [CrossRef]
70. Semenov, I.; Grigoryev, S.; Neuber, J.U.; Zemlin, C.W.; Pakhomova, O.N.; Casciola, M.; Pakhomov, A.G. Excitation and injury of adult ventricular cardiomyocytes by nano- to millisecond electric shocks. *Sci. Rep.* **2018**, *8*, 1–12. [CrossRef] [PubMed]
71. Azarov, J.E.; Semenov, I.; Casciola, M.; Pakhomov, A.G. Excitation of murine cardiac myocytes by nanosecond pulsed electric field. *J. Cardiovasc. Electrophysiol.* **2019**, *30*, 392–401. [CrossRef]
72. Xie, F.; Varghese, F.; Pakhomov, A.G.; Semenov, I.; Xiao, S.; Philpott, J.; Zemlin, C. Ablation of Myocardial Tissue With Nanosecond Pulsed Electric Fields. *PLoS ONE* **2015**, *10*, e0144833. [CrossRef]
73. Krassowska, W. Effects of Electroporation on Transmembrane Potential Induced by Defibrillation Shocks. *Pacing Clin. Electrophysiol.* **1995**, *18*, 1644–1660. [CrossRef] [PubMed]
74. Kaminska, I.; Kotulska, M.; Stecka, A.; Saczko, J.; Drag-Zalesinska, M.; Wysocka, T.; Choromanska, A.; Skolucka, N.; Nowicki, R.; Marczak, J.; et al. Electroporation-induced changes in normal immature rat myoblasts (H9C2). *Gen. Physiol. Biophys.* **2012**, *31*, 19–25. [CrossRef]
75. Hunter, D.W.; Kostecki, G.; Fish, J.M.; Jensen, J.A.; Tandri, H. In Vitro Cell Selectivity of Reversible and Irreversible Electroporation in Cardiac Tissue. *Circ. Arrhythmia Electrophysiol.* **2021**, *14*. [CrossRef] [PubMed]
76. Padmanabhan, D.; Naksuk, N.; Killu, A.K.; Kapa, S.; Witt, C.; Sugrue, A.; Desimon, C.V.; Madhavan, M.; de Groot, J.R.; O'Brien, B.; et al. Electroporation of epicardial autonomic ganglia: Safety and efficacy in medium-term canine models. *J. Cardiovasc. Electrophysiol.* **2019**, *30*, 607–615. [CrossRef] [PubMed]
77. Koruth, J.; Kuroki, K.; Iwasawa, J.; Enomoto, Y.; Viswanathan, R.; Brose, R.; Buck, E.D.; Speltz, M.; Dukkipati, S.R.; Reddy, V.Y. Preclinical Evaluation of Pulsed Field Ablation: Electrophysiological and Histological Assessment of Thoracic Vein Isolation. *Circ. Arrhythmia Electrophysiol.* **2019**, *12*. [CrossRef] [PubMed]
78. Reddy, V.Y.; Neuzil, P.; Koruth, J.S.; Petru, J.; Funosako, M.; Cochet, H.; Sediva, L.; Chovanec, M.; Dukkipati, S.R.; Jais, P. Pulsed Field Ablation for Pulmonary Vein Isolation in Atrial Fibrillation. *J. Am. Coll. Cardiol.* **2019**. [CrossRef]
79. Mercadal, B.; Arena, C.B.; Davalos, R.V.; Ivorra, A. Avoiding nerve stimulation in irreversible electroporation: A numerical modeling study. *Phys. Med. Biol.* **2017**, *62*, 8060–8079. [CrossRef] [PubMed]

80. Reddy, V.Y.; Anter, E.; Rackauskas, G.; Peichl, P.; Koruth, J.S.; Petru, J.; Funasako, M.; Minami, K.; Natale, A.; Jaïs, P.; et al. A Lattice-Tip Focal Ablation Catheter that Toggles Between Radiofrequency and Pulsed Field Energy to Treat Atrial Fibrillation: A First-in-Human Trial. *Circ. Arrhythmia Electrophysiol.* **2020**, *13*. [CrossRef]
81. Loh, P.; Van Es, R.; Groen, M.H.A.; Neven, K.; Kassenberg, W.; Wittkampf, F.H.M.; Doevendans, P.A. Pulmonary vein isolation with single pulse irreversible electroporation: A first in human study in 10 patients with atrial fibrillation. *Circ. Arrhythmia Electrophysiol.* **2020**, *13*, 1083–1091. [CrossRef]
82. Deodhar, A.; Dickfeld, T.; Single, G.W.; Hamilton, W.C.; Thornton, R.H.; Sofocleous, C.T.; Maybody, M.; Gónen, M.; Rubinsky, B.; Solomon, S.B. Irreversible electroporation near the heart: Ventricular arrhythmias can be prevented with ECG synchronization. *Am. J. Roentgenol.* **2011**, *196*, W330. [CrossRef]
83. Kim, S.C.; Vasanji, A.; Efimov, I.R.; Cheng, Y. Spatial distribution and extent of electroporation by strong internal shock in intact structurally normal and chronically infarcted rabbit hearts. *J. Cardiovasc. Electrophysiol.* **2008**, *19*, 1080–1089. [CrossRef]
84. Xie, F.; Zemlin, C.W. Effect of Twisted Fiber Anisotropy in Cardiac Tissue on Ablation with Pulsed Electric Fields. *PLoS ONE* **2016**, *11*, e0152262. [CrossRef]
85. Neven, K.; Van Driel, V.; Van Wessel, H.; Van Es, R.; Doevendans, P.A.; Wittkampf, F. Myocardial Lesion Size after Epicardial Electroporation Catheter Ablation After Subxiphoid Puncture. *Circ. Arrhythmia Electrophysiol.* **2014**, *7*, 728–733. [CrossRef]
86. Neven, K.; Van Driel, V.; Van Wessel, H.; Van Es, R.; Doevendans, P.A.; Wittkampf, F. Epicardial linear electroporation ablation and lesion size. *Hear. Rhythm* **2014**, *11*, 1465–1470. [CrossRef] [PubMed]
87. Wittkampf, F.H.M.; Van Driel, V.J.; Van Wessel, H.; Neven, K.G.E.J.; Gründeman, P.F.; Vink, A.; Loh, P.; Doevendans, P.A. Myocardial lesion depth with circular electroporation ablation. *Circ. Arrhythmia Electrophysiol.* **2012**, *5*, 581–586. [CrossRef]
88. Desimone, C.V.; Ebrille, E.; Syed, F.F.; Mikell, S.B.; Suddendorf, S.H.; Wahnschaffe, D.; Ladewig, D.J.; Gilles, E.J.; Danielsen, A.J.; Holmes, D.R.; et al. Novel balloon catheter device with pacing, ablating, electroporation, and drug-eluting capabilities for atrial fibrillation treatment - Preliminary efficacy and safety studies in a canine model. *Transl. Res.* **2014**, *164*, 508–514. [CrossRef] [PubMed]
89. Van Driel, V.J.H.M.; Neven, K.G.E.J.; Van Wessel, H.; Du Pré, B.C.; Vink, A.; Doevendans, P.A.F.M.; Wittkampf, F.H.M. Pulmonary vein stenosis after catheter ablation electroporation versus radiofrequency. *Circ. Arrhythmia Electrophysiol.* **2014**, *7*, 734–738. [CrossRef] [PubMed]
90. Kuroki, K.; Whang, W.; Eggert, C.; Lam, J.; Leavitt, J.; Kawamura, I.; Reddy, A.; Morrow, B.; Schneider, C.; Petru, J.; et al. Ostial Dimensional Changes After Pulmonary Vein Isolation: Pulsed Field Ablation vs Radiofrequency Ablation. *Hear. Rhythm* **2020**. [CrossRef]
91. Madhavan, M.; Venkatachalam, K.L.; Swale, M.J.; Desimone, C.V.; Gard, J.J.; Johnson, S.B.; Suddendorf, S.H.; Mikell, S.B.; Ladewig, D.J.; Nosbush, T.G.; et al. Novel Percutaneous Epicardial Autonomic Modulation in the Canine for Atrial Fibrillation: Results of an Efficacy and Safety Study. *PACE - Pacing Clin. Electrophysiol.* **2016**, *39*, 407–417. [CrossRef]
92. Van Driel, V.J.H.M.; Neven, K.; Van Wessel, H.; Vink, A.; Doevendans, P.A.F.M.; Wittkampf, F.H.M. Low vulnerability of the right phrenic nerve to electroporation ablation. *Hear. Rhythm* **2015**, *12*, 1838–1844. [CrossRef]
93. Witt, C.M.; Sugrue, A.; Padmanabhan, D.; Vaidya, V.; Gruba, S.; Rohl, J.; DeSimone, C.V.; Killu, A.M.; Naksuk, N.; Pederson, J.; et al. Intrapulmonary vein ablation without stenosis: A novel balloon-based direct current electroporation approach. *J. Am. Heart Assoc.* **2018**, *7*. [CrossRef]
94. Neven, K.; Van Es, R.; Van Driel, V.; Van Wessel, H.; Fidder, H.; Vink, A.; Doevendans, P.; Wittkampf, F. Acute and Long-Term Effects of Full-Power Electroporation Ablation Directly on the Porcine Esophagus. *Circ. Arrhythmia Electrophysiol.* **2017**, *10*. [CrossRef] [PubMed]
95. Jin, E.S.; Wang, P.J. Cryoballoon ablation for atrial fibrillation: A comprehensive review and practice guide. *Korean Circ. J.* **2018**, *48*, 114–123. [CrossRef]
96. Macle, L.; Weerasooriya, R.; Jais, P.; Scavee, C.; Raybaud, F.; Choi, K.-J.; Hocini, M.; Clementy, J.; Haissaguerre, M. Radiation Exposure During Radiofrequency Catheter Ablation for Atrial Fibrillation. *Pacing Clin. Electrophysiol.* **2003**, *26*, 288–291. [CrossRef]
97. Es, R.; Groen, M.H.A.; Stehouwer, M.; Doevendans, P.A.; Wittkampf, F.H.M.; Neven, K. In vitro analysis of the origin and characteristics of gaseous microemboli during catheter electroporation ablation. *J. Cardiovasc. Electrophysiol.* **2019**, *30*, 2071–2079. [CrossRef] [PubMed]
98. Groen, M.H.A.; van Es, R.; van Klarenbosch, B.R.; Stehouwer, M.; Loh, P.; Doevendans, P.A.; Wittkampf, F.H.; Neven, K. In vivo analysis of the origin and characteristics of gaseous microemboli during catheter-mediated irreversible electroporation. *EP Eur.* **2021**, *23*, 139–146. [CrossRef]
99. Neven, K.; Füting, A.; Byrd, I.; Heil, R.W.; Fish, J.M.; Feeney, D.A.; Donskoy, E.; Jensen, J.A. Absence of (sub-)acute cerebral events or lesions after electroporation ablation in the left-sided canine heart. *Hear. Rhythm* **2021**, *18*, 1004–1011. [CrossRef]
100. Bradley, C.J.; Haines, D.E. Pulsed field ablation for pulmonary vein isolation in the treatment of atrial fibrillation. *J. Cardiovasc. Electrophysiol.* **2020**, *31*, 2136–2147. [CrossRef]
101. Kambakamba, P.; Bonvini, J.M.; Glenck, M.; Castrezana López, L.; Pfammatter, T.; Clavien, P.A.; DeOliveira, M.L. Intraoperative adverse events during irreversible electroporation–a call for caution. *Am. J. Surg.* **2016**, *212*, 715–721. [CrossRef] [PubMed]
102. Koruth, J.S.; Kuroki, K.; Iwasaw1, J.; Viswanathan, R.; Richard, Brose; Buck, E.D.; Donskoy, E.; Dukkipati, S.R.; Reddy, V.Y. Endocardial Ventricular Pulsed Field Ablation: A Proof-Of-Concept Preclinical Evaluation. *EP Eur.* **2020**, *22*, 434–439. [CrossRef]
103. Livia, C.; Sugrue, A.; Witt, T.; Polkinghorne, M.D.; Maor, E.; Kapa, S.; Lehmann, H.I.; DeSimone, C.V.; Behfar, A.; Asirvatham, S.J.; et al. Elimination of Purkinje Fibers by Electroporation Reduces Ventricular Fibrillation Vulnerability. *J. Am. Heart Assoc.* **2018**, *7*, e009070. [CrossRef]

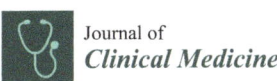

Review

Persistent Atrial Fibrillation: The Role of Left Atrial Posterior Wall Isolation and Ablation Strategies

Riyaz A. Kaba [1,2,*], Aziz Momin [1,2] and John Camm [1]

1 Cardiovascular Clinical Academic Group, Molecular and Clinical Sciences Institute, St. George's University of London and St. George's University Hospitals NHS Foundation Trust, London SW17 0QT, UK; Aziz.Momin@stgeorges.nhs.uk (A.M.); jcamm@sgul.ac.uk (J.C.)
2 Ashford and St. Peter's Hospitals NHS Foundation Trust, Surrey KT16 0PZ, UK
* Correspondence: rkaba@sgul.ac.uk; Tel.: +44-208-725-4571

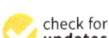

Abstract: Atrial fibrillation (AF) is a global disease with rapidly rising incidence and prevalence. It is associated with a higher risk of stroke, dementia, cognitive decline, sudden and cardiovascular death, heart failure and impairment in quality of life. The disease is a major burden on the healthcare system. Paroxysmal AF is typically managed with medications or endocardial catheter ablation to good effect. However, a large proportion of patients with AF have persistent or long-standing persistent AF, which are more complex forms of the condition and thus more difficult to treat. This is in part due to the progressive electro-anatomical changes that occur with AF persistence and the spread of arrhythmogenic triggers and substrates outside of the pulmonary veins. The posterior wall of the left atrium is a common site for these changes and has become a target of ablation strategies to treat these more resistant forms of AF. In this review, we discuss the role of the posterior left atrial wall in persistent and long-standing persistent AF, the limitations of current endocardial-focused treatment strategies, and future perspectives on hybrid epicardial–endocardial approaches to posterior wall isolation or ablation.

Keywords: persistent atrial fibrillation; posterior wall; hybrid ablation; convergent ablation

1. Introduction

Atrial fibrillation (AF) is the most commonly diagnosed sustained cardiac dysrhythmia and is characterised by rapid and irregular activation of the atria. It is associated with an increased risk of ischemic stroke, heart failure and mortality and can have a substantial impact on quality of life. Atrial fibrillation can be paroxysmal, lasting 7 days or less with or without intervention, or be continuous beyond 7 days (persistent, PersAF) or beyond 12 months (long-standing persistent, LSPersAF) [1]. Permanent AF is the term used for long-standing persistent AF when any attempt to restore sinus rhythm has been abandoned or has proved impossible. As each episode of AF continues, progressive electro-anatomical remodelling occurs that may serve to perpetuate and sustain AF, known as 'AF begets AF' [2]. Therefore, it is not surprising that treatment strategies vary in effectiveness depending on the extent and duration of AF.

Overall, optimal AF management should include a holistic, comprehensive, multidisciplinary approach that collectively considers modifiable risk factors, stroke prevention, and patient- and symptom-focused rate and rhythm control [3] (Figure 1). Using this approach, known as the AF Better Care (ABC) pathway, AF is managed with lifestyle modifications to address risk factors such as obesity and hypertension, and medical therapy which can include anticoagulation for stroke prevention as well as rate and rhythm control drugs depending on the patient and symptoms [1,3]. When antiarrhythmic drugs fail or are intolerable, ablation is recommended. This typically takes form as standalone endocardial catheter ablation or as surgical ablation if performed concomitantly with a primary cardiac surgical procedure. In both cases, pulmonary vein isolation (PVI) is paramount, although

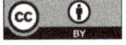

other regions often emerge as potential substrates in PersAF [4]. One of these regions, arguably the most influential after the pulmonary veins (PVs), is the posterior wall of the left atrium, which is known to generate AF triggers and is subject to electrical and structural changes that occur with the persistence of AF. However, this region is where endocardial catheter ablation is more limited in its capacity to comprehensively address the AF substrate owing to the elevated risk of collateral damage to adjacent structures such as the oesophagus. This review aims to discuss the published literature on the role of the left atrial posterior wall in PersAF and LSPersAF, outline practical limitations of endocardial catheter ablation to safely and durably isolate the posterior wall and describe the rationale for a hybrid epicardial–endocardial ablation strategy for silencing the PVI and posterior wall.

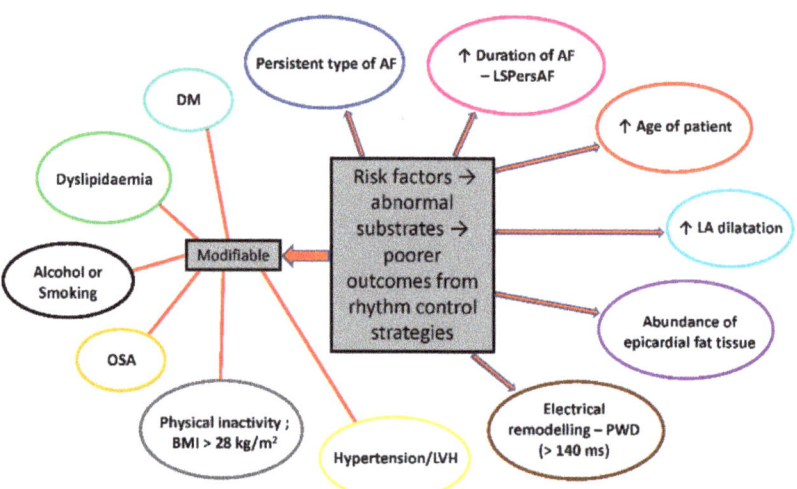

Figure 1. Risk factors for perpetuation of AF. Modifiable risk factors are highlighted separately. LSPersAF, long-standing persistent AF; LA, left atrium; PWD, p-wave duration; LVH, left ventricular hypertrophy; BMI, body mass index; OSA, obstructive sleep apnoea; DM, diabetes mellitus.

2. Burden of Atrial Fibrillation

Atrial fibrillation was estimated to affect more than 43 million people worldwide in 2016, a figure that continues to rise every year, with observed increases during the last few decades in associated disability and mortality [3]. Atrial fibrillation increases the risk of stroke around five-fold [5], more so with multiple co-existing risk factors, and is also associated with increased mortality [6] even within the first few months of diagnosis [7]. Atrial fibrillation can also overlap with heart failure in that it can exacerbate existing heart failure or lead to tachycardia-induced cardiomyopathy in patients with chronic, poorly managed AF. Therefore, the impact of AF on the global healthcare system is significant. In addition, AF is associated with a decreased quality of life, which can be attributed to the burden of symptoms, as well as the complex interplay with other patient comorbidities commonly associated with AF [8]. In effect, treating the syndrome with AF is not only aimed at reducing the risks of stroke and cardiac death but also decreasing AF burden and, consequently, AF symptoms to improve patient quality of life.

3. Treatment of Paroxysmal Atrial Fibrillation

In a seminal 1998 paper, Haïssaguerre and colleagues identified the PVs as the primary sites of arrhythmogenicity in paroxysmal AF and that these AF triggers could be destroyed or isolated with radiofrequency ablation [9]. Favourable success rates have been demonstrated for endocardial catheter ablation focused on the PVs for the treatment of drug-refractory paroxysmal AF [10], further supported by advancements in catheter-based radiofrequency, cryoballoon and other technologies [11,12].

4. Paroxysmal vs. Persistent Atrial Fibrillation: Differences in Treatment Outcomes

The consistent clinical success of endocardial catheter ablation in paroxysmal AF is not paralleled in persistent and long-standing persistent forms of AF. The discrepancy between paroxysmal and non-paroxysmal AF outcomes is well-evidenced by long-term results of endocardial radiofrequency ablation in these subgroups. With a median follow-up of 4.8 years after circumferential PVI, Ouyang et al. reported 46.6% of 161 patients with paroxysmal AF were free from atrial arrhythmia recurrence after a single procedure, and this success rose to 79.5% with multiple procedures (median 1: range 1–3) [13]. However, in long-standing PersAF, with a median follow-up of 4.7 years, the same investigators reported 20.3% of 202 patients were free from arrhythmia recurrence after PVI with additional CFAE/linear ablation [14]. After multiple procedures (median 2, range 1–5), 45% of patients with LSPersAF were in sinus rhythm. A comprehensive meta-analysis of persistent and long-standing PersAF treatment outcomes reported similarly disappointing results with much shorter follow-up times [15].

One explanation for the suboptimal effectiveness of PVI in non-paroxysmal AF is that areas outside of the PVs can drive and act as substrates as AF continues [16]. It has been well-documented that AF triggers are present outside of the PVs [17,18]. While extra-PV triggers may be present in paroxysmal AF, the majority of triggers are located in and around the PVs (Figure 2); this may, at least in part, explain why PV isolation alone is more effective in treating this type of AF [19]. However, as AF becomes persistent, there is a shift towards extra-PV triggers for atrial tachyarrhythmias and, given the progressive electrophysiological and structural changes that occur with the persistence of AF, these extra-PV regions may be appropriate substrates for ablation in PersAF and LSPersAF. Having said that, what and how to ablate in PersAF and LSPersAF is still unclear. Data from the STAR-AF II trial appeared to show that additional endocardial ablation utilising CFAEs or certain linear lesions (roof and mitral lines) adjunctive to PVI did not improve clinical outcomes over PVI alone in PersAF [20]; although, dedicated posterior wall ablation was not specifically tested in this study.

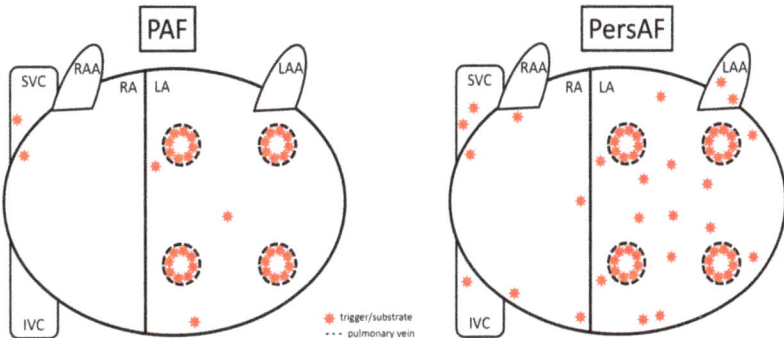

Figure 2. Triggers and substrates for PAF vs. PersAF. In PAF, the majority of these are located within and around the PVs, whereas in PersAF there are many more non-PV locations, especially in the posterior wall (between the four PVs and below the lower PVs). LA, left atrium; LAA, left atrial appendage; RA, right atrium; RAA, right atrial appendage; SVC, superior vena cava; IVC, inferior vena cava.

The left atrial posterior wall has been shown to house the highest proportion of non-PV triggers. Lin et al. reported 38% of non-PV ectopic beats emanated from the posterior wall [17]. Additionally, with continued PersAF, the left atrial posterior wall is the most common non-PV site to contain AF re-entrant drivers [16]. In the next section, we review the unique arrhythmogenic properties of the posterior wall that underscore the rationale for its role in PersAF and LSPersAF.

5. The Posterior Wall of the Left Atrium in Non-Paroxysmal Atrial Fibrillation

5.1. Intrinsic Features

The left atrial posterior wall has several inherent anatomic and electrophysiological properties that are conducive to arrhythmogenicity. When these factors are combined with the structural changes that develop with more prolonged episodes of AF (see next section on 'Effects of prolonged atrial fibrillation on posterior wall'), the posterior wall then emerges as one of the key regions in the pathophysiology of PersAF. The posterior wall is derived embryonically from the same tissue as the pulmonary veins [21]. Between approximately 6–8 weeks of gestation, the common pulmonary vein, lined with mediastinal myocardium distinct from the primary myocardium that lines systemic venous structures, bifurcates and becomes incorporated into the left atrial wall [22]. Of note, the mediastinal myocardium is composed of fast-conducting cells compared to the slower conducting cells of the primary myocardium. Given the shared tissue origin with the pulmonary veins, it is not surprising then that the posterior left atrial wall is also a site of AF triggers and plays a role in sustaining PersAF.

Myocytes within the left atrial posterior wall have unique electrophysiological properties that may be intrinsically suited to initiate or sustain AF. These cells are characterised by having larger late sodium currents and smaller potassium currents [23]. The intracellular calcium transient and content within the sarcoplasmic reticulum are high. In effect, the cells of the posterior wall have (i) a low resting membrane potential; (ii) short action potential duration; (iii) the shortest refractory period of any cell in the heart. Taken together, these cellular characteristics make the posterior wall prone to misfiring.

Other structural aspects of the posterior wall can contribute to AF initiation and facilitate re-entry. The myocardial fibres in the left atrial posterior wall, particularly near the junction with the pulmonary veins, have a heterogenous orientation with respect to each other [24]. As a consequence, non-uniform anisotropy can occur in which conduction velocity and depolarisation differ between adjacent tissues, including the transition between the epicardial and endocardial layers. Subsequently this can lead to delayed conduction, unidirectional block and, thus, local re-entry.

The autonomic nervous system is a key player in the initiation and sustainment of AF. The posterior wall of the left atrium has the highest density of autonomic neurons in the heart [25]. Ganglionated plexi are groups of autonomic neurons embedded in epicardial fat pads, and some of the ganglionated plexi are located at the posterior left atrium, near the pulmonary veins. Ganglionated plexi are thought to contribute to AF and at times are adjunctive targets in ablation procedures.

5.2. Effects of Prolonged Atrial Fibrillation on Posterior Wall

As described above, there are intrinsic functional and anatomical characteristics of the left atrial posterior wall that make it prone to the initiation and maintenance of AF. Once AF occurs and persists over time, progressive changes in the left atrium then serve to propagate and further sustain AF. As such, the left atrial posterior wall is acknowledged as a key AF substrate in persistent forms of the disease. The development of fibrosis is thought to be a contributing factor to the propagation and persistence of AF. Fibrosis can develop due to other cardiac abnormalities or health conditions that are coincident with AF, as well as aging. Fibroblasts comprise 50–70% of cardiac cells [25], and their function is to compose and dynamically maintain the heart's scaffold [26]. These fibroblasts can differentiate into myofibroblasts under various pathologic conditions, including inflammation and mechanical overload. Myofibroblasts, in turn, produce, turn over and deposit collagen and other extracellular matrix components, which lead to the hardening and scarring of cardiac tissue. This fibrotic tissue can slow conduction, serve as a unidirectional block and contribute to macro re-entry [27]. Cochet et al. demonstrated through MRI delayed enhancement that fibrosis tends to develop on the posterior left atrium [28]. This may be in part due to chronic, increased stress in the regions adjacent to the pericardial reflections that anchor the posterior heart to the chest wall [29]. Additionally, increased pressure and dilation of the left atrium due to prolonged AF leads to stretching, followed by inflammation and leading to fibrosis [30].

The accumulation of epicardial fat on the posterior wall can also contribute to AF in two ways. Firstly, adipose tissue produces inflammatory signals that support remodelling and fibrosis [31]. Secondly, animal studies have suggested infiltration of epicardial adipose tissue into the myocardium may create tissue disorganisation that can serve as a substrate for aberrant conduction [32]. Areas of abnormal conduction in the posterior left atrium have been shown to be associated with adjacent epicardial adipose tissue in obese patients with AF [33].

5.3. Difficulties with Endocardial Ablation of Posterior Wall

Given the evidence for the posterior wall as an AF substrate, both in triggering and sustaining AF, the posterior wall has been explored as a target of radiofrequency and cryoablation to improve clinical outcomes in AF, particularly PersAF and LSPersAF. This is evident from the Cox-Maze IV surgical ablation lesion set, which isolates the posterior wall of the left atrium with epicardial ablation lines on the right and left pulmonary vein antrum followed by roof and floor ablations anchored to the left atriotomy [34]. However, Cox-Maze IV is typically performed concomitantly with open cardiac surgeries, limiting its reach to patients who do not need or want an open procedure.

Endocardial catheter isolation of the left atrial posterior wall has been studied with both radiofrequency and cryothermal ablation (Table 1). The majority of these studies included only patients with PersAF and LSPersAF, which is in line with current guideline recommendations when considering posterior wall isolation in conjunction with PVI [1]. Meta-analyses of a few randomised and observational comparison studies have suggested an overall benefit of endocardial posterior wall ablation compared to pulmonary vein isolation alone in PersAF [35,36], but results of the individual studies, including the randomised clinical trials [37–39], are mixed (Table 1). This may, in part, be due to the lack of a standardised approach to posterior wall isolation, which is evidenced by the various lesion sets used in published studies. These approaches to posterior wall isolation include a single ring around the PVs and posterior left atrium [39], linear lesions (left atrial roof and posterior-inferior) to create the so-called posterior 'box' lesion [37,38,40,41], or extensive point-by-point radiofrequency [42] or segmental cryoballoon ablation [43,44] to debulk the posterior wall. Adjunctive lesions also vary among these studies.

Table 1. Summary of select studies evaluating addition of posterior wall isolation to pulmonary vein isolation.

Study	AF Type	Primary Energy Source	Ablation Strategies PVI Group	Ablation Strategies PVI + PW Group	Summarised Outcomes
Aryana et al. 2018 Non-randomised	PersAF	Cryoballoon	• PVI • >50% received CTI by irrigated RF	• PVI • Segmental LAPW ablation • >50% received CTI by irrigated RF • Point-by-point RF as needed if isolation not achieved • 32.4% had adjunct RF to complete PVI + PW	• 1-year freedom from atrial arrhythmias was 74% in PVI + PW vs. 48% in PVI ($p < 0.001$)[1]
Bai et al. 2016 Non-randomised	PersAF	Irrigated RF	• PVAI • SVC ablation if needed • Verification of PVI at 3 months and reablation if needed until isolated	• PVAI to the coronary sinus and left side of interatrial septum • Extensive PW ablation • SVC ablation if needed • Verification of PVI + PWI at 3 months and reablation if needed	• 1-year freedom from atrial arrhythmia off AADs was 65% in PVI + PW group vs. 20% in PVI group ($p < 0.001$); benefit maintained through 3 years
Tokioka et al. 2020 Non-randomised	PersAF	Irrigated RF	• Circumferential PVI • PV carina	• Circumferential PVI • PV carina • Roof line • Inferior line	• AF recurrence rate was 31.1% in PVI + PW vs. 47.3% in PVI at median 19 mths ($p = 0.35$) • Recurrence of PersAF was 5.6% vs. 20.9% ($p = 0.002$); no significant differences in recurrent PAF or atrial tachycardia
Tamborero et al. 2009 Randomised	60% PAF, 20% PersAF, 20% LSPAF	Irrigated RF	• Circumferential PVAI • MTI • Roof line	• Circumferential PVAI • MTI • Roof line • Inferior line	• Freedom from atrial arrhythmias at mean 9.8 mths follow-up was 55% in each group ($p = 0.943$) • No significant difference in outcomes between ablation strategies in Pers/LSPersAF subanalysis
Lim et al. 2012; Randomised	61% PAF, 22% PersAF, 17% LSPAF	RF	• PVAI • Roof line • MTI (54%) • CTI	• Single ring isolation • MTI (54%) • CTI	• 2-year AF-free survival was 74% in PVI + PW vs. 61% in PVI ($p = 0.031$) • 2-year atrial arrhythmia-free survival was not significantly different
Kim et al. 2015 Randomised	PersAF	Irrigated RF	• Circumferential PVI • Roof line • Anterior wall line • CTI	• Circumferential PVI • Roof line • Anterior wall line • CTI • Inferior line	• 12-month cumulative recurrence was 16.7% in PVI + PW vs. 36.7% for PVI alone ($p = 0.02$)
Lee et al. 2019 Randomised	26.7% PersAF 73.3% LSPersAF	Irrigated RF	• Circumferential PVI • CTI	• Circumferential PVI • CTI • Roof line • Inferior line • Point ablation as needed • Anterior line as per physician discretion	• Freedom from AF off AADs (mean 16.2 mths) was 55.9% in PVI + PW vs. 50.5% in PVI ($p = 0.522$) • Recurrence rate was 26.5% in PVI + PW vs. 23.8% in PVI ($p = 0.78$).

Table 1. Cont.

Study	AF Type	Primary Energy Source	Ablation Strategies		Summarised Outcomes
			PVI Group	PVI + PW Group	
Aryana et al. 2021 Randomised	65.5% PersAF; 34.5% LSPAF	Cryoballoon	• PVI • CTI by RF • Point-by-point RF as needed for PVI • 7.3% had adjunct RF ablation	• PVI • Segmental LAPW ablation • CTI by RF • Point-by-point RF as needed for PVI + PW • 45.5% had adjunct RF ablation	• 12-month AF recurrence was 25.5% in PVI + PW vs. 45.5% in PVI ($p = 0.028$) • 12-month atrial arrhythmia recurrence was 34.5% in PVI + PW vs. 49.1% in PVI ($p = 0.12$)

[1] Percentages depicted in Kaplan–Meier curve in Aryana et al. 2018 as noted in Della Rocca et al. 2020; AAD: antiarrhythmic drugs; AF: atrial fibrillation; CTI: cavotriscupid isthmus; LSPersAF: long-standing persistent AF; MTI: mitral isthmus; PAF: paroxysmal AF; PersAF: persistent AF; PVAI: pulmonary vein antrum isolation; PVI: pulmonary vein isolation; PW: posterior wall; RF: radiofrequency; SVC: superior vena cava.

In addition to a lack of standardised posterior wall ablation strategy, other practical challenges limit the extent to which endocardial posterior wall isolation can be achieved and thus may contribute to varied clinical outcomes. One major concern with endocardial catheter ablation of the left atrial posterior wall is potential collateral damage. The tissue of the posterior wall is thin, particularly at the superior aspect, in part to accommodate the stress of limited cardiac motion at the pericardial reflections [45]. It has been shown using post-mortem hearts that the posterior wall tissue is generally thinner in patients with AF, with an overall mean thickness of ≤ 3 mm [45]. Endocardial catheters apply ablative energy away from the heart towards the pericardium, therefore there are risks of cardiac perforation and tamponade as well as thermal injury to the oesophagus and other adjacent structures. Atrio-oesophageal fistula is the most devastating consequence of oesophageal thermal injury. While the documented incidence is low (<0.1%) with endocardial posterior wall ablation, the potential risk remains, and the consequences can be fatal [46]. Oesophageal temperature monitoring during ablation may be used as an alert for thermal injury; however, there are well recognised limitations such as the temperature can continue to rise after ablation is stopped and the probe may cause oesophageal damage by thermal effect. Consequently, despite the use of this device, atrio-oesophageal fistula can still develop [47], limiting the widespread use of such an approach for monitoring. Indeed, a recent randomised study demonstrated a similar rate of endoscopically-detected oesophageal lesions following endocardial catheter ablation with and without the use of an oesophageal temperature probe [48]. Additionally, aborting ablation due to an unexpected rise in temperature may result in incomplete ablation lines and gaps. Reducing the power and/or duration of energy delivery during ablation on the posterior wall is normally undertaken to reduce the risk of collateral damage, but this also reduces the efficacy of lesion formation. Taken together, active mitigation of thermal injury is important, yet it may also contribute to incomplete isolation of the posterior wall and varied clinical outcomes.

Reported rates of acute and continued isolation of the posterior wall using endocardial catheter ablation suggest there is difficulty in creating transmural and durable lesions. A meta-analysis of endocardial posterior wall isolation found an acute procedural success rate of 78% (95% CI, 59.4–94.4%) with results from box, single ring and debulking techniques combined [35]. The same meta-analysis also reported a substantial rate of posterior wall reconnections observed at repeat electrophysiology procedures for arrhythmia recurrence after endocardial catheter ablation: the pooled rate of posterior wall reconnection was 63.1% (95% CI, 42.5–82.4%) [35]. Markman et al. assessed chronic posterior wall isolation at repeat ablation after a single procedure of PVI and posterior wall ablation. They found a 40% rate of posterior wall reconnections in patients who experienced arrhythmia recurrence, with most reconnections at the atrial roof and most recurrences classified as atrial flutter in patients with failed posterior wall isolation [49]. Bai et al. reported 37.5% of patients had posterior wall reconnections three months after a single endocardial posterior wall debulking procedure [42]. In fact, four of the studies comparing PVI to PVI with posterior wall isolation discussed herein suggest suboptimal durability of posterior wall isolation using endocardial catheter ablation (Table 2).

Evidence of endocardial–epicardial dissociation in atrial fibrillation may also limit the effectiveness of endocardial posterior wall isolation, especially when considered in the context of suboptimal transmurality. Endocardial–epicardial dissociation, as evidenced by asynchronous activation of the epicardial and endocardial surfaces, was initially demonstrated in animal [50] and computational models [51]. More recently, real-time mapping has shown there may be up to 50–55% asynchronous activation between the epicardial and endocardial surfaces in patients with AF [52,53]. One contributing factor to endocardial–epicardial dissociation in AF may be the presence of fibrosis in the epicardial layer, which was first suggested by animal studies [54] and recently supported by computational modelling with validation in a small number of patients [55]. The cumulative evidence for endocardial–epicardial dissociation suggests that endocardial-only mapping and ablation may be insufficient to adequately address conduction abnormalities on both cardiac surfaces in AF.

Table 2. Posterior wall (PW) connection rates in studies comparing pulmonary vein isolation (PVI) to PVI + PW isolation.

Study	Posterior Wall Strategy	Follow-Up Time	Population Evaluated for Reconnection	Reconnection Rates in PW Ablation Group
Bai et al. 2016	Debulking with RF	3-months	All patients	37.5% [1]
Lee et al. 2015	Linear ablation with RF	16.2 ± 8.8 months	Recurrent patients	50%
Tamborero et al. 2009	Linear ablation with RF	9.8 ± 4.3 months	Recurrent patients	67%
Tokioka et al. 2020	Linear ablation with RF	1–6 months	Recurrent patients	65.2%

[1] Includes pulmonary vein and PW reconnections; PVI: pulmonary vein isolation; PW: posterior wall; RF: radiofrequency.

5.4. Hybrid Epicardial–Endocardial Approach to Address Posterior Wall Silencing

In effect, there are three main challenges in the treatment of PersAF and LSPersAF: (i) limited candidates for concomitant surgical ablation; (ii) limited effectiveness of catheter ablation in non-paroxysmal AF; (iii) challenges with endocardial catheter ablation focused on the left atrial posterior wall, which is a source of AF triggers and a substrate. These issues prompted the development of hybrid epicardial–endocardial approaches to ablation. Hybrid approaches combine minimally invasive epicardial ablation by a cardiothoracic surgeon and endocardial ablation by an electrophysiologist to complete a transmural lesion set that effectively isolates the pulmonary veins and left atrial posterior wall.

There are two general strategies for hybrid epicardial–endocardial ablation. The primary difference is the surgical epicardial ablation technique, including epicardial access, ablation tools and posterior wall lesion set. Hybrid ablation can be achieved with totally thoracoscopic (TT) epicardial ablation followed by endocardial ablation. In hybrid TT ablation, surgical access to the pericardium is achieved thoracoscopically and the epicardial lesion set is focused on PVI and creating a box lesion set across the posterior wall. Endocardial ablation is performed by an electrophysiologist to complete PVI and address gaps. The first report of this approach was published in 2011 [56]. Recent retrospective studies have reported mid-term (2–3 year) outcomes ranging from 67–79% arrhythmia-free survival off AADs in patients with PersAF and LSPersAF [57–59]. Safety and effectiveness of hybrid TT ablation are being evaluated in two randomised clinical trials (NCT02441738, NCT02695277) and one single-arm trial (NCT02393885).

In the other hybrid epicardial–endocardial approach, commonly referred to as the hybrid Convergent procedure, the surgeon uses a single, small subxiphoid incision to gain access to the pericardial space without the use of additional ports. It was initially proposed in 2009 [60] and the ablation set has evolved over time. In early studies, an ex-Maze lesion set was performed through a transabdominal, transdiaphragmatic approach [60]. A box lesion set then became the preferred method to isolate the posterior wall. Since 2012, epicardial posterior wall homogenization has been achieved with 2–3 rows of linear lesions spanning between the pulmonary veins [61], which is another distinction from the TT lesion set. Beginning in 2016, the pericardial space has been accessed via the subxiphoid incision [62], eliminating the need to divide the central tendon of the diaphragm. Endocardial mapping and ablation are subsequently performed by the electrophysiologist on the same day, sequential day, or several weeks later, with the goal of ensuring PVI and addressing any gaps following the epicardial procedure. Further, since there is recovery of electrical conduction following epicardial ablation, it remains important to undertake both components of the hybrid technique to achieve long-lasting, widespread transmurality [63]. Observational clinical outcomes from contemporary analyses have suggested favourable outcomes with this technique [64–68], which were recently corroborated by the results of the multi-centre, randomised controlled CONVERGE trial [69]. The trial compared hybrid Convergent ablation with endocardial catheter ablation in PersAF and LSPersAF and met its primary safety and effectiveness endpoints. Twelve-month freedom from atrial arrhythmias without new/increased doses of AADs was 67.7% with hybrid Convergent ablation compared to 50.0% with catheter ablation ($p = 0.036$). Significantly better effectiveness off AADs (53.5% vs. 32.0%, $p = 0.013$) and irrespective of AADs (76.8% vs. 60.0%, $p = 0.033$) were also achieved with hybrid Convergent ablation. The 30-day major adverse event rate with the hybrid Convergent procedure was 7.8% (vs 0.0% in the catheter arm, $p = 0.0525$), primarily relating to inflammatory pericardial effusions. Of note, no cardiac perforations, deaths or atrio-oesophageal fistulas occurred.

One important aspect of both hybrid ablation strategies is a collaborative, heart team approach to patient management in order to optimise clinical outcomes and safely mitigate risks [70].

6. Future Directions

Isolation of the left atrial posterior wall with a combination of epicardial and endocardial ablation to increase the likelihood of durable, transmural lesion has shown promising results in observational studies during the last decade as well as in a randomised controlled trial. More recently, these studies have described outcomes using a subxiphoid approach to reach the posterior left atrium, and additional studies dedicated to this approach will be important. Concomitant application of the AtriClip®, the most widely employed left atrial appendage exclusion device, is gaining popularity [4] and future studies should assess the precise impact on AF outcomes of including this technique. Another endpoint of interest for a hybrid approach is evaluating the length of stay for comparison with other minimally invasive surgical ablation approaches. For example, in our experience, we have seen rapid recovery after hybrid Convergent ablation, with a median length stay of 1 day, in contrast to recovery times for patients who undergo totally thoracoscopic Maze procedures, who typically require several days prior to discharge.

7. Conclusions

The left atrial posterior wall is likely an important driver and substrate as AF progresses and, as such, its isolation has been explored during AF ablation procedures to improve clinical outcomes in PersAF and LSPersAF. Surgical-only approaches to isolate the posterior wall are limited by invasiveness and patient eligibility for a concomitant procedure. Endocardial ablation alone to isolate the posterior wall has yielded mixed results in PersAF and LSPersAF. Electrophysiological differences between the endocardium and epicardium may not be safely addressable with an endocardial approach alone. The combination of the two concepts into a hybrid electrophysiological–surgical collaboration, such as in the Convergent procedure, may help to optimise lesion durability and transmurality to effectively isolate the posterior wall.

Author Contributions: All authors have contributed to the preparation of this paper, R.A.K., A.M. and J.C. All authors have read and agreed to the published version of the manuscript.

Funding: This research received no external funding.

Institutional Review Board Statement: Not applicable.

Informed Consent Statement: Not applicable.

Acknowledgments: The authors wish to thank Yashasvi Awasthi and Kristen Plasseraud for their kind assistance in the preparation of this article.

Conflicts of Interest: R. A. Kaba is a consultant for Daiichi Sankyo, Bayer, Atricure and Biotronik. A. Momin is a consultant for Atricure. A. J. Camm has received personal fees from Abbott, Boston Scientific, Medtronic and Atricure.

References

1. Calkins, H.; Hindricks, G.; Cappato, R.; Kim, Y.H.; Saad, E.B.; Aguinaga, L.; Akar, J.G.; Badhwar, V.; Brugada, J.; Camm, J.; et al. 2017 HRS/EHRA/ECAS/APHRS/SOLAECE expert consensus statement on catheter and surgical ablation of atrial fibrillation. *Heart Rhythm* **2017**, *14*, e275–e444. [CrossRef]
2. Wijffels, M.C.; Kirchhof, C.J.; Dorland, R.; Allessie, M.A. Atrial fibrillation begets atrial fibrillation. A study in awake chronically instrumented goats. *Circulation* **1995**, *92*, 1954–1968. [CrossRef]
3. Hindricks, G.; Potpara, T.; Dagres, N.; Arbelo, E.; Bax, J.J.; Blomstrom-Lundqvist, C.; Boriani, G.; Castella, M.; Dan, G.A.; Dilaveris, P.E.; et al. 2020 ESC Guidelines for the diagnosis and management of atrial fibrillation developed in collaboration with the European Association of Cardio-Thoracic Surgery (EACTS). *Eur. Heart J.* **2020**. [CrossRef]
4. Kaba, R.; Ahmed, O.; Momin, A. Electrical isolation of the left atrial appendage—A new frontier in the treatment for atrial fibrillation. *J. Cardiovasc. Dis. Diagn.* **2020**, *8*, 1–6. [CrossRef]
5. Wolf, P.A.; Abbott, R.D.; Kannel, W.B. Atrial fibrillation as an independent risk factor for stroke: The Framingham study. *Stroke* **1991**, *22*, 983–988. [CrossRef]
6. Benjamin, E.J.; Wolf, P.A.; D'Agostino, R.B.; Silbershatz, H.; Kannel, W.B.; Levy, D. Impact of atrial fibrillation on the risk of death: The Framingham heart study. *Circulation* **1998**, *98*, 946–952. [CrossRef]
7. Miyasaka, Y.; Barnes, M.E.; Bailey, K.R.; Cha, S.S.; Gersh, B.J.; Seward, J.B.; Tsang, T.S. Mortality trends in patients diagnosed with first atrial fibrillation: A 21-year community-based study. *J. Am. Coll. Cardiol.* **2007**, *49*, 986–992. [CrossRef]
8. Randolph, T.C.; Simon, D.N.; Thomas, L.; Allen, L.A.; Fonarow, G.C.; Gersh, B.J.; Kowey, P.R.; Reiffel, J.A.; Naccarelli, G.V.; Chan, P.S.; et al. Patient factors associated with quality of life in atrial fibrillation. *Am. Heart J.* **2016**, *182*, 135–143. [CrossRef] [PubMed]
9. Haissaguerre, M.; Jais, P.; Shah, D.C.; Takahashi, A.; Hocini, M.; Quiniou, G.; Garrigue, S.; Le Mouroux, A.; Le Metayer, P.; Clementy, J. Spontaneous initiation of atrial fibrillation by ectopic beats originating in the pulmonary veins. *N. Engl. J. Med.* **1998**, *339*, 659–666. [CrossRef] [PubMed]
10. Wilber, D.J.; Pappone, C.; Neuzil, P.; De Paola, A.; Marchlinski, F.; Natale, A.; Macle, L.; Daoud, E.G.; Calkins, H.; Hall, B.; et al. Comparison of antiarrhythmic drug therapy and radiofrequency catheter ablation in patients with paroxysmal atrial fibrillation: A randomized controlled trial. *JAMA* **2010**, *303*, 333–340. [CrossRef] [PubMed]
11. Kuck, K.H.; Brugada, J.; Furnkranz, A.; Metzner, A.; Ouyang, F.; Chun, K.R.; Elvan, A.; Arentz, T.; Bestehorn, K.; Pocock, S.J.; et al. Cryoballoon or radiofrequency ablation for paroxysmal atrial fibrillation. *N. Engl. J. Med.* **2016**, *374*, 2235–2245. [CrossRef]
12. Natale, A.; Reddy, V.Y.; Monir, G.; Wilber, D.J.; Lindsay, B.D.; McElderry, H.T.; Kantipudi, C.; Mansour, M.C.; Melby, D.P.; Packer, D.L.; et al. Paroxysmal AF catheter ablation with a contact force sensing catheter: Results of the prospective, multicenter SMART-AF trial. *J. Am. Coll. Cardiol.* **2014**, *64*, 647–656. [CrossRef]
13. Ouyang, F.; Tilz, R.; Chun, J.; Schmidt, B.; Wissner, E.; Zerm, T.; Neven, K.; Kokturk, B.; Konstantinidou, M.; Metzner, A.; et al. Long-term results of catheter ablation in paroxysmal atrial fibrillation: Lessons from a 5-year follow-up. *Circulation* **2010**, *122*, 2368–2377. [CrossRef] [PubMed]
14. Tilz, R.R.; Rillig, A.; Thum, A.M.; Arya, A.; Wohlmuth, P.; Metzner, A.; Mathew, S.; Yoshiga, Y.; Wissner, E.; Kuck, K.H.; et al. Catheter ablation of long-standing persistent atrial fibrillation: 5-year outcomes of the Hamburg sequential ablation strategy. *J. Am. Coll. Cardiol.* **2012**, *60*, 1921–1929. [CrossRef] [PubMed]
15. Brooks, A.G.; Stiles, M.K.; Laborderie, J.; Lau, D.H.; Kuklik, P.; Shipp, N.J.; Hsu, L.F.; Sanders, P. Outcomes of long-standing persistent atrial fibrillation ablation: A systematic review. *Heart Rhythm* **2010**, *7*, 835–846. [CrossRef]
16. Lim, H.S.; Hocini, M.; Dubois, R.; Denis, A.; Derval, N.; Zellerhoff, S.; Yamashita, S.; Berte, B.; Mahida, S.; Komatsu, Y.; et al. Complexity and distribution of drivers in relation to duration of persistent atrial fibrillation. *J. Am. Coll. Cardiol.* **2017**, *69*, 1257–1269. [CrossRef] [PubMed]
17. Lin, W.S.; Tai, C.T.; Hsieh, M.H.; Tsai, C.F.; Lin, Y.K.; Tsao, H.M.; Huang, J.L.; Yu, W.C.; Yang, S.P.; Ding, Y.A.; et al. Catheter ablation of paroxysmal atrial fibrillation initiated by non-pulmonary vein ectopy. *Circulation* **2003**, *107*, 3176–3183. [CrossRef]
18. Di Biase, L.; Burkhardt, J.D.; Mohanty, P.; Sanchez, J.; Mohanty, S.; Horton, R.; Gallinghouse, G.J.; Bailey, S.M.; Zagrodzky, J.D.; Santangeli, P.; et al. Left atrial appendage: An underrecognized trigger site of atrial fibrillation. *Circulation* **2010**, *122*, 109–118. [CrossRef] [PubMed]
19. Della Rocca, D.G.; Tarantino, N.; Trivedi, C.; Mohanty, S.; Anannab, A.; Salwan, A.S.; Gianni, C.; Bassiouny, M.; Al-Ahmad, A.; Romero, J.; et al. Non-pulmonary vein triggers in nonparoxysmal atrial fibrillation: Implications of pathophysiology for catheter ablation. *J. Cardiovasc. Electrophysiol.* **2020**, *31*, 2154–2167. [CrossRef]
20. Verma, A.; Jiang, C.Y.; Betts, T.R.; Chen, J.; Deisenhofer, I.; Mantovan, R.; Macle, L.; Morillo, C.A.; Haverkamp, W.; Weerasooriya, R.; et al. Approaches to catheter ablation for persistent atrial fibrillation. *N. Engl. J. Med.* **2015**, *372*, 1812–1822. [CrossRef]
21. Abdulla, R.; Blew, G.A.; Holterman, M.J. Cardiovascular embryology. *Pediatr. Cardiol.* **2004**, *25*, 191–200. [CrossRef] [PubMed]
22. Sherif, H.M. The developing pulmonary veins and left atrium: Implications for ablation strategy for atrial fibrillation. *Eur J. Cardiothorac. Surg.* **2013**, *44*, 792–799. [CrossRef] [PubMed]
23. Suenari, K.; Chen, Y.C.; Kao, Y.H.; Cheng, C.C.; Lin, Y.K.; Chen, Y.J.; Chen, S.A. Discrepant electrophysiological characteristics and calcium homeostasis of left atrial anterior and posterior myocytes. *Basic Res. Cardiol.* **2011**, *106*, 65–74. [CrossRef]
24. Markides, V.; Schilling, R.J.; Ho, S.Y.; Chow, A.W.; Davies, D.W.; Peters, N.S. Characterization of left atrial activation in the intact human heart. *Circulation* **2003**, *107*, 733–739. [CrossRef]

25. Stavrakis, S.; Po, S. Ganglionated plexi ablation: Physiology and clinical applications. *Arrhythmia Electrophysiol. Rev.* **2017**, *6*, 186–190. [CrossRef]
26. Souders, C.A.; Bowers, S.L.; Baudino, T.A. Cardiac fibroblast: The renaissance cell. *Circ. Res.* **2009**, *105*, 1164–1176. [CrossRef] [PubMed]
27. Rohr, S. Arrhythmogenic implications of fibroblast-myocyte interactions. *Circ. Arrhythmia Electrophysiol.* **2012**, *5*, 442–452. [CrossRef]
28. Burstein, B.; Nattel, S. Atrial fibrosis: Mechanisms and clinical relevance in atrial fibrillation. *J. Am. Coll. Cardiol.* **2008**, *51*, 802–809. [CrossRef] [PubMed]
29. Cochet, H.; Mouries, A.; Nivet, H.; Sacher, F.; Derval, N.; Denis, A.; Merle, M.; Relan, J.; Hocini, M.; Haissaguerre, M.; et al. Age, atrial fibrillation, and structural heart disease are the main determinants of left atrial fibrosis detected by delayed-enhanced magnetic resonance imaging in a general cardiology population. *J. Cardiovasc. Electrophysiol.* **2015**, *26*, 484–492. [CrossRef] [PubMed]
30. Yang, F.; Tiano, J.; Mittal, S.; Turakhia, M.; Jacobowitz, I.; Greenberg, Y. Towards a Mechanistic Understanding and Treatment of a Progressive Disease: Atrial Fibrillation. *J. Atr. Fibrillation* **2017**, *10*, 1627. [CrossRef] [PubMed]
31. Hatem, S.N.; Sanders, P. Epicardial adipose tissue and atrial fibrillation. *Cardiovasc. Res.* **2014**, *102*, 205–213. [CrossRef] [PubMed]
32. Mahajan, R.; Lau, D.H.; Brooks, A.G.; Shipp, N.J.; Manavis, J.; Wood, J.P.; Finnie, J.W.; Samuel, C.S.; Royce, S.G.; Twomey, D.J.; et al. Electrophysiological, electroanatomical, and structural remodeling of the atria as consequences of sustained obesity. *J. Am. Coll. Cardiol.* **2015**, *66*, 1–11. [CrossRef]
33. Mahajan, R.; Nelson, A.; Pathak, R.K.; Middeldorp, M.E.; Wong, C.X.; Twomey, D.J.; Carbone, A.; Teo, K.; Agbaedeng, T.; Linz, D.; et al. Electroanatomical remodeling of the atria in obesity: Impact of adjacent epicardial fat. *JACC Clin. Electrophysiol.* **2018**, *4*, 1529–1540. [CrossRef]
34. Khiabani, A.J.; MacGregor, R.M.; Bakir, N.H.; Manghelli, J.L.; Sinn, L.A.; Maniar, H.S.; Moon, M.R.; Schuessler, R.B.; Melby, S.J.; Damiano, R.J., Jr. The long-term outcomes and durability of the Cox-Maze IV procedure for atrial fibrillation. *J. Thorac. Cardiovasc. Surg.* **2020**. [CrossRef] [PubMed]
35. Thiyagarajah, A.; Kadhim, K.; Lau, D.H.; Emami, M.; Linz, D.; Khokhar, K.; Munawar, D.A.; Mishima, R.; Malik, V.; O'Shea, C.; et al. Feasibility, safety, and efficacy of posterior wall isolation during atrial fibrillation ablation: A systematic review and meta-analysis. *Circ. Arrhythmia Electrophysiol.* **2019**, *12*, e007005. [CrossRef] [PubMed]
36. Salih, M.; Darrat, Y.; Ibrahim, A.M.; Al-Akchar, M.; Bhattarai, M.; Koester, C.; Ayan, M.; Labedi, M.; Elayi, C.S. Clinical outcomes of adjunctive posterior wall isolation in persistent atrial fibrillation: A meta-analysis. *J. Cardiovasc. Electrophysiol.* **2020**, *31*, 1394–1402. [CrossRef] [PubMed]
37. Kim, J.S.; Shin, S.Y.; Na, J.O.; Choi, C.U.; Kim, S.H.; Kim, J.W.; Kim, E.J.; Rha, S.W.; Park, C.G.; Seo, H.S.; et al. Does isolation of the left atrial posterior wall improve clinical outcomes after radiofrequency catheter ablation for persistent atrial fibrillation? A prospective randomized clinical trial. *Int. J. Cardiol.* **2015**, *181*, 277–283. [CrossRef] [PubMed]
38. Tamborero, D.; Mont, L.; Berruezo, A.; Matiello, M.; Benito, B.; Sitges, M.; Vidal, B.; de Caralt, T.M.; Perea, R.J.; Vatasescu, R.; et al. Left atrial posterior wall isolation does not improve the outcome of circumferential pulmonary vein ablation for atrial fibrillation: A prospective randomized study. *Circ. Arrhythmia Electrophysiol.* **2009**, *2*, 35–40. [CrossRef]
39. Lim, T.W.; Koay, C.H.; See, V.A.; McCall, R.; Chik, W.; Zecchin, R.; Byth, K.; Seow, S.C.; Thomas, L.; Ross, D.L.; et al. Single-ring posterior left atrial (box) isolation results in a different mode of recurrence compared with wide antral pulmonary vein isolation on long-term follow-up: Longer atrial fibrillation-free survival time but similar survival time free of any atrial arrhythmia. *Circ. Arrhythmia Electrophysiol.* **2012**, *5*, 968–977. [CrossRef]
40. Lee, J.M.; Shim, J.; Park, J.; Yu, H.T.; Kim, T.H.; Park, J.K.; Uhm, J.S.; Kim, J.B.; Joung, B.; Lee, M.H.; et al. The electrical isolation of the left atrial posterior wall in catheter ablation of persistent atrial fibrillation. *JACC Clin. Electrophysiol.* **2019**, *5*, 1253–1261. [CrossRef]
41. Tokioka, S.; Fukamizu, S.; Kimura, T.; Takahashi, M.; Kitamura, T.; Hojo, R. The effect of posterior wall isolation for persistent atrial fibrillation on recurrent arrhythmia. *J. Cardiovasc. Electrophysiol.* **2021**, *32*, 597–604. [CrossRef] [PubMed]
42. Bai, R.; Di Biase, L.; Mohanty, P.; Trivedi, C.; Dello Russo, A.; Themistoclakis, S.; Casella, M.; Santarelli, P.; Fassini, G.; Santangeli, P.; et al. Proven isolation of the pulmonary vein antrum with or without left atrial posterior wall isolation in patients with persistent atrial fibrillation. *Heart Rhythm* **2016**, *13*, 132–140. [CrossRef] [PubMed]
43. Aryana, A.; Allen, S.L.; Pujara, D.K.; Bowers, M.R.; O'Neill, P.G.; Yamauchi, Y.; Shigeta, T.; Vierra, E.C.; Okishige, K.; Natale, A. Concomitant pulmonary vein and posterior wall isolation using cryoballoon with adjunct radiofrequency in persistent atrial fibrillation. *JACC Clin. Electrophysiol.* **2021**, *7*, 187–196. [CrossRef] [PubMed]
44. Aryana, A.; Baker, J.H.; Espinosa Ginic, M.A.; Pujara, D.K.; Bowers, M.R.; O'Neill, P.G.; Ellenbogen, K.A.; Di Biase, L.; d'Avila, A.; Natale, A. Posterior wall isolation using the cryoballoon in conjunction with pulmonary vein ablation is superior to pulmonary vein isolation alone in patients with persistent atrial fibrillation: A multicenter experience. *Heart Rhythm* **2018**, *15*, 1121–1129. [CrossRef] [PubMed]
45. Platonov, P.G.; Ivanov, V.; Ho, S.Y.; Mitrofanova, L. Left atrial posterior wall thickness in patients with and without atrial fibrillation: Data from 298 consecutive autopsies. *J. Cardiovasc. Electrophysiol.* **2008**, *19*, 689–692. [CrossRef] [PubMed]
46. Kim, T.H.; Park, J.; Uhm, J.S.; Kim, J.Y.; Joung, B.; Lee, M.H.; Pak, H.N. Challenging achievement of bidirectional block after linear ablation affects the rhythm outcome in patients with persistent atrial fibrillation. *J. Am. Heart Assoc.* **2016**, *5*. [CrossRef]

47. Halbfass, P.; Pavlov, B.; Muller, P.; Nentwich, K.; Sonne, K.; Barth, S.; Hamm, K.; Fochler, F.; Mugge, A.; Lusebrink, U.; et al. Progression from esophageal thermal asymptomatic lesion to perforation complicating atrial fibrillation ablation: A single-center registry. *Circ. Arrhythmia Electrophysiol.* **2017**, *10*. [CrossRef]
48. Schoene, K.; Arya, A.; Grashoff, F.; Knopp, H.; Weber, A.; Lerche, M.; Konig, S.; Hilbert, S.; Kircher, S.; Bertagnolli, L.; et al. Oesophageal probe evaluation in radiofrequency ablation of atrial fibrillation (OPERA): Results from a prospective randomized trial. *Europace* **2020**, *22*, 1487–1494. [CrossRef]
49. Markman, T.M.; Hyman, M.C.; Kumareswaran, R.; Arkles, J.S.; Santangeli, P.; Schaller, R.D.; Supple, G.E.; Frankel, D.S.; Riley, M.P.; Lin, D.; et al. Durability of posterior wall isolation after catheter ablation among patients with recurrent atrial fibrillation. *Heart Rhythm* **2020**, *17*, 1740–1744. [CrossRef]
50. Schuessler, R.B.; Kawamoto, T.; Hand, D.E.; Mitsuno, M.; Bromberg, B.I.; Cox, J.L.; Boineau, J.P. Simultaneous epicardial and endocardial activation sequence mapping in the isolated canine right atrium. *Circulation* **1993**, *88*, 250–263. [CrossRef]
51. Gharaviri, A.; Verheule, S.; Eckstein, J.; Potse, M.; Kuijpers, N.H.; Schotten, U. A computer model of endo-epicardial electrical dissociation and transmural conduction during atrial fibrillation. *Europace* **2012**, *14* (Suppl. S5), v10–v16. [CrossRef]
52. de Groot, N.; van der Does, L.; Yaksh, A.; Lanters, E.; Teuwen, C.; Knops, P.; van de Woestijne, P.; Bekkers, J.; Kik, C.; Bogers, A.; et al. Direct proof of endo-epicardial asynchrony of the atrial wall during atrial fibrillation in humans. *Circ. Arrhythmia Electrophysiol* **2016**, *9*. [CrossRef]
53. Parameswaran, R.; Kalman, J.M.; Royse, A.; Goldblatt, J.; Larobina, M.; Watts, T.; Walters, T.E.; Nalliah, C.J.; Wong, G.; Al-Kaisey, A.; et al. Endocardial-epicardial phase mapping of prolonged persistent atrial fibrillation recordings: High prevalence of dissociated activation patterns. *Circ. Arrhythmia Electrophysiol.* **2020**, *13*, e008512. [CrossRef]
54. Verheule, S.; Tuyls, E.; Gharaviri, A.; Hulsmans, S.; van Hunnik, A.; Kuiper, M.; Serroyen, J.; Zeemering, S.; Kuijpers, N.H.; Schotten, U. Loss of continuity in the thin epicardial layer because of endomysial fibrosis increases the complexity of atrial fibrillatory conduction. *Circ. Arrhythmia Electrophysiol.* **2013**, *6*, 202–211. [CrossRef]
55. Gharaviri, A.; Bidar, E.; Potse, M.; Zeemering, S.; Verheule, S.; Pezzuto, S.; Krause, R.; Maessen, J.G.; Auricchio, A.; Schotten, U. Epicardial Fibrosis explains increased endo-epicardial dissociation and epicardial breakthroughs in human atrial fibrillation. *Front. Physiol.* **2020**, *11*, 68. [CrossRef] [PubMed]
56. Mahapatra, S.; La Par, D.J.; Kamath, S.; Payne, J.; Bilchick, K.C.; Mangrum, J.M.; Ailawadi, G. Initial experience of sequential surgical epicardial-catheter endocardial ablation for persistent and long-standing persistent atrial fibrillation with long-term follow-up. *Ann. Thorac. Surg.* **2011**, *91*, 1890–1898. [CrossRef] [PubMed]
57. Maesen, B.; Pison, L.; Vroomen, M.; Luermans, J.G.; Vernooy, K.; Maessen, J.G.; Crijns, H.J.; La Meir, M. Three-year follow-up of hybrid ablation for atrial fibrillation. *Eur. J. Cardiothorac. Surg.* **2018**, *53*, i26–i32. [CrossRef] [PubMed]
58. de Asmundis, C.; Chierchia, G.B.; Mugnai, G.; Van Loo, I.; Nijs, J.; Czapla, J.; Conte, G.; Velagic, V.; Rodrigues Manero, M.; Ciconte, G.; et al. Midterm clinical outcomes of concomitant thoracoscopic epicardial and transcatheter endocardial ablation for persistent and long-standing persistent atrial fibrillation: A single-centre experience. *Europace* **2017**, *19*, 58–65. [CrossRef] [PubMed]
59. Magni, F.T.; Al-Jazairi, M.I.H.; Mulder, B.A.; Klinkenberg, T.; Van Gelder, I.C.; Rienstra, M.; Mariani, M.A.; Blaauw, Y. First-line treatment of persistent and long-standing persistent atrial fibrillation with single-stage hybrid ablation: A 2-year follow-up study. *Europace* **2021**. [CrossRef]
60. Kiser, A.C.; Landers, M.; Horton, R.; Hume, A.; Natale, A.; Gersak, B. The convergent procedure: A multidisciplinary atrial fibrillation treatment. *Heart Surg. Forum* **2010**, *13*, E317–321. [CrossRef]
61. Wats, K.; Kiser, A.; Makati, K.; Delurgio, D.; Greenberg, Y.; Sood, N.; Yang, F. The convergent AF ablation procedure: Evolution of a multidisciplinary approach to AF management. *Arrhythmia Electrophysiol. Rev.* **2020**, *9*, 88–96. [CrossRef] [PubMed]
62. Lee, L.S. Subxiphoid minimally invasive epicardial ablation (Convergent Procedure) with left thoracoscopic closure of the left atrial appendage. *Oper. Tech. Thorac. Cardiovasc. Surg. A Comp. Atlas* **2019**. [CrossRef]
63. On, Y.K.; Park, K.M.; Jeong, D.S.; Park, P.W.; Lee, Y.T.; Park, S.J.; Kim, J.S. Electrophysiologic Results After Thoracoscopic Ablation for Chronic Atrial Fibrillation. *Ann. Thorac. Surg.* **2015**, *100*, 1595–1602. [CrossRef] [PubMed]
64. Larson, J.; Merchant, F.M.; Patel, A.; Ndubisi, N.M.; Patel, A.M.; De Lurgio, D.B.; Lloyd, M.S.; El-Chami, M.F.; Leon, A.R.; Hoskins, M.H.; et al. Outcomes of convergent atrial fibrillation ablation with continuous rhythm monitoring. *J. Cardiovasc. Electrophysiol.* **2020**. [CrossRef]
65. Maclean, E.; Yap, J.; Saberwal, B.; Kolvekar, S.; Lim, W.; Wijesuriya, N.; Papageorgiou, N.; Dhillon, G.; Hunter, R.J.; Lowe, M.; et al. The convergent procedure versus catheter ablation alone in longstanding persistent atrial fibrillation: A single centre, propensity-matched cohort study. *Int. J. Cardiol.* **2020**, *303*, 49–53. [CrossRef]
66. Makati, K.J.; Sherman, A.J.; Gerogiannis, I.; Sood, N. Safety and efficacy of convergent hybrid procedure using cryo as endocardial energy source for the treatment of atrial fibrillation. *Circ. Arrhythmia Electrophysiol.* **2020**. [CrossRef]
67. Gulkarov, I.; Wong, B.; Kowalski, M.; Worku, B.; Afzal, A.; Ivanov, A.; Ramasubbu, K.; Reddy, B. Convergent ablation for persistent atrial fibrillation: Single center experience. *J. Card. Surg.* **2019**, *34*, 1037–1043. [CrossRef]
68. Tonks, R.; Lantz, G.; Mahlow, J.; Hirsh, J.; Lee, L.S. Short and intermediate term outcomes of the convergent procedure: Initial experience in a tertiary referral center. *Ann. Cardiovasc. Surg.* **2019**. [CrossRef]

69. DeLurgio, D.B.; Crossen, K.J.; Gill, J.; Blauth, C.; Oza, S.R.; Magnano, A.R.; Mostovych, M.A.; Halkos, M.E.; Tschopp, D.R.; Kerendi, F.; et al. Hybrid convergent procedure for the treatment of persistent and long-standing persistent atrial fibrillation: Results of CONVERGE clinical trial. *Circ. Arrhythmia Electrophysiol.* **2020**, *13*, e009288. [CrossRef]
70. Makati, K.J.; Sood, N.; Lee, L.S.; Yang, F.; Shults, C.C.; DeLurgio, D.B.; Melichercik, J.; Gill, J.S.; Kaba, R.A.; Ahsan, S.; et al. Combined epicardial and endocardial ablation for atrial fibrillation: Best practices and guide to hybrid convergent procedures. *Heart Rhythm* **2020**. [CrossRef]

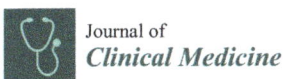

Review

Ganglionated Plexi Ablation for the Treatment of Atrial Fibrillation

Sahar Avazzadeh [1,†], Shauna McBride [1,†], Barry O'Brien [2], Ken Coffey [2], Adnan Elahi [3,4], Martin O'Halloran [3], Alan Soo [5] and Leo. R Quinlan [1,*]

1. Physiology and Human Movement Laboratory, CÚRAM SFI Centre for Research in Medical Devices, School of Medicine, Human biology building, National University of Ireland (NUI) Galway, H91 TK33 Galway, Ireland; sahar.avazzadeh@nuigalway.ie (S.A.); shauna.mcbride@nuigalway.ie (S.M.)
2. AtriAN Medical Limited, Unit 204, NUIG Business Innovation Centre, Upper Newcastle, H91 TK33 Galway, Ireland; barry.obrien@atrianmedical.com (B.O.); ken.coffey@atrianmedical.com (K.C.)
3. Translational Medical Devise Lab (TMD Lab), Lambe Institute of Translational Research, University College Hospital Galway, H91 ERW1 Galway, Ireland; adnan.elahi@nuigalway.ie (A.E.); martin.ohalloran@nuigalway.ie (M.O.)
4. Electrical & Electronic Engineering, School of Engineering, National University of Ireland Galway, H91 TK33 Galway, Ireland
5. Department of Cardiothoracic Surgery, University Hospital Galway, Saolta Hospital HealthCare Group, H91 YR71 Galway, Ireland; Alan.Soo@hse.ie
* Correspondence: leo.quinlan@nuigalway.ie; Tel.: +35-3-9149-3710
† Joint first author.

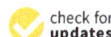

Received: 7 August 2020; Accepted: 23 September 2020; Published: 24 September 2020

Abstract: Atrial fibrillation (AF) is the most common type of cardiac arrhythmia and is associated with significant morbidity and mortality. The autonomic nervous system (ANS) plays an important role in the initiation and development of AF, causing alterations in atrial structure and electrophysiological defects. The intrinsic ANS of the heart consists of multiple ganglionated plexi (GP), commonly nestled in epicardial fat pads. These GPs contain both parasympathetic and sympathetic afferent and efferent neuronal circuits that control the electrophysiological properties of the myocardium. Pulmonary vein isolation and other cardiac catheter ablation targets including GP ablation can disrupt the fibers connecting GPs or directly damage the GPs, mediating the benefits of the ablation procedure. Ablation of GPs has been evaluated over the past decade as an adjunctive procedure for the treatment of patients suffering from AF. The success rate of GP ablation is strongly associated with specific ablation sites, surgical techniques, localization techniques, method of access and the incorporation of additional interventions. In this review, we present the current data on the clinical utility of GP ablation and its significance in AF elimination and the restoration of normal sinus rhythm in humans.

Keywords: atrial fibrillation; ganglionated plexi; autonomic nervous system; ablation

1. Introduction

Atrial Fibrillation presents clinically as chaotic electrical excitation that is detrimental to normal atrial contractility [1]. AF is the most common form of cardiac dysrhythmia and is categorized as a supraventricular tachyarrhythmia, which will affect 18 million people in Europe and 6–12 million in the United States by 2060 and 2050, respectively [2–5]. AF is generally classified as either paroxysmal, persistent, or long-standing persistent, and its presentation can in fact evolve and change over time [6]. The effects of AF can be life-threatening, as insufficient contraction of the atria results in blood stasis which promotes the formation of thromb-oemboli which effect the heart but can also propagate to other vital organs [7,8]. Despite many advances in recent years, no specific etiological factor has been pinpointed as the main cause of AF. Some epidemiological and clinical factors such as abnormalities associated with metabolism, endocrine function and genetics, are known to predispose patients to AF [6,9]. Furthermore, pathophysiological factors such as electrical and structural remodelling, inflammation, and local autonomic system regulation are also seen with AF [10]. Evidence from the literature highlights the role of the intrinsic and extrinsic autonomic nervous system (ANS) in cardiac function, the underlying mechanism of altered electrical activity in AF is not fully understood [11]. Altered autonomic activity is recognised as a significant component in both the initiation and maintenance of AF [12,13]. The incidence of atrial arrhythmias is reported to reduce when ANS innervation is significantly decreased [14,15]. The activity of the intrinsic cardiac ANS is found to be disrupted in cases of AF, with studies associating vagal interference with networks of GPs [16,17]. GPs are normally found in close proximity with epicardial fat pads and reside in discrete locations on the atria and ventricles, particularly surrounding the pulmonary veins (PV) and great vessels [18]. Numerous trials employing a variety of therapeutic interventions for cardiac disease have been completed to date, with some targeting GPs for AF treatment. The complex anatomical layout and physiological interconnectivity of these GP sites is important in understanding the pathophysiology of AF [19]. Our aim is to address the association of GPs with AF and document the extant literature reporting the impact of GP ablation procedures recorded in human clinical studies.

2. Cardiac Autonomic Nervous System

Components of the peripheral, central and intrinsic cardiac innervation systems form a complex interconnected network that manages cardiovascular function [19,20]. The cardiac ANS is organised into extrinsic and intrinsic components that are supplied by the autonomic nerves. The intrinsic ANS is comprised of clusters of neurons known as GPs that interconnect not only to the atria and ventricles, but also to the extrinsic cardiac ANS. The extrinsic sympathetic innervation arises in the grey matter of the thoracic spinal cord segments T1–T6 and are generally myelinated fibres, that increase heart rate and myocardial contractility by releasing noradrenaline, stimulating inotropy in the heart [18,20] (Figure 1). Noradrenaline (NE) binds to β1-adrenoceptors increasing sodium permeability, thereby increasing heart rate [20]. Parasympathetic fibres arise in the medulla oblongata, pons and midbrain of the brainstem, with some fibres arising from the sacral portion of the spinal cord (S2–S4). The resting heart is dominated by parasympathetic tone, which acts to reduce heart rate and slow cardiac impulses from the atria to the ventricles (Figure 1) through the release of acetylcholine (ACh). The binding of ACh to G-protein coupled muscarinic receptors (M2) activates inhibitory G proteins, reducing both the rate of depolarization and force of contraction of the atria [20]. This is achieved by reducing intracellular cyclic-AMP (cAMP) formation, reversing sympathetic effects on ion channels and Ca^{2+} handling.

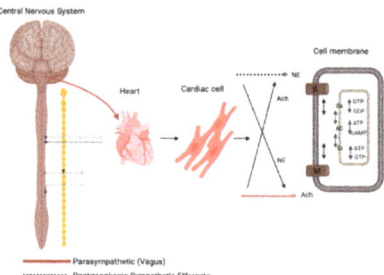

Figure 1. Sympathetic and parasympathetic mechanism in the autonomic nervous system (ANS). Parasympathetic vagal activity (in red) inhibits noradrenaline (NE) which in turn inhibit acetylcholine release (ACh). Released ACh binds to M muscarinic receptors (M) and, through the inhibition of Protein G1, coupled to adenylate cyclase (AC). Released NE from postganglionic sympathetic nerve endings (dotted line) binds to β-adrenergic receptors (β) which activate AC increasing intracellular cyclic-AMP (cAMP).

Role of the ANS in the Pathogenesis of AF

Experimental and clinical studies have reinforced the important role of the ANS in AF pathogenesis, initiation and maintenance [12]. Factors including alteration of ion currents, atrial myocardial metabolism and local autonomic regulation are responsible for the multifactorial induction of AF [21]. Reports show that pulmonary vein (PV) focal firing and AF can arise by GP stimulation at the PV-atrial junctions [22,23]. Less commonly, focal initiation of AF can be seen related to ectopic activity from the muscular sleeves of the Superior vena cava (SVC), ligament of Marshall, or regions elsewhere on the left and right atria which possibly coincide with GPs in those regions [24].

Changes in autonomic tone prior to AF onset have commonly been noted [25]. The underlying mechanism behind this is the effect of inward Ca^{2+} and/or outward K^+ current and the shortening of action potential duration observed in patients with paroxysmal AF [26]. Cervical vagal stimulation causes the release of ACh which activates outward K^+ currents in atrial myocytes, substantially shortening the action potential duration [27,28]. This has been proven to facilitate the onset and maintenance of AF in patients [29–31]. In addition, direct stimulation of GPs is commonly followed by hyperactivity and excess secretion of neurotransmitters, creating ideal conditions for AF initiation and continuation [32]. Excess release of ACh and catecholamines has been shown to result in rapid electrical firing of GPs from both PV and non-PV sites [32,33]. Studies by Po et al. investigated the effects of ACh directly injected into GPs in a canine model of AF and showed it to induce focal firing of PVs and sustained AF [23]. Thus it appears that GP stimulation not only triggers AF in patients, but also directly impacts atrial conduction properties [34]. This influence stems from both sympathetic and parasympathetic branches of the ANS, with the parasympathetic appearing as the predominant branch [34]. GPs provide a site for AF maintenance as autonomic activity was found to increase firing in six-hour rapid atrial pacing recorded from the right anterior GP, showing a decrease in the effective refractory period [35]. A shortening of atrial refractory period (AERP) is commonly seen in AF or rapid atrial pacing [36]. In a canine models of AF, GP ablation reversed electrical remodelling, implying that GP ablation may prove to be a promising strategy for the management of AF in patients [37].

3. Ganglionated Plexi

GPs are localised neural clusters of intrinsic cardiac ganglia, containing local circuits, parasympathetic neurons, and sympathetic afferent and efferent [38]. The variety of neuronal contributions associated with each ganglion reflects their complex synaptology [39]. GPs typically contain 200–1000 neurons and are variable in size, with predominantly oval-shaped soma [17,40]. Histological studies show the mean area of a human ganglia to be 0.07 ± 0.02 mm^2, with few exceeding 0.2 mm^2 [41]. Neurons within GPs vary in their projection orientation (unipolar, multipolar) (Figure 2), neurochemical profiles, and abundance on the atria (approx. 400 per GP) and ventricles (approx. 5–40) [40,42,43].

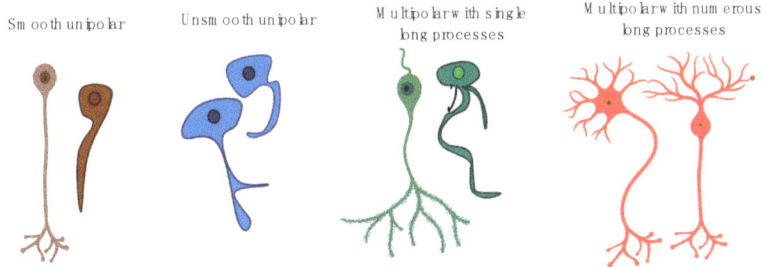

Figure 2. Different morphology of neurons found in ganglionated plexi (GP) sites in humans. There are three types of neurons that are populated in GP sites. These are either unipolar (brown, blue) or multipolar (green, red) having either single (brown, blue, green) or multiple (red) processes.

GPs are typically found embedded in epicardial adipose tissue (EAT) and have been described as having a 'raisin in bread' pattern, forming chain-like extensions onto the atria and ventricles [44]. The degree of EAT coverage varies in quantity and depth, and is generally concentrated along the coronary sulcus and interventricular and atrioventricular grooves [45,46]. The electrophysiological characteristics of three distinct epicardial fat pads have been investigated previously. These are located at the intersection of the right atrium and right superior PV (Right Pulmonary Vein-RPV fat pad), the junction of the left atrium and IVC (IVC-LA fat pad), and between the root of the aorta and SVC (SVC-Ao fat pad) superior to the right pulmonary artery [47–49] (Figure 3).

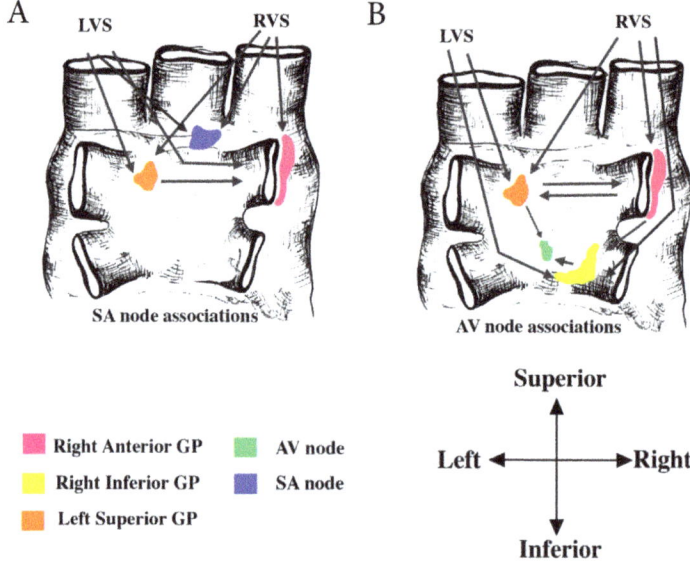

Figure 3. Posterior view of the atria showing the interactions between neural pathways. (**A**): Arrows indicate the direction of impulse and the connections of the left vagosympathetic trunk (LVS) and right vagosympathetic trunk (RVS) with the anterior right (AR) and superior left (SL) GPs. These pathways have been shown to modulate the effects of the sinoatrial node (SA) node and attenuate sinus rate slowing. (**B**): Arrows indicate the direction of impulse and connections involving the LVS and RVS trunks, with the SL, AR and inferior right (IR) GP's. These pathways have been shown to influence atrioventricular node (AV) node function and ventricular rate response. The inferior left GP (ILGP) acts as a pivotal element in the connection pathway to the AV node.

Anatomical Location of GPs

In general, GP locations are concentrated on the posterior regions of the atria and the posterior-superior aspect of the ventricles [39] (Figure 3). Knowledge of GP location and their axonal projection pathways are important when considering targeted therapeutic interventions. GPs are found in the posterior portion of the left and right atria (Figure 4), termed the dorso-atrial region, and at the transition from atria to ventricle at the level of the tricuspid and bicuspid valves, in the annular-ventricular region. They are also found around the aorta and pulmonary trunk in the peri-great vessel region, and between the aorta and superior vena cava in the aorto-caval region [50,51]. It is estimated that 75% of epicardial ganglia reside on the dorsal aspect of the heart [41].

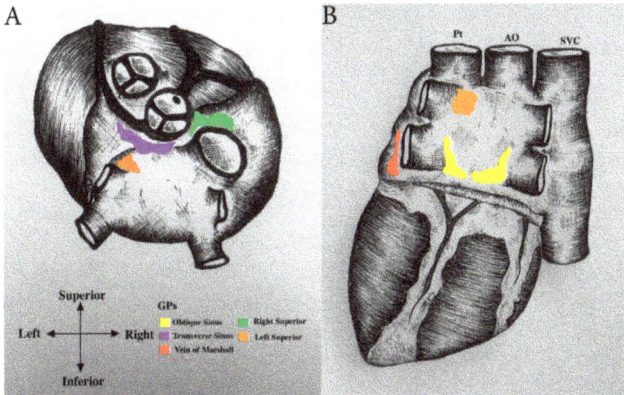

Figure 4. GP's targeted for ablation. A posterior view of the heart showing all the main ganglionated plexi sites essential for ablation. (**A**) These include the transverse sinus (in purple) and superior right (in green) located between aorta (AO) and superior vena cava (SVC). (**B**) The oblique sinus GPs (in yellow) are situated supero-anterior to the right superior pulmonary vein (PV) (ARPV) and infero-posterior region of the right inferior PV (IRPV). The left superior (in orange) can be found medial to the left superior PV (SLPV). Vein of Marshall (in red) is another target ablation region within the ligament of Marshall. Pt, pulmonary trunk.

There are four GP's found in the vicinity of the PVs that are regularly targeted in ablation procedures [52]. Each of these GPs innervate the PVs and the surrounding left atrial myocardium [52]. The superior left GP (SLGP) is located superolateral and medial to the left superior PV and extends around its root [16,44,53] (Figure 3). The SLGP is associated with both the sino-atrial (SA) and atrio-ventricular (AV) nodes, influencing sinus and ventricular rate [54,55]. The anterior right (AR) GP is situated supero-anterior to the right superior PV [52]. This GP has been found to have the most prominent interconnections converging with the SA node, where it acts as an integration center connecting the extrinsic ANS to the SA node [52]. The inferior left GP (ILGP) is located infero-posterior to the left inferior PV and has electrophysiological associations with the AV node, and can induce ventricular slowing caused by left vago-sympathetic stimulation [55]. Finally, the inferior right (IR) ganglion can be found in the infero-posterior region of the right inferior PV. The right inferior ganglion has associations with the AV node [52–54,56]. Together, the ILGPs and IRGPs are retro-atrial and termed the Oblique Sinus GPs [50].

The circuitry connecting the PV ganglia can be categorized according to the region first in contact with the vago-sympathetic trunk [54]. They can be separated into three individual pathways, with the SLGP linked to one circuit and the ARGP linked to two. The neural route, the right vago-sympathetic trunk-ARGP-SA node, is the predominant pathway and is linked to the left and right vago-sympathetic trunks where it modulates sinus rhythm and shortens the atrial refractory period, without disrupting the AV node [54,57] (Figure 3). The IRGP acts primarily on the AV node, and influences ventricular rate slowing responses induced by vago-sympathetic stimulation [54,56]. Ablation studies have shown that the SLGP does not augment sinus rhythm, but stimulation by the AR, IL and IR GPs cause an increase in rate [57].

The morphology of PVs has also been an area of interest to electrophysiologists. As the vein approaches the ostium, atrial tissue doubles over its circumference forming a fragmented myocardial sheath of pacemaker cardiomyocytes and multilayer muscles [58,59]. These myocyte layers are arranged in bundles that are predominantly spiral and circularly orientated [60]. They often associate with other bundles forming a 'mesh-like' assortment of longitudinal and oblique fibers. Ectopic foci have been found to emanate from PVs that can fire at random and induce atrial depolarization [60,61]. A number of groups have shown that the PV sites and the junction between the PVs and left atrium are abundantly enriched with innervation from both sympathetic and parasympathetic nerves, which may contribute to the frequent disruption of signals by GPs in the vicinity [59,62,63]. Experimental and clinical evaluations from some studies have suggested that the formation of spontaneous electrical discharges from PV sites is the result of abnormal automaticity, triggered activity or micro re-entry of electrical signals [60]. Other reports suggest the triggering to be due to PV-associated ganglia rather than the PV itself [64]. An influx of ACh has been touted as central to the stimulation of PV ganglia, inducing PV firing by re-entry pathways in other works [65]. The effect of Ach is to reduce action potential duration in the PV sleeves, causing them to fire until suppressed. Therefore, elimination of PV trigger sites by ablation of the associated ganglia removes the influential vagal drivers which contribute to maintaining AF [65].

The Vein of Marshall (VOM) within the Ligament of Marshall (LOM) contains another common target region for ablation procedures [50,53,66]. The VOM extends from the coronary sinus, between the left PVs and left atrial appendage, then traverses between the base of the left superior PV and pulmonary artery before attaching to the pericardium superiorly [67,68]. In this general region the VOM, myocardial sleeve and autonomic ganglia are found, with the ganglia located in a fat pad between the left PVs and left atrial appendage [67–69] Studies have shown that the LOM may act as a conduit of sympathetic innervation between the ventricles and the left superior ganglia [67]. In some patients, the LOM is an electrically active bypass of the left atrium/PV junction, rendering PV isolation ineffective [53].

There is growing interest in some of the more anatomically inaccessible GPs for ablation purposes. The Transverse Sinus GP (TSGP) resides between the pulmonary artery and base of the aorta, within the transverse sinus. It is sometimes referred to as the Great Artery GP in accordance with its associations [39]. The Aorto-caval or Superior Vena Caval-Aortic ganglion (SVC-Ao) is found along the posteromedial wall of the superior vena cava, the anterolateral wall of the ascending aorta and superior to the right pulmonary artery [70]. It is also referred to as the Superior Right (SR) GP. The SVC-Ao GP was believed to be a large, sprawling GP expanding from the anterolateral aspect of the aorta to the posterior portion of the aorta [71]. However, more recently it is suggested that two separate GPs reside in this area, the TS GP and the SVC-Ao GP. The TS GP and SVC-Ao GP are not as commonly targeted for ablation compared to other GPs and have mainly been targeted in canine studies [72,73] (Table 1). This is owing primarily to the difficulty in accessing them, with an epicardial approach preferred over an endocardial approach to avoid ablation within the great vessels [66]. The aorto-caval ganglion receives preganglionic parasympathetic innervation from the vagus nerve, while its postganglionic neurons send impulses to the atrium and superior vena cava. The SVC-Ao GP is believed to be the 'head station' for extrinsic cardiac ANS innervation to the heart [73]. Previous studies have shown this GP to shorten the effective refractory period and increase the window of vulnerability to arrhythmias at all atrial and PV sites influenced by stimulation of the vagal trunk [73]. It is also known to act as a trigger of SVC [73] (Figure 4). Hyperactivity of the SVC-Ao GP is also known induce ACh injection which acts as a trigger for SVC firing, but the exact mechanism is not entirely understood and requires further study [72,73] (Figure 4).

Table 1. Ganglionated plexi as main target for AF.

Author, Year	GP Sites Ablated	Localization of GPs	Additional Intervention	Number of Patients	Control Group	Method of Access	Follow Up Period (Max)	Outcome
Iso K et al., 2019	Ligament of Marshall (LOM,) SL, AR, IL, IR	High frequency stimulation (HFS)	Pulmonary vein isolation (PVI)	42	-	Endocardial	N/A	(1) R-R interval was longer in patients with AF. (2) More active GPs were found in patients with AF.
Garibelli P et al., 2018	SL, LL, RL, AR	HFS	PVI	18	-	Endocardial	1.8 ± 0.8 years	(1) 48% freedom from AF in GP ablation alone. (2) 74% freedom of AF in in GP ablation + PVI.
Budera P et al., 2018	LOM, SL, AR, IL, IR	HFS	PVI (Box lesion)	38	-	Epicardial	12 months	(1) 82% AF free using two-staged hybrid ablation of non-paroxysmal AF.
Bagge L et al., 2017	LA GP + LOM (if identified (96%))	HFS	PVI	42	-	Epicardial	12 months	(1) 76% AF free after 12 months.
Budera P et al., 2017	LA GPs	Anatomical	PVI (Box lesion)/cavotricuspid isthmus ablation	41	-	Epicardial/endocardial	507.2 ± 201.1 days	(1) 80% AF free without ADD/re-ablation in 2 staged hybrid procedure after 1.5 years. (2) 65% AF free with ADD/re-ablation at last follow-ups.
Barta J et al., 2017	SL, AR, IR, IL, LOM	HFS	Box lesion, R + L PV isolation, lesion of LA isthmus, resection of LAA + connecting lesion of appendage base with LSPV	35	65	Epicardial	12 months	(1) GP ablation alone showed 97.5% in NSR with ADD, 50% in NSR without ADD.
Suwalski G et al., 2017	SL, AR, IL, IR	HFS	PVI, LAA	34	-	Epicardial	3 months	(1) 85% success of GP detection based on preoperative heart rate.
Saini A et al., 2017	SL, AR, IL, IR, LOM	HFS	PVI	109	-	Epicardial	5 years	(1) 79.6% AF free without interventions (ADD, cardioversion, CA).
Baykaner T et al., 2017	SL, AR, IL, IR	HFS	N/A	97	-	Endocardial	N/A	(1) Sources of AF were found in: 47% at the SLGP site, 34% at ILCP, 14% at ARGP and 19% at IRGP sites.
Nagamoto Y et al., 2017	SL, AR, IR, IL	HFS	PVI	1	-	Endocardial	Not specified	(1) Inferior GP ablation itself did not eliminate PV potentials. (2) PVI had possibly helped eliminate PV potentials by cumulative effect.
Xhaet O et al., 2017	AR, IR, SL	HFS	PVI	20	-	Epicardial	N/A	(1) GPs are a mandatory link to the right vagus and AV node.
Romanov A et al., 2017	GPs of left atrium	HFS	N/A	1	-	Epicardial	6 months	(1) Using D-SPECT™ SUMO image acquisition created 3D cardiac electro-anatomical mapping system for GP ablation. (2) Patient was AF free with no ADD.
Takahashi K et al., 2016	LOM, SL, AR, IL, IR	HFS	PVI	40	-	Epicardial	18.6 months	(1) >80% Complex fractionated atrial electrograms (CFAE) overlay GP sites while 100% of epicardial adipose tissue (EAT) overlay GP sites.
Sharma P et al., 2016	10 sites each side	HSF + anatomical	Mini maze	67	-	Epicardial	4.5 ± 2.3 years	(1) Selective ablation of right GPs first is linked to higher rate of AF recurrence. (2) Lower number of GPs on the left side observed.
Antoine H.G. et al., 2016	SL, AR, IL, IR, LOM	HFS	PVI	117	123	Epicardial	12 months	(1) GP ablation alone did not reduce the AF occurrence during thoracoscopic surgery (70% vs. 68%).
Jiang et al., 2016	SL, AR, IL, IR	Anatomical	PVI	12	-	Epicardial	Not specified	(1) Majority of PV firing ceased after targeting GP outside of circumferential line or addition ablation along previous circular lesion.
Gelsomino S et al., 2015	SL, AR, IL, IR, LOM + Waterston groove	HSF	PVI (cox maze IV)	306	213	Epicardial	7 years	(1) GP ablations with or without cox maze IV showed no significant difference on AF recurrence NSR.
Sakamoto S et al., 2014	SL, AR, IL, IR, LOM	HSF + anatomical	Modified cox maze	30	-	Endocardial	3 months	(1) Most active GP sites were located in the Right PV antrum. (2) Anatomic GP ablation showed a greater decrease in sympathetic and parasympathetic tone.
Mamchur S et al., 2014	GPs of left atrium	Anatomical	PVI (Hybrid)	10	-	Epicardial & Endocardial	12 months	(1) 100% restoration of sinus rhythm with all patients free from arrhythmia in 6–9 months.
Zheng S et al., 2014	SL, AR, IL, IR,	HFS	PVI	89	-	Epicardial	60 months	(1) Single-procedure success rate is 56.3% for paroxysmal AF, 27.3% for persistent AF, and 25% for long-term persistent AF.
Katritsis D et al., 2013	SL, AR, IL, IR	Anatomic	PVI	242	-	Endocardial	24 months	(1) PVI group 56%, GP 48%, PVI + GP 74% maintained sinus rhythm/free from AF. (2) PVI + GP ablation is best strategy.
Kondo Y et al., 2013	SL, AR, IL, IR	HFS	PVI (Maze IV)	16	-	Epicardial	3 months	(1) 81% maintained NSR. (2) For those with active GPs, 92% maintained SR. (3) IRGP is an important pathway between other GPs and the AV node.
Malcolme-Lawes L et al., 2013	SL, AR, IL, IR	HFS	PVI (Cryoablation)	30	-	Endocardial	N/A	(1) Presence of a LA neural network with a common entry to the AV node via the IRGP.

71

Table 1. Cont.

Author, Year	GP Sites Ablated	Localization of GPs	Additional Intervention	Number of Patients	Control Group	Method of Access	Follow Up Period (Max)	Outcome
Pokushalov E et al., 2013	SL, AR, IL, IR, LOM	HPS	PVI	132	132	Endocardial	36 months	(1) 34% of patients without GP ablation were in sinus rhythm. (2) 49% of patients with GP ablation were in sinus rhythm.
Kasirajan V et al., 2012	Not specified	Not specified	PVI	118	-	Epicardial	12 months	(1) Additional ablation needed in 5% of patients. (2) 80% had freedom from AF after single procedure with no need for antiarrhythmics.
Santini M et al., 2012	Left atrial GPs and LOM	Not specified	PVI	22	-	Epicardial	22 months	(1) Ablation was successful in 73% of patients. (2) Freedom from AF was 91% without ADD.
Calo L et al., 2011	Left & Right atrial GPs	HPS and Anatomic	N/A	34	-	Endocardial	19.7 ± 5.2 months	(1) AF recurred in 29% of patients with anatomic ablation and in 76% of patients with the selective approach.
Krul S et al., 2011	SL, AR	HPS	PVI (Hybrid)	31	-	Epicardial	12 months	(1) 86% AF free after 1 year follow up without use of ADD.
Lim P et al., 2011	SL, AR, IL, IR	HPS	N/A	12	-	Endocardial	N/A	(1) Direct link between activation of the intrinsic cardiac ANS and PV ectopy.
Katrisis D et al., 2011	SL, AR, IL, IR	HPS	PVI	34	33	Endocardial	5 ± 1.3 months	(1) PVI group had 54.5% recurrence rate and re-ablation rate of 21.2%. (2) PVI + GP group had 26.5% recurrence and 17.6% re-ablation.
Mikhaylov E et al., 2011	SL, AR, IL, IR	HPS and Anatomic	PVI	35	35	Endocardial	36 months	(1) Freedom from arrhythmia without drugs at 12 months was 54.3% for GP group and 74.3% for CPVI group. (2) Re-ablation was done in 17% of GP group.
Ware A.L et al., 2011	GPs of Left and Right atrium, LOM	HPS	PVI (Maze)	20	-	Epicardial	25 months	(1) 89% of patients were free of AF. (2) 79% were in NSR. 3) 11% were in a paced rhythm.
Lim et al., 2011	GPs of Left and Right atrium	HPS	N/A	25	-	Endocardial	N/A	(1) 16% reduction in AF cycle length was found in PV adjacent to HPS site. (2) 9% reduction at PV-atrial junction.
Pokushalov E et al., 2010	SL, AR, IL, IR	No specific mapping	N/A	56	-	Endocardial	12 months	(1) 71% of patients free from AF.
Pokushalov E et al., 2010	SL, AR, IL, IR	Anatomic	N/A	89	-	Endocardial	24 ± 3 months	(1) 38.2% freedom from AF after single ablation.
Pokushlov E et al., 2009	SL, AR, IL, IR and Active GP areas	Anatomic and HPS	N/A	80	-	Endocardial	12 months	(1) Recurrence of AF was 57.5% in selective and 22.5% in anatomic.
Po S et al., 2009	SL, AR, IL, IR	HPS	PVI	83	-	Endocardial	22 months	(1) GP ablation alone decreased incidence of spontaneous PV firing from 65.1% to 14.5%. (2) Freedom from AF after first procedure was 80%.
Ohkubo K et al., 2008	SL, AR, IL, IR	HPS	PVI	21	-	Endocardial	8 months	(1) 69% of patients free from AF.
Danik S et al., 2008	SL, AR, IL, IR	HPS	PVI	18	-	Endocardial	6 weeks	(1) Early AF recurrence in 22% of patients.
Ononati F et al., 2008	Left and Right PVs, LOM	HPS	PVI (Maze)	31	44	Epicardial	12 months	(1) Freedom from AF was higher in group with GP ablation (92.9±6.9%) when compared to group without (62.5 ± 6.9%).
Pokushalov E et al., 2008	SL, AR, IL, IR	Anatomic	N/A	58	-	Endocardial	7.2 ± 0.4 months	(1) Transient vagal bradycardia was seen in 93% of patients. (2) 86.2% of patients free from AF.
Matsutani N et al., 2008	GP around Waterson's + left side + LOM	N/A	PVI	17	-	Epicardial	16.6 ± 5.7 months	(1) 90% of patients free at months 1, 3 or 6. (2) 85% weaned from AADs after 3 months.
Puskas J et al., 2007	LOM	HPS	PVI	1	-	Epicardial	6 months	(1) No AF revealed at months 1, 3 or 6. (2) Patient reported as no symptomatic AF.
Sherlag B et al., 2005	SL, AR, IL, IR	HPS	PVI	33	27	Endocardial	10 months	(1) 91% of patients were free from AF in PVI + GP ablation group, PVI alone group was 70%.

Normal sinus rhythm (NSR), Anti-arrhythmic drugs (ADD), left atrial (LA), left atrial appendage, (LAA), catheter ablation (CA), heart rate variability (HRV).

4. GP Ablation for AF

Therapeutic interventions for AF have been adapted to target the pathophysiological state involved in structural remodeling or to influence the excitation of ion channels and adrenergic receptors [21,74]. Many therapeutic approaches are employed to serve as a preventative measure, aiming to inhibit the primary occurrence of new-onset AF or secondary recurrence of AF, and are less effective in cases of persistent AF or AF with a prolonged duration [21,75,76]. Many invasive techniques have been adapted to target symptomatic drug refractory AF [77]. Surgical ablation such as the classical 'cut and sew' Cox-Maze procedures, claim a 97–99% success rate and have been deemed by some to be more effective than catheter-based approaches [78–80]. The drive to develop less aggressive techniques has encouraged the development of minimally invasive catheter-based procedures [81]. In the last 20 years, catheter cardiac ablation has become an established, fundamental treatment strategy for AF. Catheter ablation aims to relieve symptoms of AF, by eliminating the trigger of AF or altering the arrhythmogenic tissue underlying AF [80,82].

4.1. GP Localization and Its Importance for Effective Ablation

The active area of all GP sites, i.e., the GP areas where the vagal response is mostly elicited, appears significantly higher in AF compared to non-AF patients [83]. Additionally, the maximum R-R interval is significantly longer in AF patients after high frequency stimulation (HFS), when compared to non-AF groups [83]. Active GP areas are more prevalent on the right side of the PVs, with no considerable difference observed between paroxysmal, persistent and long-standing persistent AF patients [84–87] (Table 1). Ablation of active GPs on the right side of the PVs resulted in 92% sinus rhythm maintenance in patients at three month follow-up [86]. Zheng et al. reported that there are a mean of 2.8 active GP sites on the right side (Waterson's grove and LOM) compared to 1.4 on the left side [84]. A reduced number of active GPs is associated with cardiac and neural remodelling and subsequent development of AF [84]. 95% of GPs are cholinergic and when activated a local release of ACh leads to bradycardia [62]. In chronic AF, there is a down regulation in the number of available ACh receptors, weakening the vagal response from GP areas upon stimulation [62]. This suggests that the strength of the vagal response is associated with a number of active GP areas before ablation, and higher numbers of GP sites ablated are significantly correlated with reduced AF recurrence at 12-month follow-up [84]. Similar findings are reported by others where 5 active GPs were identified on the right and 2.7 on the left side [88,89]. Again, this was directly linked to higher long-term success rates in patients with a mean number of active GPs over five [84].

A recent study by Hu et al. indicates that endocardial ablation of the right anterior GPs produced a significant increase in heart rate in 93% of patients [16]. In addition, there appears to be an essential role for the right anterior GP which inhibits positive vagal responses and increases heart rate during pulmonary vein isolation (PVI) [90]. These findings demonstrate the importance of GP ablation of specific sites between the PVs and interatrial groove when targeting AF. While ablation of right-sided GPs is a significant factor in minimizing and reducing AF recurrences, active GPs on the left have also been targeted for ablation in some studies (Table 1).

The modulation of SA and AV nodal function is governed by the extrinsic cardiac ANS. Animal studies have demonstrated that GPs on the right side act as "integration centers" and are capable of modulating the effect of stimulated left-sided GPs on AV and SA nodal responses [91]. HFS of the right inferior GPs has shown how they selectively innervate the AV node in humans [92]. As previously demonstrated in animal studies, ablation and mapping of right-sided GPs in humans with HFS can lower the number and magnitude of GP activity on the left side [93]. Neural pathways between left atrial GPs and the AV node have been shown to pass through the lower right GPs [94]. In support of this, there was significantly higher AF and atrial tachyarrhythmia (AT) recurrence rates reported in patients who underwent selective GP ablation of the right side first [93]. This study also implied that ablation of one active GP out of sequential pacing is insufficient for vagal denervation [95]. It is worth noting that no significant difference was observed between patients who underwent extensive anatomical mapping instead of HFS [93].

Despite our growing understanding of the anatomical map and location of GPs, the extent to which GPs are hyperactive and are viable targets for ablation is still largely unknown. GPs can be identified and targeted by applying HFS [44,96] or by ablating at presumed anatomic sites [97,98] (Table 1). The vagal response of GPs to HFS is found to be very specific, but the sensitivity of HFS in portraying the full extent of GPs is still lacking [52]. The first comparative study was carried out by Pokushalov et al. in which they demonstrated that the AF freedom rate after 13 month follow-up was 42.5% and 77.5% in HFS-induced and anatomical mapping ablation groups, respectively [97]. An explanation for this may be the greater extent to which ablation (RF ablation in this case) targets anatomical GP regions in comparison to specific HFS mapped areas. Synchronized HFS serves as an alternative method and involves the delivery of current during the atrial refractory period. This helps identify GP ablation sites based on the activation of autonomic neural elements and has been associated with better outcomes [94]. However, this technology is only applicable for patients in sinus rhythm and further research is required for its use for persistent AF. A case report study by Romanov et al. showed that using D-SPECTTM SUMO image acquisition after injection of I-mIBG provides a 3D cardiac electro-anatomical map that can be used to identify target sites [99]. This approach can potentially increase the efficacy of the ablation procedure by accurately identifying GPs that are verified by HFS [100]. Furthermore, GPs can be identified with additional complex fractioned atrial electrograms (CFAE) around the GP area [101,102].

An additional factor is that the efficacy of GP ablation can be diminished by the surroundings, e.g., the epicardial adipose tissue (EAT) and epicardial fat pads. The location and amount (>5 mm) of EAT may act as a protective covering of the coronary vessels to prevent vascular damage, serving as an insulating cushion to targeted epicardial sites, and minimizing the efficiency of thermal-based ablation strategies [103]. 80% and 100% of the major five anatomical GP sites are found and overlaid at CFAE sites and left atrium-EAT respectively [104]. GP ablation through positive vagal response by HFS stimulation on CFAE areas has shown sinus rhythm maintenance in 71% of patients with paroxysmal AF [102]. Extensive ablation of these CFAE areas defines the boundaries for GP ablation [102,104]. Left atrium-EAT and CFAE areas have similar distribution, and are adjacent to vagal response sites [101,104]. Ablation of the anterior fat pads has also been investigated, with many contradictory results recorded [105,106].

4.2. Technical Procedures for GP Ablation

RF ablation is a well-established technique for GP ablation and is employed in many ablation procedures (Table 1) [107]. Cryoablation is not as commonly used, despite being found to significantly reduce the surface area of GPs, with the SL and ARGPs most dramatically reduced overall [108]. However, with increased reports of its efficacy in treating AF, interest is growing in cryoablation as a stand-alone ablation modality and in the development of cryoablation devices [109]. Cryoablation can also be used in conjunction with RF to target GPs and achieve PVI [107,108]. One study presented a comparison between a group (35 patients) with PVI treated with cryoablation and an additional GP ablation and a group (65 patients) with only PVI, which showed comparable results of sinus rhythm maintenance at 94% and 89% at 12 months, respectively [107].

The extent to whether GP ablation alone contributes to successful abolition of AF is not clear and early experiments by Pokushalov et al. conducted using RF show freedom from AF in 77.5% of patients with paroxysmal AF [97]. A similar outcome was recorded in another of their studies that included 56 patients with paroxysmal AF which yielded a 71% success rate upon ablation of GPs [110]. Furthermore, the same group demonstrated that GP ablation alone over the course of 24 months resulted in freedom of AF in 38.2% of patients with persistent AF, in comparison to higher success rate in 12 months follow up studies [111]. This work also revealed that the success rate increased substantially (59.6%) after performing additional ablation procedures, suggesting that GP ablation may be most effective when accompanied by other ablative procedures such as PVI, rather than a single-shot approach. Interestingly, comparison of results from a single ablation procedure at 13 months and 24 months in two studies by the Pokushalov group showed success to be 77.5% and 38.2%, respectively. Patient numbers were similar in these two studies which may stand as a good comparison for incorporating the long-term effects of GP ablation; however, the types of AF did vary [97,111]. It is plausible that the different success rates may be influenced by the type of AF with a typically lower success related to persistent AF and a higher rate associated with paroxysmal AF [97,111].

PVI is associated with denervation of the ANS and a significant reduction in AF recurrence [82]. Most studies have incorporated PVI into their GP ablation procedures. Investigation of comparative studies of PVI and GP ablation alone or as combined procedures present intriguing results. Studies have shown that a stand-alone PVI yields higher success rates than GP ablation procedures alone [112,113]. However, in studies comparing PVI alone with PVI + GP, the success rate increases from anywhere between 20% and 28% in short-term follow-up of less than 12 months [114,115]. Success of PVI + GP ablation procedures can range from anywhere between 50% and 91% in studies involving all types of AF (paroxysmal, persistent and long-standing persistent) [116,117]. Higher success rates have been associated with paroxysmal AF patients in comparison to long-standing persistent patients at 86% and 50%, respectively [116]. However, some studies recorded high success rates in patients with persistent and long-standing AF, showing an incoherence between AF subtypes [118]. Typically, PVI with GP ablation are carried out in one session or in two stages, giving the patient time to recover between procedures. Hybrid procedures involving initial endocardial PVI followed by GP ablation at a later stage have been trialed on patients with persistent or long-standing persistent AF. The outcome of these procedures shows a high success rate of 93% and 82% at 12 month follow-up, respectively [119,120]. It is plausible that hybrid procedures may be more appropriate in treating these types of AF. The addition of PVI to GP ablation procedures increases the success rate regardless of AF type; however, more testing would be required throughout AF groups to delineate the most appropriate and efficient procedure.

The 'mini-Maze' procedure and Dallas lesion set are examples of adaptations that have been made to some procedures where epicardial PVI is incorporated into lesion sets, with promising results. RF energy is used as an adaption from the original Cox Maze 'cut and sew' methods. These methods can either intentionally or unintentionally integrate the ablation or intersection of GPs into their lesion sets [93]. Mini-maze procedures with intentional GP ablation has proved to be successful in treating AF in previous work. Outcomes recorded from two studies over sixteen months conducted by Onorati et al. and Matsutani et al. showed 83 ± 7.9% freedom from AF (75 patients) and 90% of (18) patients in sinus rhythm [118,121]. A Dallas lesion set modified from the Cox Maze III procedure also shows some potential for AF treatment [122]. A long-term two year follow-up has shown the Dallas lesion set to bring freedom from AF in 80.6% of patients with long-standing persistent AF [123,124]. These are similar data to those reported in Cox Maze studies that incorporated both paroxysmal and persistent AF in their study population [123]. It is possible that the extensive lesions formed during these procedures may in fact be important for treating particularly difficult and advanced AF cases and may inadvertently have included GPs in the lesions. Endocardial and epicardial access during PVI procedures have been associated with unintentional damage and incidental ablation at GP sites [125]. PVI via thermal epicardial approaches can result in overlap of ablation lesions with numerous GP sites, while the endocardial thermal approaches may induce collateral damage by conductive heating. For PVI with GP ablation, mapping can be used to locate gaps in ablation lines to test for electrical block in targeted areas [124]. Epicardial access for GP ablation with PVI yielded a rate of freedom from AF ranging from anywhere between 65% and 90% [121,126]. Similarly, the endocardial approach yielded 73.5%–91% freedom from AF [115,117]. Success rates involving GP ablation mainly appear to be similar, whether procedures are done via epicardial or endocardial approach.

4.3. GP Ablation for Non-AF Cardiovascular Conditions

GP ablation may offer an alternative way of treating other conditions that are related to an imbalance of cardiac ANS activity. Post operational AF (POAF) typically appears two–five days after cardiac surgery and can be associated with serious complications including cardiac failure, stroke and death [100]. Ablation of GP sites has been shown to significantly lower the incidence of POAF by 93% in a randomized controlled trial after coronary artery bypass grafting [88]. However, this approach is sometimes not clinically desirable. To avoid ablation with its destruction of anatomical structures and capacity for collateral damage, alternative measures have been examined, for example involving the neurotoxin Botulism produced by the bacterium Clostridium Botulinum [127]. Studies have shown that the intraoperative injection of Botulism toxin into epicardial fat pads can significantly reduce instances of POAF [127]. The neurotoxin temporarily blocks the exocytotic release of ACh and diminishes sympathetic and parasympathetic activity, highlighting the involvement of autonomic imbalance and GP activation in the mechanism of POAF. The effects of the Botulism toxin can last anywhere between one and six months and provide a better, untaxing alternative to the use of β-blocker medication. In studies by Pokushalov et al. and Romanov et al. the number of AF recurrences in patients administered Botulism injections showed a decrease of AF instances (7% Botulism group, 30% Placebo group, and 23.3% Botulism group, 50% Placebo group) at 12 and 36 months, respectively [127,128]. The Botulism toxin was found to induce a pronounced alteration of heart rate variability (HRV) in patients at six months, with heart rate parameters remaining significantly reduced during follow-up [127].

5. Discussion

The ablation of GPs appears to be an efficacious technique for improving outcomes of patients with paroxysmal, persistent and long-standing persistent forms of AF. Nonetheless, some very important questions remain unanswered. The long-term outcomes of GP ablation, the precise location and depth of GPs, and the exact mechanism in which GP ablation results in improved outcomes for AF are still not fully understood. Similarly, the ablation techniques used pose a risk of damaging the myocardium and surrounding structures.

Collateral damage is a significant drawback to current thermal ablation techniques. Cardiac tamponade, PV stenosis, oesophageal fistula and thrombi are among the associated risks with current ablation energies [1]. Another drawback to thermal ablation is the difficulty in delivering precise, appropriate energy to GPs. While GPs in association with PVs are accessed with relative ease, others are found in concealed locations. Overall, there is also significant complexity involved in catheter positioning from both within the pericardial space and the heart itself. Additionally a more efficient and effective visualization of GPs using imaging techniques such as SPECT™ SUMO (Spectrum Dynamics Medical Limited, Caesarea, Israel) and I-mIBG may provide additional information for a much better localization before ablation [99]. These advances have significantly propelled research over the last decade. While the understanding of GP location is sometimes obscure, this may be due to the degree of anatomical variability between individuals [125]. However, the specifics in terms of report accuracy of the GPs that are targeted in some research papers remain ambiguous, with some studies not including nor clearly describing which GPs, or where they ablated [123,124]. This causes difficulty when comparing results from different studies targeting specific GPs associated with the maintenance of neural pathways and their subsequent effects on the SA and AV nodes [86,94]. Similarly, in some procedures with PVI + GP ablation, no clear reference is made to which GPs are ablated or whether there is an overlap of PVI lesions with targeted GP sites, making it challenging to compare success rates linked to GP ablation [120].

Augmented success rates (by 21%, 20% or 28%) with combined procedures is evident thus far only in short term follow-up (12 months or under) and with small patient numbers [61,115,118]. The added success of the PVI + GP ablation procedures in comparison to PVI alone is much lower (8%, 2.5% and 5%) in long-term follow ups (two–five years); however these studies include many more patients [107,114,129]. Due to the different techniques and study designs in clinical studies in the literature, it is difficult to assess and make a true comparison of success. HRV has been found to be a predictor of ablation success and is a useful, non-invasive tool for investigating cardiac autonomic tone [130,131]. HRV measures the fluctuations of time intervals between consecutive heartbeats [132]. An increased heart rate has been found to have positive associations with freedom from AF [130]. A recent study by Goff et al. showed a correlation between HRV in patients with paroxysmal AF who previously underwent PVI and the recurrence of AF [130]. While HRV is not always associated with PVI, an average increase of 60.6 ± 11.3 to 70.7 ± 12.0 beats per minute was recorded in 53% of patients at 12 months follow-up in this study [130]. Overall, it is evident that sufficient disruption of vagal responses results in an increased HR and freedom from AF. Coinciding with an adjusted HR is a shortening of AERP [133]. This has been found to facilitate the genesis and coexistence of numerous signals linked to AF [134]. Studies have shown the relationship between shortening of fibrillation intervals and AERP [36,135]. Additionally, the mean AERP has been reported to be shorter in persistent AF than those with paroxysmal AF due to electrical remodelling [136]. Reports by Lee et al. have also linked prolonged AERP with future development of AF with possible induction of remodelling over a twelve year follow-up [133,137]. Dispute remains over the relationship of action potential and refractory period in AF initiation, despite extensive animal and human studies [133]. Despite its importance, AERP is not a common parameter measured by clinicians. This may be owing to the technicalities associated with the recording of AERP in humans, in particular its inability to be recorded during AF [138].

In addition, it is possible that the positive post-procedural effects of GP ablation may only persist for a short amount of time. It may also be plausible that the GPs are not entirely ablated, enabling regeneration and the formation of new re-entrant pathways around the proximity of the GP, due to thermal myocardial damage caused by RF for example. Another reason for a low, long-term success rate may be the internal or external factors influencing remodeling of the heart over time. Concern exists regarding the proarrhythmic relationship between GP ablation without PVI. This approach carries the risk of inducing increased atrial parasympathetic and sympathetic innervation, coupled with a decreased atrial effective refractory period [139]. Similarly, selective GP ablation has been linked to the formation of macro-re-entrant atrial tachycardias which may be associated with autonomic reinnervation [139]. Animal studies have linked reinnervation at four weeks post-GP ablation with the selectivity of the regions targeted [140,141]. Therefore, further study must be carried out to understand what may or may not cause this relapse to AF and what changes can be made to increase the denervation time induced by GP ablation, and reduce the occurrence of pro-arrhythmia. Currently sample size is a major limitation in many studies with numbers ranging from individual case studies to research including up to 306 patients [142,143]. Evidently, variation in patient population will significantly influence success percentages, making it difficult to draw accurate comparisons.

Despite our evolving understanding of the physiology and success associated with GP ablation in AF treatment, the complications and challenges are not yet fully understood. Most patients involved in GP ablation procedures experience paroxysmal, persistent or long-standing persistent AF with some studies comparing all three [116]. Patients with symptomatic AF or AF associated with valvular disease are also included in research studies [95,144]. Similarly, investigations into specific AF types are not consistent, which leads to difficulty in assessing the extent to which GP ablation is effective. In a large randomized control during thoracoscopic surgery, there were no reported benefits of GP ablation in patients exhibiting advanced AF [114]. This may further suggest that the role of the ANS in the disease progression of AF may diminish over time [64]. Therefore, while varying degrees of AF have been examined, the true success of GP ablation for each type remains ambiguous. Nevertheless, from the expansive research and meta-analysis undergone on GP ablation, results show that it does give relief from AF in most cases, both initially and in the long term [145,146]. While much work is required to provide consistency between experiments, it is evident that the potential exists for significant advances in the treatment of AF through targeted ablation of GP sites.

Author Contributions: S.A. and S.M. for Conceptualization, investigation, resources, writing—original draft preparation, writing—review and editing. B.O. for writing—review and editing, funding acquisition. K.C. for writing—review and editing, funding acquisition. A.E., M.O. and A.S. for writing—review and editing. L.R.Q. for Conceptualization, investigation, resources, writing—review and editing, supervision. All authors have read and agreed to the published version of the manuscript.

Funding: This research was funded by Enterprise Ireland Disruptive technology (DTIF) grant number [DT20180123].

Conflicts of Interest: The authors declare no conflict of interest.

References

1. Safaei, N.; Montazerghaem, H.; Azarfarin, R.; Alizadehasl, A.; Alikhah, H. Radiofrequency ablation for treatment of atrial fibrillation. *BioImpacts* **2011**, *1*, 171–177.
2. De Bakker, J.M.T.; Ho, S.Y.; Hocini, M. Basic and clinical electrophysiology of pulmonary vein ectopy. *Cardiovasc. Res.* **2002**, *54*, 287–294. [CrossRef]
3. Wang, T.J.; Parise, H.; Levy, D.; D'Agostino, R.B.; Wolf, P.A.; Vasan, R.S.; Benjamin, E.J. Obesity and the risk of new-onset atrial fibrillation. *J. Am. Med. Assoc.* **2004**, *292*, 2471–2477. [CrossRef] [PubMed]
4. Kim, M.H. Concepts in Disease Progression of Atrial Fibrillation and Implications for Medical Management. *J. Innov. Card. Rhythm Manag.* **2012**, *3*, 697–712.
5. Morillo, C.A.; Banerjee, A.; Perel, P.; Wood, D.; Jouven, X. Atrial fibrillation: The current epidemic. *J. Geriatr. Cardiol.* **2017**, *14*, 195–203. [PubMed]
6. Fuster, V.; Rydén, L.E.; Cannom, D.S.; Crijns, H.J.; Curtis, A.B.; Ellenbogen, K.A.; Halperin, J.L.; Kay, G.N.; Le Huezey, J.Y.; Lowe, J.E.; et al. 2011 ACCF/AHA/HRS focused updates incorporated into the ACC/AHA/ESC 2006 guidelines for the management of patients with atrial fibrillation: A report of the American College of Cardiology Foundation/American Heart Association Task Force on Practice Guidel. *Circulation* **2011**, *123*, e269–e367. [CrossRef]
7. Nattel, S. New ideas about atrial fibrillation 50 years on. *Nature* **2002**, *415*, 219–226. [CrossRef]
8. Patten, M.; Pecha, S.; Aydin, A. Atrial fibrillation in hypertrophic cardiomyopathy: Diagnosis and considerations for management. *J. Atr. Fibrillation* **2018**, *10*, 1556. [CrossRef]
9. Allessie, M.A.; Boyden, P.A.; Camm, A.J.; Kléber, A.G.; Lab, M.J.; Legato, M.J.; Rosen, M.R.; Schwartz, P.J.; Spooner, P.M.; Van Wagoner, D.R.; et al. Pathophysiology and prevention of atrial fibrillation. *Circulation* **2001**, *103*, 769–777. [CrossRef]
10. Kourliouros, A.; Savelieva, I.; Kiotsekoglou, A.; Jahangiri, M.; Camm, J. Current concepts in the pathogenesis of atrial fibrillation. *Am. Heart J.* **2009**, *157*, 243–252. [CrossRef]
11. Calkins, H.; Hindricks, G.; Cappato, R.; Kim, Y.H.; Saad, E.B.; Aguinaga, L.; Akar, J.G.; Badhwar, V.; Brugada, J.; Camm, J.; et al. 2017 HRS/EHRA/ECAS/APHRS/SOLAECE expert consensus statement on catheter and surgical ablation of atrial fibrillation. *Heart Rhythm* **2017**, *14*, e275–e444. [CrossRef] [PubMed]
12. Schauerte, P.; Scherlag, B.J.; Patterson, E.; Scherlag, M.A.; Matsudaria, K.; Nakagawa, H.; Lazzara, R.; Jackman, W.M. Focal atrial fibrillation: Experimental evidence for a pathophysiologic role of the autonomic nervous system. *J. Cardiovasc. Electrophysiol.* **2001**, *12*, 592–599. [CrossRef] [PubMed]
13. Shen, M.J.; Choi, E.K.; Tan, A.Y.; Lin, S.F.; Fishbein, M.C.; Chen, L.S.; Chen, P.S. Neural mechanisms of atrial arrhythmias. *Nat. Rev. Cardiol.* **2012**, *9*, 30–39. [CrossRef]
14. Shen, M.J.; Shinohara, T.; Park, H.-W.; Frick, K.; Ice, D.S.; Choi, E.-K.; Han, S.; Maruyama, M.; Sharma, R.; Shen, C.; et al. Continuous Low-Level Vagus Nerve Stimulation Reduces Stellate Ganglion Nerve Activity and Paroxysmal Atrial Tachyarrhythmias in Ambulatory Canines. *Circulation* **2011**, *123*, 2204–2212. [CrossRef] [PubMed]
15. Leiria, T.L.L.; Glavinovic, T.; Armour, J.A.; Cardinal, R.; de Lima, G.G.; Kus, T. Longterm effects of cardiac mediastinal nerve cryoablation on neural inducibility of atrial fibrillation in canines. *Auton. Neurosci. Basic Clin.* **2011**, *161*, 68–74. [CrossRef]
16. Hu, F.; Zheng, L.; Liang, E.; Ding, L.; Wu, L.; Chen, G.; Fan, X.; Yao, Y. Right anterior ganglionated plexus: The primary target of cardioneuroablation? *Heart Rhythm* **2019**, *16*, 1545–1551. [CrossRef]
17. Choi, E.K.; Zhao, Y.; Everett, T.H.; Chen, P.S. Ganglionated plexi as neuromodulation targets for atrial fibrillation. *J. Cardiovasc. Electrophysiol.* **2017**, *28*, 1485–1491. [CrossRef]

18. Hasan, W. Autonomic cardiac innervation: Development and adult plasticity. *Organogenesis* **2013**, *9*, 176–193. [CrossRef]
19. Kapa, S.; Venkatachalam, K.L.; Asirvatham, S.J. The Autonomic Nervous System in Cardiac Electrophysiology. *Cardiol. Rev.* **2010**, *18*, 275–284. [CrossRef]
20. Gordan, R.; Gwathmey, J.K.; Xie, L.-H. Autonomic and endocrine control of cardiovascular function. *World J. Cardiol.* **2015**, *7*, 204. [CrossRef]
21. Savelieva, I.; Kakouros, N.; Kourliouros, A.; Camm, A.J. Upstream Therapies for Management of Atrial Fibrillation: Review of Clinical Evidence and Implications for European Society of Cardiology Guidelines. Part II: Secondary Prevention. *Europace* **2011**, *13*, 610–625. [CrossRef] [PubMed]
22. Zhou, J.; Scherlag, B.J.; Edwards, J.; Jackman, W.M.; Lazzara, R.; Po, S.S. Gradients of Atrial Refractoriness and Inducibility of Atrial Fibrillation due to Stimulation of Ganglionated Plexi. *J. Cardiovasc. Electrophysiol.* **2007**, *18*, 83–90. [CrossRef]
23. Po, S.S.; Scherlag, B.J.; Yamanashi, W.S.; Edwards, J.; Zhou, J.; Wu, R.; Geng, N.; Lazzara, R.; Jackman, W.M. Experimental model for paroxysmal atrial fibrillation arising at the pulmonary vein-atrial junctions. *Heart Rhythm* **2006**, *3*, 201–208. [CrossRef] [PubMed]
24. Markides, V.; Schilling, R.J. Atrial fibrillation: Classification, pathophysiology, mechanism and drug treatment. *Heart* **2003**, *89*, 939–943. [CrossRef] [PubMed]
25. Bettoni, M.; Zimmermann, M. Autonomic tone variations before the onset of paroxysmal atrial fibrillation. *Circulation* **2002**, *105*, 2753–2759. [CrossRef]
26. Patterson, E.; Po, S.S.; Scherlag, B.J.; Lazzara, R. Triggered firing in pulmonary veins initiated by in vitro autonomic nerve stimulation. *Heart Rhythm* **2005**, *2*, 624–631. [CrossRef]
27. Zaza, A.; Malfatto, G.; Schwartz, P.J. Effects on atrial repolarization of the interaction between K^+ channel blockers and muscarinic receptor stimulation. *J. Pharmacol. Exp. Ther.* **1995**, *273*, 1095–1104.
28. Krapivinsky, G.; Gordon, E.A.; Wickman, K.; Velimirović, B.; Krapivinsky, L.; Clapham, D.E. The G-protein-gated atrial K^+ channel IKAch is a heteromultimer of two inwardly rectifying K^+-channel proteins. *Nature* **1995**, *374*, 135–141. [CrossRef]
29. Krummen, D.E.; Bayer, J.D.; Ho, J.; Ho, G.; Smetak, M.R.; Clopton, P.; Trayanova, N.A.; Narayan, S.M. Mechanisms of human atrial fibrillation initiation clinical and computational studies of repolarization restitution and activation latency. *Circ. Arrhythm. Electrophysiol.* **2012**, *5*, 1149–1159. [CrossRef]
30. Roney, C.H.; Siong Ng, F.; Debney, M.T.; Eichhorn, C.; Nachiappan, A.; Chowdhury, R.A.; Qureshi, N.A.; Cantwell, C.D.; Tweedy, J.H.; Niederer, S.A.; et al. Determinants of new wavefront locations in cholinergic atrial fibrillation. *Europace* **2018**, *20*, iii3–iii15. [CrossRef]
31. Quan, K.J.; Lee, J.H.; Geha, A.S.; Biblo, L.A.; Hare, G.F.; Mackall, J.A.; Carlson, M.D. Characterization of Sinoatrial Parasympathetic Innervation in Humans. *J. Cardiovasc. Electrophysiol.* **1999**, *10*, 1060–1065. [CrossRef] [PubMed]
32. Kurotobi, T.; Shimada, Y.; Kino, N.; Ito, K.; Tonomura, D.; Yano, K.; Tanaka, C.; Yoshida, M.; Tsuchida, T.; Fukumoto, H. Features of intrinsic ganglionated plexi in both atria after extensive pulmonary isolation and their clinical significance after catheter ablation in patients with atrial fibrillation. *Heart Rhythm* **2015**, *12*, 470–476. [CrossRef] [PubMed]
33. Ogawa, M.; Zhou, S.; Tan, A.Y.; Song, J.; Gholmieh, G.; Fishbein, M.C.; Luo, H.; Siegel, R.J.; Karagueuzian, H.S.; Chen, L.S.; et al. Left Stellate Ganglion and Vagal Nerve Activity and Cardiac Arrhythmias in Ambulatory Dogs with Pacing-Induced Congestive Heart Failure. *J. Am. Coll. Cardiol.* **2007**, *50*, 335–343. [CrossRef]
34. Krul, S.P.J.; Meijborg, V.M.F.; Berger, W.R.; Linnenbank, A.C.; Driessen, A.H.G.; Van Boven, W.J.; Wilde, A.A.M.; De Bakker, J.M.; Coronel, R.; De Groot, J.R. Disparate response of high-frequency ganglionic plexus stimulation on sinus node function and atrial propagation in patients with atrial fibrillation. *Heart Rhythm* **2014**, *11*, 1743–1751. [CrossRef] [PubMed]
35. Yu, L.; Scherlag, B.J.; Sha, Y.; Li, S.; Sharma, T.; Nakagawa, H.; Jackman, W.M.; Lazzara, R.; Jiang, H.; Po, S.S. Interactions between atrial electrical remodeling and autonomic remodeling: How to break the vicious cycle. *Heart Rhythm* **2012**, *9*, 804–809. [CrossRef]
36. Wijffels, M.C.E.F.; Kirchhof, C.J.H.J.; Dorland, R.; Allessie, M.A. Atrial fibrillation begets atrial fibrillation: A study in awake chronically instrumented goats. *Circulation* **1995**, *92*, 1954–1968. [CrossRef] [PubMed]

37. Lu, Z.; Scherlag, B.J.; Lin, J.; Niu, G.; Fung, K.M.; Zhao, L.; Ghias, M.; Jackman, W.M.; Lazzara, R.; Jiang, H.; et al. Atrial fibrillation begets atrial fibrillation: Autonomic mechanism for atrial electrical remodeling induced by short-term rapid atrial pacing. *Circ. Arrhythm. Electrophysiol.* **2008**, *1*, 184–192. [CrossRef]
38. Hanna, P.; Shivkumar, K. Targeting the Cardiac Ganglionated Plexi for Atrial Fibrillation: Modulate or Destroy? *JACC Clin. Electrophysiol.* **2018**, *4*, 1359–1361. [CrossRef]
39. Armour, J.A.; Murphy, D.A.; Yuan, B.X.; Macdonald, S.; Hopkins, D.A. Gross and microscopic anatomy of the human intrinsic cardiac nervous system. *Anat. Rec.* **1997**, *247*, 289–298. [CrossRef]
40. Pauza, D.H.; Pauziene, N.; Pakeltyte, G.; Stropus, R. Comparative quantitative study of the intrinsic cardiac ganglia and neurons in the rat, guinea pig, dog and human as revealed by histochemical staining for acetylcholinesterase. *Ann. Anat.* **2002**, *184*, 125–136. [CrossRef]
41. Pauza, D.H.; Skripka, V.; Pauziene, N.; Stropus, R. Morphology, distribution, and variability of the epicardiac neural ganglionated subplexuses in the human heart. *Anat. Rec.* **2000**, *259*, 353–382. [CrossRef]
42. Mesiano Maifrino, L.B.; Liberti, E.A.; Castelucci, P.; Rodrigues de Souza, R. NADPH-diaphorase positive cardiac neurons in the atria of mice. A morphoquantitative study. *BMC Neurosci.* **2006**, *7*, 10. [CrossRef]
43. Jurgaitienė, R.; Paužienė, N.; Aželis, V.; Žurauskas, E. Morphometric study of age-related changes in the human intracardiac ganglia. *Medicina* **2004**, *40*, 574–581.
44. Po, S.S.; Nakagawa, H.; Jackman, W.M. Localization of left atrial ganglionated plexi in patients with atrial fibrillation: Techniques and technology. *J. Cardiovasc. Electrophysiol.* **2009**, *20*, 1186–1189. [CrossRef]
45. D'Avila, A.; Scanavacca, M.; Sosa, E.; Ruskin, J.N.; Reddy, V.Y. Pericardial anatomy for the interventional electrophysiologist. *J. Cardiovasc. Electrophysiol.* **2003**, *14*, 422–430. [CrossRef]
46. Abbara, S.; Desai, J.C.; Cury, R.C.; Butler, J.; Nieman, K.; Reddy, V. Mapping epicardial fat with multi-detector computed tomography to facilitate percutaneous transepicardial arrhythmia ablation. *Eur. J. Radiol.* **2006**, *57*, 417–422. [CrossRef]
47. Randall, W.C.; Ardell, J.L. Selective parasympathectomy of automatic and conductile tissues of the canine heart. *Am. J. Physiol.-Heart Circ. Physiol.* **1985**, *248*, H61–H68. [CrossRef]
48. Ardell, J.L.; Randall, W.C. Selective vagal innervation of sinoatrial and atrioventricular nodes in canine heart. *Am. J. Physiol.-Heart Circ. Physiol.* **1986**, *251*, H764–H773. [CrossRef]
49. Chiou, C.W.; Eble, J.N.; Zipes, D.P. Efferent vagal innervation of the canine atria and sinus and atrioventricular nodes: The third fat pad. *Circulation* **1997**, *95*, 2573–2584. [CrossRef]
50. Lachman, N.; Syed, F.F.; Habib, A.; Kapa, S.; Bisco, S.E.; Venkatachalam, K.L.; Asirvatham, S.J. Correlative anatomy for the electrophysiologist, part II: Cardiac ganglia, phrenic nerve, coronary venous system. *J. Cardiovasc. Electrophysiol.* **2011**, *22*, 104–110. [CrossRef]
51. Kapa, S.; DeSimone, C.V.; Asirvatham, S.J. Innervation of the heart: An invisible grid within a black box. *Trends Cardiovasc. Med.* **2016**, *26*, 245–257. [CrossRef] [PubMed]
52. Stavrakis, S.; Po, S. Ganglionated plexi ablation: Physiology and clinical applications. *Arrhythm. Electrophysiol. Rev.* **2017**, *6*, 186–190. [CrossRef] [PubMed]
53. Zipes, D.P.; Knope, R.F. Electrical properties of the thoracic veins. *Am. J. Cardiol.* **1972**, *29*, 372–376. [CrossRef]
54. Hou, Y.; Scherlag, B.J.; Lin, J.; Zhang, Y.; Lu, Z.; Truong, K.; Patterson, E.; Lazzara, R.; Jackman, W.M.; Po, S.S. Ganglionated Plexi Modulate Extrinsic Cardiac Autonomic Nerve Input. Effects on Sinus Rate, Atrioventricular Conduction, Refractoriness, and Inducibility of Atrial Fibrillation. *J. Am. Coll. Cardiol.* **2007**, *50*, 61–68. [CrossRef]
55. Lin, J.; Scherlag, B.J.; Niu, G.; Lu, Z.; Patterson, E.; Liu, S.; Lazzara, R.; Jackman, W.M.; Po, S.S. Autonomic elements within the ligament of marshall and inferior left ganglionated plexus mediate functions of the atrial neural network. *J. Cardiovasc. Electrophysiol.* **2009**, *20*, 318–324. [CrossRef]
56. Chen, P.S.; Chen, L.S.; Fishbein, M.C.; Lin, S.F.; Nattel, S. Role of the autonomic nervous system in atrial fibrillation: Pathophysiology and therapy. *Circ. Res.* **2014**, *114*, 1500–1515. [CrossRef]
57. Qin, M.; Zhang, Y.; Liu, X.; Jiang, W.F.; Wu, S.H.; Po, S. Atrial Ganglionated Plexus Modification: A Novel Approach to Treat Symptomatic Sinus Bradycardia. *JACC Clin. Electrophysiol.* **2017**, *3*, 950–959. [CrossRef]
58. Jiang, R.-H.; Hu, G.-S.; Liu, Q.; Sheng, X.; Sun, Y.-X.; Yu, L.; Zhang, P.; Zhang, Z.-W.; Chen, S.-Q.; Ye, Y.; et al. Impact of Anatomically Guided Ganglionated Plexus Ablation on Electrical Firing from Isolated Pulmonary Veins. *Pacing Clin. Electrophysiol.* **2016**, *39*, 1351–1358. [CrossRef]

59. Chevalier, P.; Tabib, A.; Meyronnet, D.; Chalabreysse, L.; Restier, L.; Ludman, V.; Aliès, A.; Adeleine, P.; Thivolet, F.; Burri, H.; et al. Quantitative study of nerves of the human left atrium. *Heart Rhythm* **2005**, *2*, 518–522. [CrossRef]
60. Kircher, S.; Sommer, P. Electrophysiological Evaluation of Pulmonary Vein Isolation. *J. Atr. Fibrillation* **2013**, *6*, 934. [CrossRef]
61. Scherlag, B.J.; Yamanashi, W.; Patel, U.; Lazzara, R.; Jackman, W.M. Autonomically induced conversion of pulmonary vein focal firing into atrial fibrillation. *J. Am. Coll. Cardiol.* **2005**, *45*, 1878–1886. [CrossRef] [PubMed]
62. Tan, A.Y.; Li, H.; Wachsmann-Hogiu, S.; Chen, L.S.; Chen, P.S.; Fishbein, M.C. Autonomic Innervation and Segmental Muscular Disconnections at the Human Pulmonary Vein-Atrial Junction. Implications for Catheter Ablation of Atrial-Pulmonary Vein Junction. *J. Am. Coll. Cardiol.* **2006**, *48*, 132–143. [CrossRef] [PubMed]
63. Chou, C.C.; Nihei, M.; Zhou, S.; Tan, A.; Kawase, A.; Macias, E.S.; Fishbein, M.C.; Lin, S.F.; Chen, P.S. Intracellular calcium dynamics and anisotropic reentry in isolated canine pulmonary veins and left atrium. *Circulation* **2005**, *111*, 2889–2897. [CrossRef] [PubMed]
64. Stavrakis, S.; Nakagawa, H.; Po, S.S.; Scherlag, B.J.; Lazzara, R.; Jackman, W.M. The role of the autonomic ganglia in atrial fibrillation. *JACC Clin. Electrophysiol.* **2015**, *1*, 1–13. [CrossRef]
65. Lemola, K.; Chartier, D.; Yeh, Y.H.; Dubuc, M.; Cartier, R.; Armour, A.; Ting, M.; Sakabe, M.; Shiroshita-Takeshita, A.; Comtois, P.; et al. Pulmonary vein region ablation in experimental vagal atrial fibrillation: Role of pulmonary veins versus autonomic ganglia. *Circulation* **2008**, *117*, 470–477. [CrossRef]
66. Lachman, N.; Syed, F.F.; Habib, A.; Kapa, S.; Bisco, S.E.; Venkatachalam, K.L.; Asirvatham, S.J. Correlative anatomy for the electrophysiologist, part I: The pericardial space, oblique sinus, transverse sinus. *J. Cardiovasc. Electrophysiol.* **2010**, *21*, 1421–1426. [CrossRef]
67. Rodríguez-Mañero, M.; Schurmann, P.; Valderrábano, M. Ligament and vein of Marshall: A therapeutic opportunity in atrial fibrillation. *Heart Rhythm* **2016**, *13*, 593–601. [CrossRef]
68. Nakagawa, H.; Scherlag, B.J.; Patterson, E.; Ikeda, A.; Lockwood, D.; Jackman, W.M. Pathophysiologic basis of autonomic ganglionated plexus ablation in patients with atrial fibrillation. *Heart Rhythm* **2009**, *6*, S26–S34. [CrossRef]
69. Liu, S.; Yu, X.; Luo, D.; Qin, Z.; Wang, X.; He, W.; Ma, R.; Hu, H.; Xie, J.; He, B.; et al. Ablation of the Ligament of Marshall and Left Stellate Ganglion Similarly Reduces Ventricular Arrhythmias during Acute Myocardial Infarction. *Circ. Arrhythm. Electrophysiol.* **2018**, *11*, e005945. [CrossRef]
70. Hu, T.Y.; Kapa, S.; Cha, Y.M.; Asirvatham, S.J.; Madhavan, M. Swallow-induced syncope: A case report of atrial tachycardia originating from the SVC. *Heart Case Rep.* **2016**, *2*, 83–87. [CrossRef]
71. Padmanabhan, D.; Naksuk, N.; Killu, A.K.; Kapa, S.; Witt, C.; Sugrue, A.; Desimon, C.V.; Madhavan, M.; de Groot, J.R.; O'Brien, B.; et al. Electroporation of epicardial autonomic ganglia: Safety and efficacy in medium-term canine models. *J. Cardiovasc. Electrophysiol.* **2019**, *30*, 607–615. [CrossRef]
72. Lo, L.W.; Scherlag, B.J.; Chang, H.Y.; Lin, Y.J.; Chen, S.A.; Po, S.S. Paradoxical long-term proarrhythmic effects after ablating the head station ganglionated plexi of the vagal innervation to the heart. *Heart Rhythm* **2013**, *10*, 751–757. [CrossRef]
73. Lu, Z.; Scherlag, B.J.; Niu, G.; Lin, J.; Fung, K.M.; Zhao, L.; Yu, L.; Jackman, W.M.; Lazzara, R.; Jiang, H.; et al. Functional properties of the superior Vena Cava (SVC)-aorta ganglionated plexus: Evidence suggesting an autonomic basis for rapid SVC firing. *J. Cardiovasc. Electrophysiol.* **2010**, *21*, 1392–1399. [CrossRef] [PubMed]
74. Pellman, J.; Sheikh, F. Atrial Fibrillation: Mechanisms, Therapeutics, and Future Directions. In *Comprehensive Physiology*; John Wiley & Sons, Inc.: Hoboken, NJ, USA, 2015; Volume 5, pp. 649–665.
75. Hohnloser, S.H.; Kuck, K.H.; Lilienthal, J. Rhythm or rate control in atrial fibrillation—Pharmacological intervention in atrial fibrillation (PIAF): A randomised trial. *Lancet* **2000**, *356*, 1789–1794. [CrossRef]
76. Heist, E.K.; Mansour, M.; Ruskin, J.N. Rate control in atrial fibrillation: Targets, methods, resynchronization considerations. *Circulation* **2011**, *124*, 2746–2755. [CrossRef] [PubMed]
77. Scherr, D.; Khairy, P.; Miyazaki, S.; Aurillac-Lavignolle, V.; Pascale, P.; Wilton, S.B.; Ramoul, K.; Komatsu, Y.; Roten, L.; Jadidi, A.; et al. Five-year outcome of catheter ablation of persistent atrial fibrillation using termination of atrial fibrillation as a procedural endpoint. *Circ. Arrhythm. Electrophysiol.* **2015**, *8*, 18–24. [CrossRef] [PubMed]

78. Khargi, K.; Hutten, B.A.; Lemke, B.; Deneke, T. Surgical treatment of atrial fibrillation; a systematic review. *Eur. J. Cardio-Thorac. Surg.* **2005**, *27*, 258–265. [CrossRef] [PubMed]
79. Cox, J.; Ad, N.; Palazzo, T.; Fitzpatrick, S.; Suyderhoud, J.P.; DeGroot, K.W.; Pirovic, E.A.; Lou, H.G.; Duvall, W.Z.; Kim, Y.D. Current status of the Maze procedure for the treatment of atrial fibrillation. *Elsevier* **2000**, *12*, 15–19. [CrossRef]
80. Kearney, K.; Stephenson, R.; Phan, K.; Chan, W.Y.; Huang, M.Y.; Yan, T.D. A systematic review of surgical ablation versus catheter ablation for atrial fibrillation. *Ann. Cardiothorac. Surg.* **2014**, *3*, 15–29. [CrossRef]
81. Marescaux, J.; Rubino, F. The ZEUS robotic system: Experimental and clinical applications. *Surg. Clin. N. Am.* **2003**, *83*, 1305–1315. [CrossRef]
82. Pappone, C.; Santinelli, V.; Manguso, F.; Vicedomini, G.; Gugliotta, F.; Augello, G.; Mazzone, P.; Tortoriello, V.; Landoni, G.; Zangrillo, A.; et al. Pulmonary Vein Denervation Enhances Long-Term Benefit after Circumferential Ablation for Paroxysmal Atrial Fibrillation. *Circulation* **2004**, *109*, 327–334. [CrossRef] [PubMed]
83. Iso, K.; Okumura, Y.; Watanabe, I.; Nagashima, K.; Takahashi, K.; Arai, M.; Watanabe, R.; Wakamatsu, Y.; Otsuka, N.; Yagyu, S.; et al. Is vagal response during left atrial ganglionated plexi stimulation a normal phenomenon? Comparison between patients with and without atrial fibrillation. *Circ. Arrhythm. Electrophysiol.* **2019**, *12*, 1–9. [CrossRef]
84. Zheng, S.; Zeng, Y.; Li, Y.; Han, J.; Zhang, H.; Meng, X. Active ganglionated plexi is a predictor of atrial fibrillation recurrence after minimally invasive surgical ablation. *J. Card. Surg.* **2014**, *29*, 279–285. [CrossRef] [PubMed]
85. Bagge, L.; Blomström, P.; Jidéus, L.; Lönnerholm, S.; Blomström-Lundqvist, C. Left atrial function after epicardial pulmonary vein isolation in patients with atrial fibrillation. *J. Interv. Card. Electrophysiol.* **2017**, *50*, 195–201. [CrossRef]
86. Kondo, Y.; Ueda, M.; Watanabe, M.; Ishimura, M.; Kajiyama, T.; Hashiguchi, N.; Kanaeda, T.; Nakano, M.; Hiranuma, Y.; Ishizaka, T.; et al. Identification of left atrial ganglionated plexi by dense epicardial mapping as ablation targets for the treatment of concomitant atrial fibrillation. *PACE—Pacing Clin. Electrophysiol.* **2013**, *36*, 1336–1341. [CrossRef]
87. Suwalski, G.; Marczewska, M.M.; Kaczejko, K.; Mróz, J.; Gryszko, L.; Cwetsch, A.; Skrobowski, A. Left atrial ganglionated plexi detection is related to heart rate and early recurrence of atrial fibrillation after surgical ablation. *Braz. J. Cardiovasc. Surg.* **2017**, *32*, 118–124. [CrossRef]
88. Al-Atassi, T.; Toeg, H.; Malas, T.; Lam, B.K. Mapping and ablation of autonomic ganglia in prevention of postoperative atrial fibrillation in coronary surgery: Maappafs atrial fibrillation randomized controlled pilot study. *Can. J. Cardiol.* **2014**, *30*, 1202–1207. [CrossRef]
89. Mehall, J.R.; Kohut, R.M.; Schneeberger, E.W.; Taketani, T.; Merrill, W.H.; Wolf, R.K. Intraoperative Epicardial Electrophysiologic Mapping and Isolation of Autonomic Ganglionic Plexi. *Ann. Thorac. Surg.* **2007**, *83*, 538–541. [CrossRef]
90. Hu, F.; Zheng, L.; Liu, S.; Shen, L.; Liang, E.; Ding, L.; Wu, L.; Chen, G.; Fan, X.; Yao, Y. Avoidance of Vagal Response during Circumferential Pulmonary Vein Isolation: Effect of Initiating Isolation From Right Anterior Ganglionated Plexi. *Circ. Arrhythm. Electrophysiol.* **2019**, *12*, e007811. [CrossRef]
91. Hou, Y.; Scherlag, B.J.; Lin, J.; Zhou, J.; Song, J.; Zhang, Y.; Patterson, E.; Lazzara, R.; Jackman, W.M.; Po, S.S. Interactive atrial neural network: Determining the connections between ganglionated plexi. *Heart Rhythm* **2007**, *4*, 56–63. [CrossRef]
92. Xhaet, O.; De Roy, L.; Floria, M.; Deceuninck, O.; Blommaert, D.; Dormal, F.; Ballant, E.; La Meir, M. Integrity of the Ganglionated Plexi Is Essential to Parasympathetic Innervation of the Atrioventricular Node by the Right Vagus Nerve. *J. Cardiovasc. Electrophysiol.* **2017**, *28*, 432–437. [CrossRef] [PubMed]
93. Sharma, P.S.; Kasirajan, V.; Ellenbogen, K.A.; Koneru, J.N. Interconnections between Left Atrial Ganglionic Plexi: Insights from Minimally Invasive Maze Procedures and Their Outcomes. *PACE—Pacing Clin. Electrophysiol.* **2016**, *39*, 427–433. [CrossRef] [PubMed]
94. Malcolme-Lawes, L.C.; Lim, P.B.; Wright, I.; Kojodjojo, P.; Koa-Wing, M.; Jamil-Copley, S.; Dehbi, H.M.; Francis, D.P.; Davies, D.W.; Peters, N.S.; et al. Characterization of the left atrial neural network and its impact on autonomic modification procedures. *Circ. Arrhythm. Electrophysiol.* **2013**, *6*, 632–640. [CrossRef]

95. Sakamoto, S.I.; Fujii, M.; Watanabe, Y.; Hiromoto, A.; Ishii, Y.; Morota, T.; Nitta, T. Exploration of theoretical ganglionated plexi ablation technique in atrial fibrillation surgery. *Ann. Thorac. Surg.* **2014**, *98*, 1598–1604. [CrossRef]
96. Lim, P.B.; Malcolme-Lawes, L.C.; Stuber, T.; Wright, I.; Francis, D.P.; Davies, D.W.; Peters, N.S.; Kanagaratnam, P. Intrinsic cardiac autonomic stimulation induces pulmonary vein ectopy and triggers atrial fibrillation in humans. *J. Cardiovasc. Electrophysiol.* **2011**, *22*, 638–646. [CrossRef] [PubMed]
97. Pokushalov, E.; Romanov, A.; Shugayev, P.; Artyomenko, S.; Shirokova, N.; Turov, A.; Katritsis, D.G. Selective ganglionated plexi ablation for paroxysmal atrial fibrillation. *Heart Rhythm* **2009**, *6*, 1257–1264. [CrossRef]
98. Katritsis, D.; Giazitzoglou, E.; Sougiannis, D.; Goumas, N.; Paxinos, G.; Camm, A.J. Anatomic Approach for Ganglionic Plexi Ablation in Patients with Paroxysmal Atrial Fibrillation. *Am. J. Cardiol.* **2008**, *102*, 330–334. [CrossRef]
99. Romanov, A.; Minin, S.; Breault, C.; Pokushalov, E. Visualization and ablation of the autonomic nervous system corresponding to ganglionated plexi guided by D-SPECT 123I-mIBG imaging in patient with paroxysmal atrial fibrillation. *Clin. Res. Cardiol.* **2017**, *106*, 76–78. [CrossRef]
100. Stirrup, J.; Gregg, S.; Baavour, R.; Roth, N.; Breault, C.; Agostini, D.; Ernst, S.; Underwood, S.R. Hybrid solid-state SPECT/CT left atrial innervation imaging for identification of left atrial ganglionated plexi: Technique and validation in patients with atrial fibrillation. *J. Nucl. Cardiol.* **2019**. [CrossRef]
101. Katritsis, D.; Giazitzoglou, E.; Sougiannis, D.; Voridis, E.; Po, S.S. Complex fractionated atrial electrograms at anatomic sites of ganglionated plexi in atrial fibrillation. *Europace* **2009**, *11*, 308–315. [CrossRef]
102. Pokushalov, E.; Romanov, A.; Artyomenko, S.; Shirokova, N.; Turov, A.; Karaskov, A.; Katritsis, D.G.; Po, S.S. Ganglionated Plexi Ablation Directed by High-Frequency Stimulation and Complex Fractionated Atrial Electrograms for Paroxysmal Atrial Fibrillation. *Pacing Clin. Electrophysiol.* **2012**, *35*, 776–784. [CrossRef] [PubMed]
103. D'Avila, A.; Gutierrez, P.; Scanavacca, M.; Reddy, V.; Lustgarten, D.L.; Sosa, E.; Ramires, J.A.F. Effects of radiofrequency pulses delivered in the vicinity of the coronary arteries: Implications for nonsurgical transthoracic epicardial catheter ablation to treat ventricular tachycardia. *PACE—Pacing Clin. Electrophysiol.* **2002**, *25*, 1488–1495. [CrossRef] [PubMed]
104. Takahashi, K.; Okumura, Y.; Watanabe, I.; Nagashima, K.; Sonoda, K.; Sasaki, N.; Kogawa, R.; Iso, K.; Kurokawa, S.; Ohkubo, K.; et al. Anatomical proximity between ganglionated plexi and epicardial adipose tissue in the left atrium: Implication for 3D reconstructed epicardial adipose tissue-based ablation. *J. Interv. Card. Electrophysiol.* **2016**, *47*, 203–212. [CrossRef] [PubMed]
105. White, C.M.; Sander, S.; Coleman, C.I.; Gallagher, R.; Takata, H.; Humphrey, C.; Henyan, N.; Gillespie, E.L.; Kluger, J. Impact of Epicardial Anterior Fat Pad Retention on Postcardiothoracic Surgery Atrial Fibrillation Incidence: The AFIST-III Study. *J. Am. Coll. Cardiol.* **2007**, *49*, 298–303. [CrossRef]
106. Cummings, J.E.; Gill, I.; Akhrass, R.; Dery, M.; Biblo, L.A.; Quan, K.J. Preservation of the anterior fat pad paradoxically decreases the incidence of postoperative atrial fibrillation in humans. *J. Am. Coll. Cardiol.* **2004**, *43*, 994–1000. [CrossRef]
107. Bárta, J.; Brát, R. Assessment of the effect of left atrial cryoablation enhanced by ganglionated plexi ablation in the treatment of atrial fibrillation in patients undergoing open heart surgery. *J. Cardiothorac. Surg.* **2017**, *12*, 69. [CrossRef]
108. Garabelli, P.; Stavrakis, S.; Kenney, J.F.A.; Po, S.S. Effect of 28-mm Cryoballoon Ablation on Major Atrial Ganglionated Plexi. *JACC Clin. Electrophysiol.* **2018**, *4*, 831–838. [CrossRef]
109. Baust, J.M.; Robilotto, A.; Snyder, K.; Van Buskirk, R.; Baust, J.G. Evaluation of a new epicardial cryoablation system for the treatment of Cardiac Tachyarrhythmias. *Trends Med.* **2018**, *18*. [CrossRef]
110. Pokushalov, E.; Romanov, A.; Artyomenko, S.; Turov, A.; Shirokova, N.; Katritsis, D.G. Left atrial ablation at the anatomic areas of ganglionated plexi for paroxysmal atrial fibrillation. *PACE—Pacing Clin. Electrophysiol.* **2010**, *33*, 1231–1238. [CrossRef]
111. Pokushalov, E.; Romanov, A.; Artyomenko, S.; Turov, A.; Shugayev, P.; Shirokova, N.; Katritsis, D.G. Ganglionated plexi ablation for longstanding persistent atrial fibrillation. *Europace* **2010**, *12*, 342–346. [CrossRef]
112. Mikhaylov, E.; Kanidieva, A.; Sviridova, N.; Abramov, M.; Gureev, S.; Szili-Torok, T.; Lebedev, D. Outcome of anatomic ganglionated plexi ablation to treat paroxysmal atrial fibrillation: A 3-year follow-up study. *Europace* **2011**, *13*, 362–370. [CrossRef]

113. Pantos, I.; Katritsis, G.; Zografos, T.; Camm, A.J.; Katritsis, D.G. Temporal stability of atrial electrogram fractionation in patients with paroxysmal atrial fibrillation. *Am. J. Cardiol.* **2013**, *111*, 863–868. [CrossRef]
114. Driessen, A.H.G.; Berger, W.R.; Krul, S.P.J.; van den Berg, N.W.E.; Neefs, J.; Piersma, F.R.; Yin, D.R.C.P.; de Jong, J.S.S.G.; van Boven, W.J.P.; de Groot, J.R. Ganglion Plexus Ablation in Advanced Atrial Fibrillation: The AFACT Study. *J. Am. Coll. Cardiol.* **2016**, *68*, 1155–1165. [CrossRef]
115. Katritsis, D.G.; Giazitzoglou, E.; Zografos, T.; Pokushalov, E.; Po, S.S.; Camm, A.J. Rapid pulmonary vein isolation combined with autonomic ganglia modification: A randomized study. *Heart Rhythm* **2011**, *8*, 672–678. [CrossRef]
116. Edgerton, J.R.; McClelland, J.H.; Duke, D.; Gerdisch, M.W.; Steinberg, B.M.; Bronleewe, S.H.; Prince, S.L.; Herbert, M.A.; Hoffman, S.; Mack, M.J. Minimally invasive surgical ablation of atrial fibrillation: Six-month results. *J. Thorac. Cardiovasc. Surg.* **2009**, *138*, 109–114. [CrossRef]
117. Scherlag, B.J.; Nakagawa, H.; Jackman, W.M.; Yamanashi, W.S.; Patterson, E.; Po, S.; Lazzara, R. Electrical stimulation to identify neural elements on the heart: Their role in atrial fibrillation. *J. Interv. Card. Electrophysiol.* **2005**, *13*, 37–42. [CrossRef]
118. Onorati, F.; Curcio, A.; Santarpino, G.; Torella, D.; Mastroroberto, P.; Tucci, L.; Indolfi, C.; Renzulli, A. Routine ganglionic plexi ablation during Maze procedure improves hospital and early follow-up results of mitral surgery. *J. Thorac. Cardiovasc. Surg.* **2008**, *136*, 408–418. [CrossRef]
119. Budera, P.; Osmancik, P.; Talavera, D.; Kraupnerova, A.; Fojt, R.; Zdarska, J.; Vanek, T.; Straka, Z. Two-staged hybrid ablation of non-paroxysmal atrial fibrillation: Clinical outcomes and functional improvements after 1 year. *Interact. Cardiovasc. Thorac. Surg.* **2018**, *26*, 77–83. [CrossRef]
120. Kurfirst, V.; Mokráček, A.; Bulava, A.; Čanádyová, J.; Haniš, J.; Pešl, L. Two-staged hybrid treatment of persistent atrial fibrillation: Short-term single-centre results. *Interact. Cardiovasc. Thorac. Surg.* **2014**, *18*, 451–456. [CrossRef]
121. Matsutani, N.; Takase, B.; Ozeki, Y.; Maehara, T.; Lee, R. Minimally Invasive Cardiothoracic Surgery for Atrial Fibrillation. *Circ. J.* **2008**, *72*, 434–436. [CrossRef]
122. Edgerton, J.R.; Jackman, W.M.; Mack, M.J. A New Epicardial Lesion Set for Minimal Access Left Atrial Maze: The Dallas Lesion Set. *Ann. Thorac. Surg.* **2009**, *88*, 1655–1657. [CrossRef]
123. Wang, J.G.; Xin, M.; Han, J.; Li, Y.; Luo, T.G.; Wang, J.; Meng, F.; Meng, X. Ablation in selective patients with long-standing persistent atrial fibrillation: Medium-term results of the Dallas lesion set. *Eur. J. Cardio-Thorac. Surg.* **2014**, *46*, 213–220. [CrossRef] [PubMed]
124. Lockwood, D.; Nakagawa, H.; Peyton, M.D.; Edgerton, J.R.; Scherlag, B.J.; Sivaram, C.A.; Po, S.S.; Beckman, K.J.; Abedin, M.; Jackman, W.M. Linear left atrial lesions in minimally invasive surgical ablation of persistent atrial fibrillation: Techniques for assessing conduction block across surgical lesions. *Heart Rhythm* **2009**, *6*, S50–S63. [CrossRef] [PubMed]
125. Zdarska, J.; Osmancik, P.; Budera, P.; Herman, D.; Prochazkova, R.; Talavera, D.; Straka, Z. The absence of effect of ganglionated plexi ablation on heart rate variability parameters in patients after thoracoscopic ablation for atrial fibrillation. *J. Thorac. Dis.* **2017**, *9*, 4997–5007. [CrossRef]
126. Han, F.T.; Kasirajan, V.; Kowalski, M.; Kiser, R.; Wolfe, L.; Kalahasty, G.; Shepard, R.K.; Wood, M.A.; Ellenbogen, K.A. Results of a minimally invasive surgical pulmonary vein isolation and ganglionic plexi ablation for atrial fibrillation: Single-center experience with 12-month follow-up. *Circ. Arrhythm. Electrophysiol.* **2009**, *2*, 370–377. [CrossRef]
127. Pokushalov, E.; Kozlov, B.; Romanov, A.; Strelnikov, A.; Bayramova, S.; Sergeevichev, D.; Bogachev-Prokophiev, A.; Zheleznev, S.; Shipulin, V.; Lomivorotov, V.V.; et al. Long-Term Suppression of Atrial Fibrillation by Botulinum Toxin Injection into Epicardial Fat Pads in Patients Undergoing Cardiac Surgery: One-Year Follow-Up of a Randomized Pilot Study. *Circ. Arrhythm. Electrophysiol.* **2015**, *8*, 1334–1341. [CrossRef]
128. Romanov, A.; Pokushalov, E.; Ponomarev, D.; Bayramova, S.; Shabanov, V.; Losik, D.; Stenin, I.; Elesin, D.; Mikheenko, I.; Strelnikov, A.; et al. Long-term suppression of atrial fibrillation by botulinum toxin injection into epicardial fat pads in patients undergoing cardiac surgery: Three-year follow-up of a randomized study. *Heart Rhythm* **2019**, *16*, 172–177. [CrossRef]
129. Katritsis, D.G.; Pokushalov, E.; Romanov, A.; Giazitzoglou, E.; Siontis, G.C.M.; Po, S.S.; Camm, A.J.; Ioannidis, J.P.A. Autonomic denervation added to pulmonary vein isolation for paroxysmal atrial fibrillation: A randomized clinical trial. *J. Am. Coll. Cardiol.* **2013**, *62*, 2318–2325. [CrossRef]

130. Goff, Z.D.; Laczay, B.; Yenokyan, G.; Sivasambu, B.; Sinha, S.K.; Marine, J.E.; Ashikaga, H.; Berger, R.D.; Akhtar, T.; Spragg, D.D.; et al. Heart rate increase after pulmonary vein isolation predicts freedom from atrial fibrillation at 1 year. *J. Cardiovasc. Electrophysiol.* **2019**, *30*, 2818–2822. [CrossRef]
131. Vesela, J.; Osmancik, P.; Herman, D.; Prochazkova, R. Changes in heart rate variability in patients with atrial fibrillation after pulmonary vein isolation and ganglionated plexus ablation. *Physiol. Res.* **2019**, *68*, 49–57. [CrossRef]
132. Shaffer, F.; Ginsberg, J.P. An Overview of Heart Rate Variability Metrics and Norms. *Front. Public Health* **2017**, *5*. [CrossRef]
133. Lee, J.M.; Lee, H.; Janardhan, A.H.; Park, J.; Joung, B.; Pak, H.N.; Lee, M.H.; Kim, S.S.; Hwang, H.J. Prolonged atrial refractoriness predicts the onset of atrial fibrillation: A 12-year follow-up study. *Heart Rhythm* **2016**, *13*, 1575–1580. [CrossRef]
134. Tamargo, J.; Delpón, E. Vagal Stimulation and Atrial Electrical Remodeling. *Rev. Española Cardiol.* **2009**, *62*, 729–732. [CrossRef]
135. Daoud, E.G.; Bogun, F.; Goyal, R.; Harvey, M.; Man, K.C.; Strickberger, S.A.; Morady, F. Effect of Atrial Fibrillation on Atrial Refractoriness in Humans. *Circulation* **1996**, *94*, 1600–1606. [CrossRef]
136. Uhm, J.-S.; Mun, H.-S.; Wi, J.; Shim, J.; Joung, B.; Lee, M.-H.; Pak, H.-N. Prolonged Atrial Effective Refractory Periods in Atrial Fibrillation Patients Associated with Structural Heart Disease or Sinus Node Dysfunction Compared with Lone Atrial Fibrillation. *Pacing Clin. Electrophysiol.* **2013**, *36*, 163–171. [CrossRef]
137. Li, D.; Fareh, S.; Leung, T.K.; Nattel, S. Promotion of Atrial Fibrillation by Heart Failure in Dogs. *Circulation* **1999**, *100*, 87–95. [CrossRef]
138. Sahadevan, J.; Ryu, K.; Matsuo, K.; Khrestian, C.M.; Waldo, A.L. Characterization of Atrial Activation (A-A) Intervals during Atrial Fibrillation Due to a Single Driver: Do They Reflect Atrial Effective Refractory Periods? *J. Cardiovasc. Electrophysiol.* **2011**, *22*, 310–315. [CrossRef]
139. Mao, J.; Yin, X.; Zhang, Y.; Yan, Q.; Dong, J.; Ma, C.; Liu, X. Ablation of epicardial ganglionated plexi increases atrial vulnerability to arrhythmias in dogs. *Circ. Arrhythm. Electrophysiol.* **2014**, *7*, 711–717. [CrossRef]
140. Sakamoto, S.I.; Schuessler, R.B.; Lee, A.M.; Aziz, A.; Lall, S.C.; Damiano, R.J. Vagal denervation and reinnervation after ablation of ganglionated plexi. *J. Thorac. Cardiovasc. Surg.* **2010**, *139*, 444–452. [CrossRef]
141. Oh, S.; Zhang, Y.; Bibevski, S.; Marrouche, N.F.; Natale, A.; Mazgalev, T.N. Vagal denervation and atrial fibrillation inducibility: Epicardial fat pad ablation does not have long-term effects. *Heart Rhythm* **2006**, *3*, 701–708. [CrossRef]
142. Puskas, J.; Lin, E.; Bailey, D.; Guyton, R. Thoracoscopic Radiofrequency Pulmonary Vein Isolation and Atrial Appendage Occlusion. *Ann. Thorac. Surg.* **2007**, *83*, 1870–1872. [CrossRef] [PubMed]
143. Gelsomino, S.; Lozekoot, P.; La Meir, M.; Lorusso, R.; Lucà, F.; Rostagno, C.; Renzulli, A.; Parise, O.; Matteucci, F.; Gensini, G.F.; et al. Is ganglionated plexi ablation during Maze IV procedure beneficial for postoperative long-term stable sinus rhythm? *Int. J. Cardiol.* **2015**, *192*, 40–48. [CrossRef] [PubMed]
144. Mamchur, S.E.; Mamchur, I.N.; Khomenko, E.A.; Gorbunova, E.V.; Sizova, I.N.; Odarenko, Y.N. Catheter ablation for atrial fibrillation after an unsuccessful surgical ablation and biological prosthetic mitral valve replacement: A pilot study. *J. Chin. Med. Assoc.* **2014**, *77*, 409–415. [CrossRef] [PubMed]
145. Kampaktsis, P.N.; Oikonomou, E.K.; Choi, D.Y.; Cheung, J.W. Efficacy of ganglionated plexi ablation in addition to pulmonary vein isolation for paroxysmal versus persistent atrial fibrillation: A meta-analysis of randomized controlled clinical trials. *J. Interv. Card. Electrophysiol.* **2017**, *50*, 253–260. [CrossRef]
146. Zhang, Y.; Wang, Z.; Zhang, Y.; Wang, W.; Wang, J.; Gao, M.; Hou, Y. Efficacy of Cardiac Autonomic Denervation for Atrial Fibrillation: A Meta-Analysis. *J. Cardiovasc. Electrophysiol.* **2012**, *23*, 592–600. [CrossRef] [PubMed]

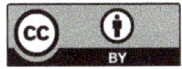

© 2020 by the authors. Licensee MDPI, Basel, Switzerland. This article is an open access article distributed under the terms and conditions of the Creative Commons Attribution (CC BY) license (http://creativecommons.org/licenses/by/4.0/).

Article

Pre-Stroke Statin Therapy Improves In-Hospital Prognosis Following Acute Ischemic Stroke Associated with Well-Controlled Nonvalvular Atrial Fibrillation

Paweł Wańkowicz [1,*], Jacek Staszewski [2], Aleksander Dębiec [2], Marta Nowakowska-Kotas [3], Aleksandra Szylińska [1], Agnieszka Turoń-Skrzypińska [1] and Iwona Rotter [1]

1. Department of Medical Rehabilitation and Clinical Physiotherapy, Pomeranian Medical University in Szczecin, Żołnierska 48, 71-210 Szczecin, Poland; aleksandra.szylinska@gmail.com (A.S.); agi.skrzypinska@gmail.com (A.T.-S.); iwrot@wp.pl (I.R.)
2. Department of Neurology, Military Medical Institute, Szaserów 128, 04-141 Warszawa, Poland; jacekstaszewski@wp.pl (J.S.); adebiec@wim.mil.pl (A.D.)
3. Department of Neurology, Medical University of Wrocław, Borowska 213, 50-566 Wrocław, Poland; marnow64@interia.pl
* Correspondence: pawel.wankowicz@pum.edu.pl; Tel.: +48-9148-00914

Abstract: Many studies have confirmed the positive effect of statins in the secondary prevention of ischemic stroke. Although several studies have concluded that statins may also be beneficial in patients with atrial fibrillation-related stroke, the results of those studies are inconclusive. Therefore, the aim of this study was to analyze the effect of pre-stroke statin therapy on atrial fibrillation-related stroke among patients with a well-controlled atrial fibrillation. This retrospective multicenter analysis comprised 2309 patients with acute stroke, with a total of 533 patients meeting the inclusion criteria. The results showed a significantly lower neurological deficit on the National Institutes of Health Stroke Scale at hospital admission and discharge in the group of atrial fibrillation-related stroke patients who took statins before hospitalization compared with those who did not ($p < 0.001$). In addition, in-hospital mortality was significantly higher in the atrial fibrillation-related stroke patients not taking statins before hospitalization than in those who did ($p < 0.001$). Based on the results of our previous research and this current study, we postulate that the addition of a statin to the oral anticoagulants may be helpful in the primary prevention of atrial fibrillation-related stroke.

Keywords: ischemic stroke; atrial fibrillation; NOAC; VKA; statin; outcome; mortality

1. Introduction

Atrial fibrillation (AF) is the main cardiac rhythm disorder. An inadequate treatment or late detection may result in serious health complications such as ischemic stroke (IS). Currently, the prevalence of AF in the general population is age-dependent and varies from 4% to 15% [1–3]. As a result of systematic developments in medicine and the consequent increase in the lifespan of the general population, these percentages are expected to increase dramatically in the next decade [4,5].

Old-generation oral anticoagulants (vitamin K antagonists, VKAs) or non-vitamin K antagonist oral anticoagulant (NOACs) are the most popular therapeutic options used to prevent embolic events in patients with AF. The use of VKAs reduces the risk of IS by 65% and reduces subsequent mortality by 25% compared with a placebo group [6–8]. The main reason behind failures in this therapy are reductions in the international normalized ratio (INR), which can affect its efficacy and increase the risk of bleeding complications. These difficulties were the reason for initiating research on NOACs. These drugs have at least the same efficacy in the prevention of IS as VKAs, but at a reduced risk of life-threatening hemorrhages compared with VKAs, relaxing the requirement for continuous monitoring of blood levels [9–15].

Non-modifiable AF risk factors include gender, age, ethnicity, and genetic factors, while modifiable risk factors include heart failure, coronary artery disease, hypertension, atherosclerosis, or diabetes [16–20]. Significantly, all these AF risk factors are also recognized risk factors for IS [21]. Despite this, the latest ESC guidelines for the diagnosis and management of AF, developed in collaboration with the European Association for Cardio-Thoracic Surgery (EACTS), still mainly focus on the embolic mechanism and the implementation of an oral anticoagulant in the presence of an appropriate constellation of modifiable and non-modifiable risk factors based on the CHADS2, CHA2DS2-VASc, or ABC pathway, but with marginal attention paid to prothrombotic, atherogenic, and proinflammatory risk factors [22]. In the literature, only a few studies have addressed the co-occurrence of embolic and prothrombotic risk factors in IS patients with coexisting AF.

In an earlier study, we examined the configuration of ischemic stroke risk factors in patients with nonvalvular atrial fibrillation (NVAF) and therapeutic INR levels. Based on a univariable and multivariable logistic regression model, we found that there were more smokers (OR = 20.337; OR = 147.589), patients with a previous ischemic stroke (OR = 6.556; OR = 11.094), patients with hypertension (OR = 3.75; OR = 2.75), and patients with dyslipidemia (OR = 2.318; OR = 2.294) with these factors [23]. In a following multicenter study, we examined the configuration of IS risk factors in patients with NVAF that had been treated with NOACs, finding that AF patients treated with the NOACs displayed higher thrombotic, proatherogenic, and proinflammatory risk factors, in addition to the embolic risk closely associated with AF [24]. Based on the aforementioned observations, statins appear to be ideal candidates to complement the anticoagulant effects of VKAs and NOACs, with a broad-spectrum of positive clinical effects on thrombotic, proatherogenic, and proinflammatory factors. Numerous studies in diverse patient populations have shown that statins (HMG-CoA reductase inhibitors) exhibit effects beyond just lowering lipid levels—they improve endothelial dysfunction, increase nitric oxide bioavailability, have antioxidant properties, inhibit the inflammatory response, and stabilize atherosclerotic plaque. Moreover, an increasing number of studies also mention the positive role of statins in the recruitment of endothelial progenitor cells, immunosuppressive activity, or inhibition of myocardial hypertrophy [25–27]. A large meta-analysis has confirmed the positive effect of statins in the secondary prevention of IS [28]. Although several studies have concluded that statins may also be beneficial in patients with AF-related stroke, the results of those studies are inconclusive [29–32]. Therefore, the aim of this study was to analyze the effect of pre-stroke statin therapy on AF-related stroke among patients with a well-controlled AF.

2. Materials and Methods

This retrospective multicenter analysis comprised 2309 patients hospitalized at three Neurology Clinics in Poland (Department of Neurology at the Pomeranian Medical University in Szczecin, Department of Neurology at the Military Medical Institute in Warsaw, and Department of Neurology at the Medical University in Wroclaw) with acute ischemic stroke between 2014 and 2020.

Inclusion criteria for the study were as follows: (1) aged 18 years or older, (2) NVAF treated with VKA and a therapeutic INR (2.0–3.0) on admission, (3) NVAF treated with a NOACs, and (4) information regarding the use of statins before the acute IS. Exclusion criteria were as follows: (1) no data regarding the use, or not, of statins before acute IS; (2) no or irregular intake of NOACs; and (3) non-therapeutic levels of INR (<2.0).

In total, 533 patients with acute IS, with NVAF treated with NOACs and VKAs, and a therapeutic level of INR were eligible for this study after meeting the inclusion criteria. These patients were divided into two groups based on receiving information on using statins, or not, before their IS. Group one comprised 191 patients who were not using statins, with group two comprising 342 patients who were using statins (Figure 1).

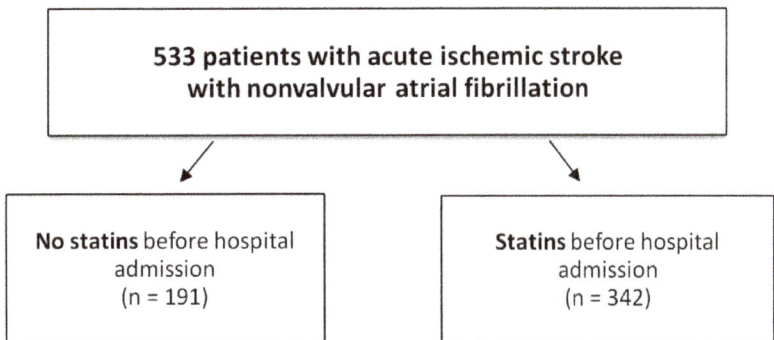

Figure 1. Study flowchart.

All patients with IS had undergone neurological examination, ECG, neuroimaging, and vascular and biochemical testing according to the guidelines of the American Heart Association and American Stroke Association.

The neurological status of the patients was assessed on the day of admission and on the day of discharge, according to the National Institutes of Health Stroke Scale (NIHSS) used to assess the severity of neurological deficit in a patient with ischemic stroke. The NIHSS was designed around the traditional neurological examination to assesses consciousness, eye movements, visual fields, motor and sensory impairments, ataxia, speech, cognition, and inattention. A score of 0 usually indicates normal functioning, with a higher score indicating the degree of deficit. The individual scores for each item are added together to calculate a total personal NIHSS score. The maximum possible score is 42 and the minimum score is 0. Importantly, a score of 0 does not indicate a valid neurological examination because it does not account for subtle neurological deficits [33].

Basic demographic data such as age, gender, information on common risk factors for IS such as hypertension, dyslipidemia, diabetes, coronary artery disease, peripheral artery disease, hemodynamically significant stenosis of the internal carotid artery, and smoking, as well as information on mortality during hospitalization, were collected on the basis of the medical interview and analysis of medical records. The Bioethics Committee of the Pomeranian Medical University issued a consent to conduct the study (KB-0012/49/07/2020/Z).

Diagnosis of atrial fibrillation was based on either ECG or medical records at admission [34]. The diagnosis of hypertension was based on an analysis of medical records, patient history, and hypotensive medication intake. Hypertension was defined as a systolic blood pressure of 140 mmHg or higher and/or a diastolic blood pressure of 90 mmHg or higher in repeated measurements [35]. The diagnosis of diabetes mellitus was based on an analysis of medical records, patient history, and p/diabetic medication intake. Diabetes was defined as a fasting blood glucose level of 126 mg/dL or higher, or a blood glucose level of 200 mg/dl or higher measured throughout the day [36]. The diagnosis of dyslipidemia was based on an analysis of medical records, patient history, and hypolipemic medication intake. Dyslipidemia was defined as a serum cholesterol concentration of >190 mg/dL, low-density lipoprotein cholesterol > 115 mg/dL, serum triglyceride concentration > 150 mg/dL, and high-density lipoprotein cholesterol < 40 mg/dL in males and <45 mg/dL in females. The diagnosis of coronary artery disease was based on an analysis of medical records, patient history, and cardiovascular medication intake. The diagnosis of significant internal carotid artery stenosis was based on vascular examination (Doppler ultrasound/angio-tomography or angio-resonance imaging) [37,38]. The diagnosis of peripheral artery disease was based on an analysis of medical records, patient history, and intake of cardiovascular medications. The definition of cigarette smoking was determined by current smoking of any number of cigarettes, an analysis of medical records, or from medical interviews with the patient.

Statistical Analysis

Statistica v13.0 software (StatSoft, Inc., Tulsa, OK, USA) was used to perform the statistical analysis.

The null hypothesis stated that there were no significant improvement in patients with AF-related stroke who had taken statins in the prehospital period. The alternative hypothesis stated that the use of statins in the prehospital period in patients with AF-related stroke does positively affect in-hospital outcomes and mortality. The distribution of the data was tested using a Shapiro–Wilk test. Quantitative data were analyzed using a Mann–Whitney U test. Qualitative data were analyzed based on the X^2 test. If the subgroup size was insufficient, a Yates's correction was used. The relationship between the analyzed parameters was evaluated using univariable and multivariable logistic regression model analysis. The multivariable logistic regression was corrected for potentially distorting data (age, dyslipidemia, diagnosed hypertension, and smoking). Differences were statistically significant at $p \leq 0.05$.

3. Results

The median age of all patients was 79.0 years (77.9 ± 8.8 years). One hundred and seventy-four patients (32.65%) were male and 359 patients (67.35%) were female. Hypertension was present in 504 patients (94.56%), diabetes mellitus in 239 (44.84%), dyslipidemia in 393 (73.73%), internal carotid artery significant stenosis/occlusion in 64 (12%), coronary heart disease in 338 (63.41%), and peripheral arterial disease in 77 (14.44%), and 242 patients (45.40%) were smokers.

3.1. Comparison of Variables in Patients with AF-Related Stroke Who Were Taking Statins before Hospitalization versus Those Not Taking Statins before Hospitalization

Compared with the patients with AF-related stroke who did not take statins before hospitalization, the patients with AF-related stroke who took statins before hospitalization were significantly younger (83 vs. 77 years; $p < 0.001$) and were also much more likely to have hypertension (99.42% vs. 85.86%; $p < 0.001$) and dyslipidemia (100% vs. 26.98%; $p < 0.001$), and to smoke cigarettes (51.75% vs. 34.03%; $p < 0.001$). We also observed a significantly lower neurological deficit on the NIHSS scale at admission and at hospital discharge in the group of AF-related stroke patients who took statins before hospitalization compared with those who did not. We also found that in-hospital neurological improvement was significantly more common in patients with AF-related stroke who took statins before hospitalization (Figure 2). In-hospital mortality was significantly higher in the AF-related stroke patients not taking statins before hospitalization than in those AF-related stroke patients taking statins before hospitalization (50.26% vs. 2.92%; $p < 0.001$). A comparison of both groups is shown in Table 1.

3.2. Prognosis in Patients with Acute AF-Related Stroke Who Were Taking Statins before Hospitalization

After adjusting the results for age, hypertension, dyslipidemia, and smoking, we confirmed that the prehospital use of statins in patients with AF-related stroke was related to a reduced risk of death and a milder stroke course. The results are presented in Table 2.

Table 1. Comparison of patients taking and not taking statins.

Variables.		No Statins before Hospital Admission n = 191	Statins before Hospital Admission n = 342	p
Age [years], mean ± SD; median		81.86 ± 8.67; 83.0	75.76 ± 8.18; 77.0	<0.001
Gender	male	55 (28.80%)	119 (34.80%)	0.157
	female	136 (71.20%)	223 (65.20%)	
Hypertension	no	27 (14.14%)	2 (0.58%)	<0.001
	yes	164 (85.86%)	340 (99.42%)	
Coronary heart disease	no	70 (36.65%)	125 (36.55%)	0.982
	yes	121 (63.35%)	217 (63.45%)	
Peripheral arterial disease	no	165 (86.39%)	291 (85.09%)	0.682
	yes	26 (13.61%)	51 (14.91%)	
Diabetes mellitus	no	106 (55.50%)	188 (54.97%)	0.907
	yes	85 (44.50%)	154 (45.03%)	
Smoking	no	126 (65.97%)	165 (48.25%)	<0.001
	yes	65 (34.03%)	177 (51.75%)	
Dyslipidemia	no	138 (73.02%)	0 (0.00%)	<0.001
	yes	51 (26.98%)	342 (100.00%)	
Stenosis/occlusion	no	167 (87.43%)	302 (88.30%)	0.767
	yes	24 (12.57%)	40 (11.70%)	
NIHSS at hospital admission, mean ± SD; median		19.27 ± 6.71; 20.0	7.36 ± 5.29; 6.0	<0.001
NIHSS at discharge, mean ± SD; median		21.81 ± 12.01; 23.0	3.51 ± 5.29; 2.0	<0.001
Delta NIHSS, mean ± SD; median		3.25 ± 8.52; 4.0	−3.73 ± 3.77; −3.0	<0.001
Death	no	95 (49.74%)	332 (97.08%)	<0.001
	yes	96 (50.26%)	10 (2.92%)	

Abbreviations: p—level of statistical significance, n—number of patients, Me—median, SD—standard deviation, NIHSS—National Institutes of Health Stroke Scale.

Table 2. Multivariate regression model for patients taking statins.

Variables	No Adjusted				Adjusted *			
	p	OR	CI OR− 95%	CI + OR 95%	p	OR	CI OR− 95%	CI + OR 95%
Death	<0.001	0.030	0.015	0.059	<0.001	0.022	0.008	0.060
NIHSS on admission to hospital	<0.001	0.766	0.734	0.799	<0.001	0.790	0.742	0.843
NIHSS at discharge	<0.001	0.818	0.791	0.846	<0.001	0.840	0.804	0.877
Delta NIHSS	<0.001	0.824	0.791	0.858	<0.001	0.775	0.718	0.836

Abbreviations: p—level of statistical significance, OR—odds ratio, CI—confidence interval, NIHSS—National Institutes of Health Stroke Scale. Notes: * adjusted by age, hypertension, dyslipidemia, smoking.

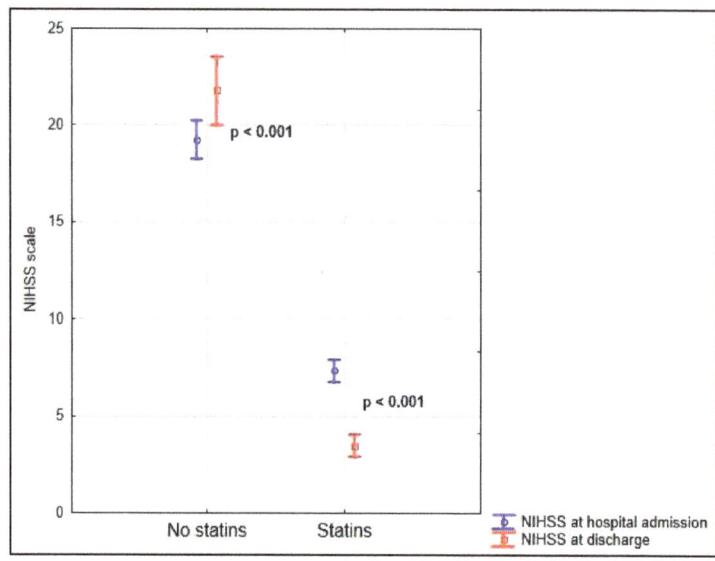

Figure 2. Change in NIHSS scores before hospital admission and at hospital discharge.

4. Discussion

In a previous study, we showed that (a) both non-modifiable and modifiable AF risk factors are also recognized risk factors for IS; and (b) AF patients treated with VKAs and who had therapeutic INR levels, as well as AF patients treated with NOACs, have a higher prevalence of thrombotic, proatherogenic, and pro-inflammatory risk factors. In another study conducted by Yang et al., it was observed that the presence of cardioembolic risk factors was independently associated with left atrial volume index, persistent atrial fibrillation, heart failure, and body mass index. In contrast, the presence of non-cardioembolic risk factors was independently associated with coronary artery calcium score, hypertension, diabetes, and age [39]. This indicates that statins may be the ideal candidates to complement the anticoagulation effects of VKAs and NOACs, with their broad-spectrum positive clinical effect on thrombotic, proatherogenic, and proinflammatory risk factors. However, cardiologists do not recommend the routine use of statins in all patients with atrial fibrillation as a primary prophylaxis for ischemic stroke, rather relying solely on the prescription of older or new-generation oral anticoagulants. Neurologists recommend statins only for the prevention of atherosclerotic strokes [22,40].

The available literature includes studies reporting the beneficial effects of statins on the prognosis of patients with AF-related stroke, as well as studies showing no such association. In a meta-analysis by Biffi et al., the use of statins prior to a stroke is shown to be correlated with better outcomes for small vessel strokes than any other stroke subtype [41]. Another meta-analysis by Eun et al. shows that the use of statins before AF-related stroke is associated with a lower risk of poor short-term functional outcomes [42].

The results of the current study indicate that, among the entire studied group of patients with well-controlled AF, those who were medicating with statins before the onset of IS had a higher prevalence of thrombotic, proatherogenic, and proinflammatory risk factors than those patients not taking statins. In other words, the patients treated with statins were at a higher risk of adverse vascular complications compared with the patients who did not receive such treatment before the onset of IS. Despite the higher prevalence of thrombotic, proatherogenic, and proinflammatory risk factors, those patients treated with statins achieved better NIHSS scores (both at admission and discharge) compared with those patients not taking statins before their stroke. This indicates the pleiotropic effect of statins that goes beyond a mere reduction of lipid levels [43].

Statin therapy in the pre-stroke period increases cerebral collateral circulation, which is crucial in the acute phase of AF-related stroke when a large artery is suddenly blocked by an embolus and the effective collateral circulation is needed rapidly. In this way, statins may reduce the risk of large cortical infarcts and severe neurological deficits usually associated with an AF-related stroke [44]. This is all the more significant as the recanalization in this type of stroke is lower compared with an atherosclerotic stroke [45]. The neovascularization potential of rosuvastatin and atorvastatin has been confirmed in animal models [46].

Previous research investigating the association of pre-stroke statin medication in patients with AF-related stroke has shown better survival in these patients [29,30]. These findings are consistent with the results of our study, in which we demonstrated that, in the entire group of patients with well-controlled AF, those who were not treated with statins before IS had a significantly higher in-hospital mortality compared with those patients medicating with statins in the pre-stroke period (50.26% vs. 2.92%; $p < 0.001$).

The mechanisms by which statins reduce mortality in AF-related stroke are related to their pleiotropic effects on the cardiovascular and endocardial circulatory systems [47,48]. Statins have also been found to improve left ventricular function, reduce levels of interleukin-6 and C-reactive protein, increase nitric oxide bioavailability, increase antioxidant properties, and inhibit inflammatory response and plaque stabilization. Potential mechanisms that may mediate the beneficial effects of statins on the circulatory system include modulation of endothelial function, anti-inflammatory effects, antioxidant properties, stabilize atherosclerotic plaque, and angiogenesis [49]. The cardioprotective potential of statins has been confirmed in a wide range of studies on cardiovascular pathology, in which statins have been shown to inhibit myocardial remodeling, prevent AF and life-threatening ventricular arrhythmias, preserve nitric oxide production in heart failure, reduce small G-protein activity in myocardial hypertrophy, and contribute to myocardial repair after ischemia by mobilizing endothelial progenitor cells and protecting the myocardium from damage [50–52].

Our study has several limitations. First, it is a retrospective study. Second, reference to specific types of statins was not possible because of the limited number of cases. Third, the absence of stroke type (embolic or atherosclerotic) data. Fourth, the absence of echo data, such as LA size, LV function, and spontaneous echo contrast (SEC). Fifth, the absence of data on AF temporal type (paroxysmal/persistent). Despite these limitations, our study seems to be the first multicenter study focusing on the effect of pre-stroke medication with statins in a selected group of patients with AF-related stroke who were also taking NOACs or maintaining therapeutic levels of INR.

5. Conclusions

Statin therapy before IS is associated with a reduced risk of mortality and improved functional outcome in the acute phase of AF-related stroke. Based on the results of our previous research and this current study, we postulate that the addition of a statin to the oral anticoagulants may be helpful in the primary prevention of AF-related stroke, although further well-designed randomized controlled trials are necessary to confirm this association.

Author Contributions: Conceptualization, P.W.; Formal analysis, P.W., J.S., A.D., M.N.-K., A.S., A.T.-S. and I.R.; Investigation, P.W., J.S., A.D., M.N.-K., A.S., A.T.-S. and I.R.; Methodology, P.W.; Supervision, I.R.; Writing—original draft, P.W., J.S., A.D., M.N.-K., A.S., A.T.-S. and I.R.; Writing—review and editing, P.W., J.S., A.D., M.N.-K., A.S., A.T.-S. and I.R. All authors have read and agreed to the published version of the manuscript.

Funding: This research received no external funding.

Institutional Review Board Statement: The study was conducted according to the guidelines of the Declaration of Helsinki, and approved by the Bioethics Committee of the Pomeranian Medical University in Szczecin (KB-0012/49/07/2020/Z).

Informed Consent Statement: Informed consent was obtained from all subjects involved in the study.

Data Availability Statement: All data that support the findings of this study are available upon request from the corresponding author.

Conflicts of Interest: The authors have declared that no competing interests exist.

References

1. Wolowacz, S.E.; Samuel, M.; Brennan, V.K.; Jasso-Mosqueda, J.-G.; Van Gelder, I.C. The cost of illness of atrial fibrillation: A systematic review of the recent literature. *Europace* **2011**, *13*, 1375–1385. [CrossRef]
2. Friberg, L.; Bergfeldt, L. Atrial fibrillation prevalence revisited. *J. Intern. Med.* **2013**, *274*, 461–468. [CrossRef]
3. Zoni-Berisso, M.; Lercari, F.; Carazza, T.; Domenicucci, S. Epidemiology of atrial fibrillation: European perspective. *Clin. Epidemiol.* **2014**, *6*, 213–220. [CrossRef]
4. Go, A.S.; Hylek, E.M.; Phillips, K.A.; Chang, Y.; Henault, L.E.; Selby, J.V.; Singer, D.E. Prevalence of diagnosed atrial fibrillation in adults: National implications for rhythm management and stroke prevention: The AnTicoagulation and Risk Factors in Atrial Fibrillation (ATRIA) Study. *JAMA* **2001**, *285*, 2370–2375. [CrossRef] [PubMed]
5. Krijthe, B.P.; Kunst, A.; Benjamin, E.; Lip, G.Y.; Franco, O.H.; Hofman, A.; Witteman, J.C.; Stricker, B.H.; Heeringa, J. Projections on the number of individuals with atrial fibrillation in the European Union, from 2000 to 2060. *Eur. Heart J.* **2013**, *34*, 2746–2751. [CrossRef]
6. EAFT (European Atrial Fibrillation Trial) Study Group. Secondary prevention in non-rheumatic atrial fibrillation after transient ischaemic attack or minor stroke. *Lancet* **1993**, *342*, 1255–1262. [CrossRef]
7. Laupacis, A. Risk factors for stroke and efficacy of antithrombotic therapy in atrial fibrillation. Analysis of pooled data from five randomized controlled trials. *Arch. Intern. Med.* **1994**, *154*, 1449–1457.
8. Undas, A.; Pasierski, T.; Windyga, J.; Crowther, M. Practical aspects of new oral anticoagulant use in atrial fibrillation. *Pol. Arch. Intern. Med.* **2014**, *124*, 124–135. [CrossRef] [PubMed]
9. Connolly, S.J.; Ezekowitz, M.D.; Yusuf, S.; Eikelboom, J.; Oldgren, J.; Parekh, A.; Pogue, J.; Reilly, P.A.; Themeles, E.; Varrone, J.; et al. Dabigatran versus Warfarin in Patients with Atrial Fibrillation. *N. Engl. J. Med.* **2009**, *361*, 1139–1151. [CrossRef] [PubMed]
10. Patel, M.R.; Mahaffey, K.W.; Garg, J.; Pan, G.; Singer, D.E.; Hacke, W.; Breithardt, G.; Halperin, J.L.; Hankey, G.J.; Piccini, J.P.; et al. Rivaroxaban versus warfarin in nonvalvular atrial fibrillation. *N. Engl. J. Med.* **2011**, *365*, 883–891. [CrossRef]
11. Granger, C.B.; Alexander, J.H.; McMurray, J.J.V.; Lopes, R.D.; Hylek, E.M.; Hanna, M.; Al-Khalidi, H.R.; Ansell, J.; Atar, D.; Avezum, A.; et al. Apixaban versus Warfarin in Patients with Atrial Fibrillation. *N. Engl. J. Med.* **2011**, *365*, 981–992. [CrossRef]
12. Giugliano, R.; Ruff, C.T.; Braunwald, E.; Murphy, A.; Wiviott, S.D.; Halperin, J.L.; Waldo, A.L.; Ezekowitz, M.D.; Weitz, J.I.; Špinar, J.; et al. Edoxaban versus Warfarin in Patients with Atrial Fibrillation. *N. Engl. J. Med.* **2013**, *369*, 2093–2104. [CrossRef]
13. Heidbuchel, H.; Verhamme, P.; Alings, M.; Antz, M.; Hacke, W.; Oldgren, J.; Sinnaeve, P.; Camm, A.J.; Kirchhof, P. European Heart Rhythm Association Practical Guide on the use of new oral anticoagulants in patients with non-valvular atrial fibrillation. *Europace* **2013**, *15*, 625–651. [CrossRef] [PubMed]
14. Ciurus, T.; Sobczak, S.; Cichocka-Radwan, A.; Lelonek, M. New oral anticoagulants—A practical guide. *Pol. J. Cardio-Thoracic Surg.* **2015**, *12*, 111–118. [CrossRef]
15. Raval, A.N.; Cigarroa, J.E.; Chung, M.K.; Diaz-Sandoval, L.J.; Diercks, D.; Piccini, J.P.; Jung, H.S.; Washam, J.B.; Welch, B.G.; Zazulia, A.R.; et al. Management of Patients on Non–Vitamin K Antagonist Oral Anticoagulants in the Acute Care and Periprocedural Setting: A Scientific Statement From the American Heart Association. *Circulation* **2017**, *135*, e604–e633. [CrossRef] [PubMed]
16. Benjamin, E.J.; Levy, D.; Vaziri, S.M.; D'Agostino, R.B.; Belanger, A.J.; Wolf, P.A. Independent risk factors for atrial fibrillation in a population-based cohort. The Framingham Heart Study. *JAMA* **1994**, *271*, 840–844. [CrossRef] [PubMed]
17. Psaty, B.M.; Manolio, T.A.; Kuller, L.H.; Kronmal, R.A.; Cushman, M.; Fried, L.P.; White, R.; Furberg, C.D.; Rautaharju, P.M. Incidence of and risk factors for atrial fibrillation in older adults. *Circulation* **1997**, *96*, 2455–2461. [CrossRef]
18. Conen, D.; Tedrow, U.B.; Koplan, B.A.; Glynn, R.J.; Buring, J.E.; Albert, C.M. Response to Letter Regarding Article, "Influence of Systolic and Diastolic Blood Pressure on the Risk of Incident Atrial Fibrillation in Women". *Circulation* **2010**, *121*, 2146–2152. [CrossRef]
19. Huxley, R.R.; Lopez, F.L.; Folsom, A.R.; Agarwal, S.K.; Loehr, L.R.; Soliman, E.Z.; Maclehose, R.; Konety, S.; Alonso, A. Absolute and attributable risks of atrial fibrillation in relation to optimal and borderline risk factors: The Atherosclerosis Risk in Communities (ARIC) study. *Circulation* **2011**, *123*, 1501–1508. [CrossRef]
20. Nalliah, C.J.; Sanders, P.; Kottkamp, H.; Kalman, J.M. The role of obesity in atrial fibrillation. *Eur. Heart J.* **2016**, *37*, 1565–1572. [CrossRef]
21. Wańkowicz, P.; Nowacki, P.; Gołąb-Janowska, M. Atrial fibrillation risk factors in patients with ischemic stroke. *Arch. Med. Sci.* **2021**, *17*, 19–24. [CrossRef]
22. Hindricks, G.; Potpara, T.; Dagres, N.; Arbelo, E.; Bax, J.J.; Blomström-Lundqvist, C.; Boriani, G.; Castella, M.; Dan, G.A.; Dilaveris, P.E.; et al. 2020 ESC Guidelines for the diagnosis and management of atrial fibrillation developed in collabora-tion with the European Association of Cardio-Thoracic Surgery (EACTS): The Task Force for the diagnosis and management of atrial fibrillation of the European Society of Cardiology (ESC) Developed with the special contribution of the European Heart Rhythm Association (EHRA) of the ESC. *Eur. Heart J.* **2021**, *42*, 373–489. [CrossRef]

23. Wańkowicz, P.; Nowacki, P.; Gołąb-Janowska, M. Risk factors for ischemic stroke in patients with non-valvular atrial fibrillation and therapeutic international normalized ratio range. *Arch. Med. Sci.* **2019**, *15*, 1217–1222. [CrossRef]
24. Wańkowicz, P.; Staszewski, J.; Dębiec, A.; Nowakowska-Kotas, M.; Szylińska, A.; Rotter, I. Ischemic Stroke Risk Factors in Patients with Atrial Fibrillation Treated with New Oral Anticoagulants. *J. Clin. Med.* **2021**, *10*, 1223. [CrossRef] [PubMed]
25. Liao, J.K.; Laufs, U. Pleiotropic Effects of Statins. *Annu. Rev. Pharmacol. Toxicol.* **2005**, *45*, 89–118. [CrossRef] [PubMed]
26. Kavalipati, N.; Shah, J.; Ramakrishan, A.; Vasnawala, H. Pleiotropic effects of statins. *Indian J. Endocrinol. Metab.* **2015**, *19*, 554–562. [PubMed]
27. Oesterle, A.; Laufs, U.; Liao, J.K. Pleiotropic Effects of Statins on the Cardiovascular System. *Circ. Res.* **2017**, *120*, 229–243. [CrossRef]
28. Tramacere, I.; Boncoraglio, G.B.; Banzi, R.; Del Giovane, C.; Kwag, K.H.; Squizzato, A.; Moja, L. Comparison of statins for secondary prevention in patients with ischemic stroke or transient ischemic attack: A systematic review and network meta-analysis. *BMC Med.* **2019**, *17*, 67. [CrossRef]
29. Ntaios, G.; Papavasileiou, V.; Makaritsis, K.; Milionis, H.; Manios, E.; Michel, P.; Lip, G.; Vemmos, K. Statin treatment is associated with improved prognosis in patients with AF-related stroke. *Int. J. Cardiol.* **2014**, *177*, 129–133. [CrossRef]
30. Choi, K.; Seo, W.; Park, M.; Kim, J.; Chung, J.; Bang, O.Y.; Kim, G.; Song, T.; Kim, B.J.; Heo, S.H.; et al. Effect of Statin Therapy on Outcomes of Patients With Acute Ischemic Stroke and Atrial Fibrillation. *J. Am. Heart Assoc.* **2019**, *8*, e013941. [CrossRef]
31. Ingrid, L.; Von Euler, M.; Sunnerhagen, K.S. Association of prestroke medicine use and health outcomes after ischaemic stroke in Sweden: A registry-based cohort study. *BMJ Open* **2020**, *10*, e036159. [CrossRef] [PubMed]
32. Ishikawa, H.; Wakisaka, Y.; Matsuo, R.; Makihara, N.; Hata, J.; Kuroda, J.; Ago, T.; Kitayama, J.; Nakane, H.; Kamouchi, M.; et al. Influence of Statin Pretreatment on Initial Neurological Severity and Short-Term Functional Outcome in Acute Ischemic Stroke Patients: The Fukuoka Stroke Registry. *Cerebrovasc. Dis.* **2016**, *42*, 395–403. [CrossRef]
33. Lyden, P. Using the National Institutes of Health Stroke Scale: A Cautionary Tale. *Stroke* **2017**, *48*, 513–519. [CrossRef] [PubMed]
34. Steinberg, J.S.; O'Connell, H.; Li, S.; Ziegler, P.D. Thirty-Second Gold Standard Definition of Atrial Fibrillation and Its Relationship with Subsequent Arrhythmia Patterns: Analysis of a Large Prospective Device Database. *Circ. Arrhythm. Electrophysiol.* **2018**, *11*, e006274. [CrossRef]
35. Mancia, G.; Laurent, S.; Agabiti-Rosei, E.; Ambrosioni, E.; Burnier, M.; Caulfield, M.J.; Cifkova, R.; Clement, D.; Coca, A.; Dominiczak, A.; et al. 2007 Guidelines for the Management of Arterial Hypertension: The Task Force for the Management of Arterial Hypertension of the European Society of Hypertension (ESH) and of the European Society of Cardiology (ESC). *J. Hypertens.* **2007**, *25*, 1105–1187. [CrossRef]
36. Tahrani, A.A.; Bailey, C.J.; Del Prato, S.; Barnett, A.H. Management of type 2 diabetes: New and future developments in treatment. *Lancet* **2011**, *378*, 182–197. [CrossRef]
37. Inzitari, D.; Eliasziw, M.; Gates, P.; Sharpe, B.L.; Chan, R.K.; Meldrum, H.E.; Barnett, H.J. The Causes and Risk of Stroke in Patients with Asymptomatic Internal-Carotid-Artery Stenosis. *N. Engl. J. Med.* **2000**, *342*, 1693–1701. [CrossRef]
38. Halliday, A.; Harrison, M.; Hayter, E. Ten-Year Stroke Prevention after Successful Carotid Endarterectomy for Asymptomatic Stenosis (ACST-1): A Multicentre Randomised Trial. *J. Vasc. Surg.* **2011**, *53*, 246. [CrossRef]
39. Yang, P.-S.; Pak, H.-N.; Park, D.-H.; Yoo, J.; Kim, T.-H.; Uhm, J.-S.; Kim, Y.D.; Nam, H.S.; Joung, B.; Lee, M.-H.; et al. Non-cardioembolic risk factors in atrial fibrillation-associated ischemic stroke. *PLoS ONE* **2018**, *13*, e0201062. [CrossRef] [PubMed]
40. Powers, W.J.; Rabinstein, A.A.; Ackerson, T.; Adeoye, O.M.; Bambakidis, N.C.; Becker, K.; Biller, J.; Brown, M.; Demaerschalk, B.M.; Hoh, B.; et al. Guidelines for the Early Management of Patients With Acute Ischemic Stroke: 2019 Update to the 2018 Guidelines for the Early Management of Acute Ischemic Stroke: A Guideline for Healthcare Professionals From the American Heart Association/American Stroke Association. *Stroke* **2019**, *50*, e344–e418.
41. Biffi, A.; Devan, W.J.; Anderson, C.D.; Cortellini, L.; Furie, K.L.; Rosand, J.; Rost, N.S. Statin treatment and functional outcome after ischemic stroke: Case-control and meta-analysis. *Stroke* **2011**, *42*, 1314–1319. [CrossRef]
42. Eun, M.Y.; Jung, J.M.; Choi, K.H.; Seo, W.K. Statin Effects in Atrial Fibrillation-Related Stroke: A Systematic Review and Meta-Analysis. *Front. Neurol.* **2020**, *11*, 589684. [CrossRef]
43. Endres, M. Statins and Stroke. *Br. J. Pharmacol.* **2005**, *25*, 1093–1110. [CrossRef]
44. Tu, H.T.; Campbell, B.; Christensen, S.; Collins, M.; De Silva, D.A.; Butcher, K.S.; Parsons, M.W.; Desmond, P.M.; Barber, P.A.; Levi, C.R.; et al. Pathophysiological Determinants of Worse Stroke Outcome in Atrial Fibrillation. *Cerebrovasc. Dis.* **2010**, *30*, 389–395. [CrossRef] [PubMed]
45. Kimura, K.; Iguchi, Y.; Yamashita, S.; Shibazaki, K.; Kobayashi, K.; Inoue, T. Atrial fibrillation as an independent predictor for no early recanalization after IV-t-PA in acute ischemic stroke. *J. Neurol. Sci.* **2008**, *267*, 57–61. [CrossRef]
46. Pecoraro, V.; Moja, L.; Dall'Olmo, L.; Cappellini, G.; Garattini, S. Most appropriate animal models to study the efficacy of statins: A systematic review. *Eur. J. Clin. Investig.* **2014**, *44*, 848–871. [CrossRef] [PubMed]
47. Horwich, T.B.; Middlekauff, H.R. Potential Autonomic Nervous System Effects of Statins in Heart Failure. *Heart Fail. Clin.* **2008**, *4*, 163–170. [CrossRef] [PubMed]
48. Tacoy, G.; Akboga, M.K.; Yayla, C.; Akyel, A.; Turkoglu, S.; Ozdemir, M.; Yalcin, R. The effect of statin treatment on P-wave characteristics and atrial conduction time. *Kardiol. Polska* **2015**, *73*, 747-452. [CrossRef]

49. Loppnow, H.; Zhang, L.; Buerke, M.; Lautenschlager, M.; Chen, L.; Frister, A.; Schlitt, A.; Luther, T.; Song, N.; Hofmann, B.; et al. Statins potently reduce the cytokine-mediated IL-6 release in SMC/MNC cocultures. *J. Cell. Mol. Med.* **2011**, *15*, 994–1004. [CrossRef] [PubMed]
50. Dimmeler, S.; Aicher, A.; Vasa, M.; Mildner-Rihm, C.; Adler, K.; Tiemann, M.; Rutten, H.; Fichtlscherer, S.; Martin, H.; Zeiher, A.M. HMG-CoA reductase inhibitors (statins) increase endothelial progenitor cells via the PI 3-kinase/Akt pathway. *J. Clin. Investig.* **2001**, *108*, 391–397. [CrossRef]
51. Suzuki, G.; Iyer, V.; Cimato, T.; Canty, J.J.M. Pravastatin Improves Function in Hibernating Myocardium by Mobilizing CD133 + and cKit + Bone Marrow Progenitor Cells and Promoting Myocytes to Reenter the Growth Phase of the Cardiac Cell Cycle. *Circ. Res.* **2009**, *104*, 255–264. [CrossRef] [PubMed]
52. Porter, K.E.; Turner, N.A. Statins and myocardial remodelling: Cell and molecular pathways. *Expert Rev. Mol. Med.* **2011**, *13*, e22. [CrossRef] [PubMed]

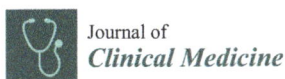

Article

What Is the Ideal Blood Pressure Threshold for the Prevention of Atrial Fibrillation in Elderly General Population?

Yoon Jung Park [1,†], Pil-Sung Yang [2,†], Hee Tae Yu [1], Tae-Hoon Kim [1], Eunsun Jang [1], Jae-Sun Uhm [1], Hui-Nam Pak [1], Moon-Hyoung Lee [1], Gregory Y.H. Lip [1,3,*] and Boyoung Joung [1,*]

1. Division of Cardiology, Department of Internal Medicine, Severance Cardiovascular Hospital, Yonsei University College of Medicine, Seoul 03722, Korea; PYJ221@yuhs.ac (Y.J.P.); HEETYU@yuhs.ac (H.T.Y.); THKIMCARDIO@yuhs.ac (T.-H.K.); SUNNY_JES@yuhs.ac (E.J.); JASON@yuhs.ac (J.-S.U.); HNPAK@yuhs.ac (H.-N.P.); MHLEE@yuhs.ac (M.-H.L.)
2. Department of Cardiology, CHA Bundang Medical Centre, CHA University, Seongnam 13496, Korea; psyang01@cha.ac.kr
3. Liverpool Centre for Cardiovascular Science, University of Liverpool and Liverpool Heart & Chest Hospital, Liverpool L14 3PE, UK
* Correspondence: Gregory.Lip@liverpool.ac.uk (G.Y.H.L.); cby6908@yuhs.ac (B.J.); Tel.: +82-2-2228-846 (B.J.)
† The first two authors contributed equally to this work.

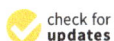

Received: 25 August 2020; Accepted: 11 September 2020; Published: 16 September 2020

Abstract: Intensive blood pressure (BP) lowering in patients with hypertension at increased risk of cardiovascular disease has been associated with a lowered risk of incident atrial fibrillation (AF). It is uncertain whether maintaining the optimal BP levels can prevent AF in the general elderly population. We included 115,866 participants without AF in the Korea National Health Insurance Service-Senior (≥60 years) cohort from 2002 to 2013. We compared the influence of BP on the occurrence of new-onset AF between octogenarians (≥80 years) and non-octogenarians (<80 years) subjects. With up to 6.7 ± 1.7 years of follow-up, 4393 incident AF cases occurred. After multivariable adjustment for potentially confounding clinical covariates, the risk of AF in non-octogenarians was significantly higher in subjects with BP levels of <120/<80 and ≥140/90 mm Hg, with hazard ratios of 1.15 (95% confidence interval (CI), 1.03–1.28; $p < 0.001$) and 1.14 (95% CI, 1.04–1.26; $p < 0.001$), compared to the optimal BP levels (120–129/<80 mm Hg). In octogenarians, the optimal BP range was 130–139/80–89 mm Hg, higher than in non-octogenarians. A U-shaped relationship for the development of incident AF was evident in non-octogenarians, and BP levels of 120–129/<80 mm Hg were associated the lowest risk of incident AF. Compared to non-octogenarians, the lowest risk of AF was associated with higher BP levels of 130–139/80–89 mm Hg amongst octogenarians.

Keywords: atrial fibrillation; hypertension; elderly; prevention

1. Introduction

Hypertension is the most common comorbidity in patients with atrial fibrillation (AF) and is highly prevalent in patients with AF, especially those aged over 60 years [1]. Elevated blood pressure (BP) is associated with a greater burden of AF [2] and every 20 mm Hg increase in systolic blood pressure (SBP) has a 21% higher risk of AF [3]. The high incidence of hypertension with AF has prompted the argument that AF is another sign of hypertensive target organ damage [4–6].

Several epidemiological studies have shown that the levels of SBP 130–139 mm Hg are also associated with increased risk of AF, compared to normal SBP (<120 mm Hg) [7–10]. Several randomized controlled trials also showed the relationship between BP and risk of AF. In the Cardio-Sis trial (Controllo della Pressione Arteriosa Sistolica trial), the risk of new-onset AF was reduced in the tight control group (SBP < 130 mm Hg) compared to the usual control group (SBP < 140 mm Hg) in patients with hypertension without diabetes [11]. Other report have shown that the intensive therapy group (target SBP < 120 mm Hg) did not show statistical significance with respect to the incidence of AF in patients with hypertension and diabetes [12]. A recent study, using data from Systolic Blood Pressure Intervention Trial (SPRINT) found that intensive treatment with a target SBP of <120 mm Hg in patients with hypertension at high risk of cardiovascular disease reduced the risk of AF [13]. However, the relationship of BP and incident AF has not been established in older subjects.

However, strict BP control can induce serious adverse events such as hypotension, syncope, electrolyte imbalance, and acute kidney injury [14]. The Elderly population is more likely have other risk factors and target organ damage that may be worsened by lowering BP than the younger population [15]. Exacerbation of postural hypotension could be associated with injurious falls, and a low BP targets could be related to an increased risk of reduced renal function amongst octogenarians (age > 80 years) [16]. Of note, the 2018 European Society of Cardiology (ESC) and the European Society of Hypertension (ESH) guidelines recommend less strict BP control for the elderly (age ≥ 65 years) and close monitoring of adverse effects. Additionally, a previous study suggests that intensive BP control had no more benefit than harm in patients with a 10 year-cardiovascular risk of <18.2% [17].

It remains uncertain whether intensive BP lowering to a target SBP of <120 mm Hg results in further lowering of the risk of new-onset AF in octogenarians with hypertension. In this study using the nationwide population-based National Health Insurance Service (NHIS)-senior cohort (NHIS-Senior), we aimed to investigate the optimal BP levels for the prevention of incident AF, defining the ideal BP threshold for the prevention of AF in the general elderly population. Second, we evaluated whether these associations were observed in different age groups and were influenced by strict BP control.

2. Experimental Section

Data were collected from the NHIS-Senior, which included about 558,147 individuals, accounting for approximately 10% of the total elderly population over 60 years old in South Korea (approximately 5.1 million) in 2002 [18]. The NHIS-Senior database included the following parameters: sociodemographic and socioeconomic information, insurance status, health checkup examinations, and records of patients' medical and dental history. These parameters have been stratified to cover 12 years (2002–2013) and anonymized in the cohort study to protect the privacy of individuals. This study was approved by the Institutional Review Board of Yonsei University Health System (4-2016-0179). Informed consent was waived. The NHIS-Senior database used in this study (NHIS-2016-2-171) was made by the NHIS of Korea. The authors declare no conflict of interest with the NHIS.

2.1. BP Measurement

BP measurements were obtained at local hospitals and clinics certified for medical health examination centers by the Korean National Health Insurance Corporation. After the patient rested for 5 min in the sitting position, brachial BP was measured by qualified medical personnel at each health examination center. A blood pressure (BP) measurement was repeated if the first measurement was >120/80 mm Hg. Automatic oscillometric devices and mercury sphygmomanometers were used for BP measurements, with the choice of device being at the discretion of individual examination centers. The preferred recommendation stipulated the use of mercury sphygmomanometers until 2015, when the sale of mercury sphygmomanometers was banned. The average of the BP measured at the first and second medical examinations was used for analysis.

2.2. Study Population

From the Korean NHIS-Senior, a total of 312,736 patients who had a health checkup between 2005 and 2012 were enrolled, and follow-up data were reviewed until December 2013. The exclusion criteria were as follows: (i) patients who had AF before enrollment ($n = 8873$); (ii) those who had heart failure (HF) before enrollment ($n = 26{,}210$); (iii) those who had ischemic stroke or transient ischemic attack before enrollment ($n = 32{,}344$); (iv) those who had myocardial infarction (MI) before enrollment ($n = 3944$); (v) those who had hemorrhagic stroke before enrollment ($n = 1149$); (vi) those who had malignancy before enrollment ($n = 25{,}436$); (vii) those who had missing data ($n = 120$); and (viii) those who check BP once ($n = 98{,}794$). Finally, we included 115,866 patients with repeated BP measurement (Figure 1).

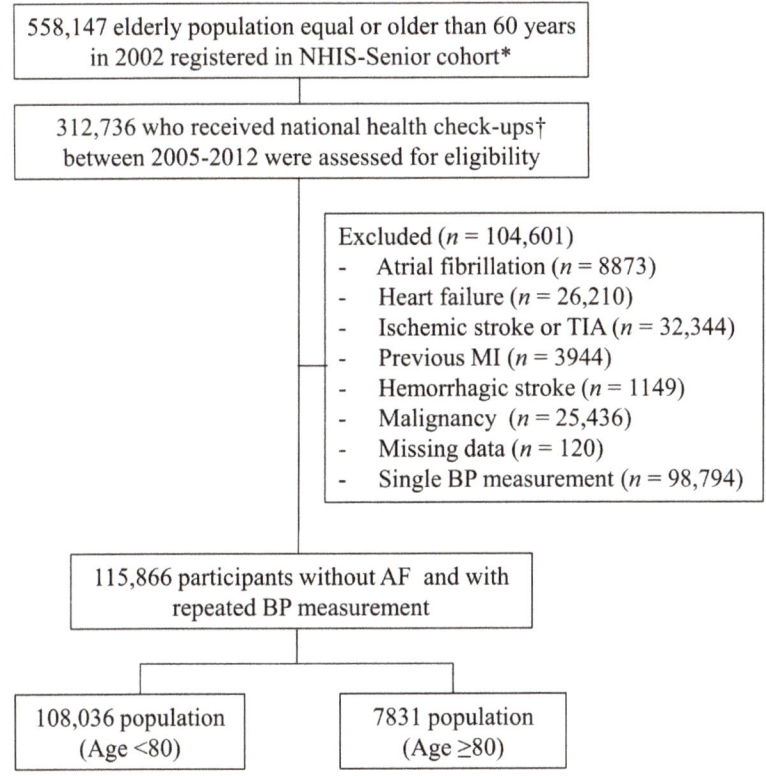

Figure 1. Flowchart of the study population enrollment and analyses. NHIS, National Health Insurance Service; TIA, transient ischemic attack; MI, myocardial infarction; BP, blood pressure; AF, atrial fibrillation. * Korean National Health Insurance Service (NHIS)-Senior cohort. † Complete checkup includes smoking, physical activity, alcohol, BMI, Total cholesterol, blood pressure, fasting glucose.

2.3. Covariates

We obtained information on selected comorbidities in inpatient and outpatient hospital diagnoses. Baseline comorbidities were defined using the medical claims and information about prescription medication prior to the index date. To ensure the accuracy of diagnosis, the patients were considered to have comorbid condition when the condition was a discharge diagnosis or confirmed at least twice in an outpatient setting according to previous studies using the NHIS (Supplementary Materials Table S1) [19,20]. For the status of standard income, the total amount of national health insurance premiums paid by the insured in the year was evaluated in proportion to personal income.

2.4. Hypertension and Atrial Fibrillation

Hypertension was defined as the combination of previous hypertension diagnosis (International Classification of Disease-10th Revision (ICD-10) codes) and use of one or more antihypertensive drugs. The hypertension onset date for duration calculations was determined using information on the first date of hypertension diagnosis. The BP status was divided into four groups: (i) SBP of <120 mm Hg and diastolic blood pressure (DBP) of <80 mm Hg; (ii) SBP of 120–129 mm Hg and DBP of <80 mm Hg; (iii) SBP of 130–139 mm Hg or DBP of 80–90 mm Hg; and (iv) SBP of ≥140 mm Hg or DBP of ≥90 mm Hg. The study also compared the SBP status and incidence of AF. Furthermore, the relationship between the DBP status and incidence of AF was analyzed.

AF was diagnosed using the ICD-10, code I48. To ensure diagnostic accuracy, the patients were defined as having AF only when it was a discharge diagnosis or had been confirmed at least twice in the outpatient department. This AF diagnosis definition has been previously validated in the NHIS database with a positive predictive value of 94.1% [19,21].

2.5. Statistical Analysis

The baseline characteristics of participants with age over and under 80 years were compared using Student's *t*-test and Pearson's chi-square test. The incidence rates of events were calculated by dividing the number of events by person-times at risk, with the 95% confidence intervals (CI) estimated by exact Poisson distributions. Cox proportional hazards regressions were used to compare the incidence of AF with BP status. Two-sided *p*-values <0.05 were considered statistically significant. Statistical analyses were conducted using Statistical Package for Social Sciences (SPSS) version 23.0 (Chicago, IL, USA) and R version 3.3.2 (The R Foundation, www.R-project.org).

3. Results

3.1. Baseline Characteristics

Compared with non-octogenarians, the octogenarians were predominantly female and had more comorbidities, including hypertension, chronic kidney disease (CKD), anemia, chronic obstructive pulmonary disease, and osteoporosis (Table 1). The low rates of CKD and diabetes for ages in this study might be related with the rigid exclusion criteria of this study. The comparisons of baseline characteristics among patients with different BP levels in non-octogenarians and octogenarians are presented in Supplementary Materials Table S2.

Table 1. Comparison of clinical characteristics between the non-octogenarian and the octogenarian populations.

	All Population (N = 115,866)	Age < 80 (n = 108,035)	Age ≥ 80 (n = 7831)	p-Value
Age, years	71.7 (69.5–74.6)	71.2 (69.3–74.0)	82.2 (81.0–84.5)	<0.001
Male	53,609 (46.3)	50,391 (46.6)	3218 (41.1)	<0.001
Systolic BP	130.5 (122.5–140.0)	130.0 (122.5–140.0)	132.5 (124.5–142.5)	<0.001
Diastolic BP *	79.5 (74.0–85.0)	79.5 (74.0–85.0)	79.5 (73.5–85.0)	0.017
Economic state *	7.0 (4.0–9.0)	7.0 (4.0–9.0)	7.0 (3.0–9.0)	0.001
Alcohol				<0.001
No drinking	64,681 (80.9)	60,075 (80.6)	4606 (85.8)	
Moderate drinking	5982 (7.5)	5673 (7.6)	309 (5.8)	
Heavy drinking †	9243 (11.6)	8789 (11.8)	454 (8.5)	

Table 1. *Cont.*

	All Population (N = 115,866)	Age < 80 (n = 108,035)	Age ≥ 80 (n = 7831)	p-Value
Smoking				<0.001
Non-smoker or quit ≥12 months	63,389 (79.3)	58,993 (79.1)	4396 (81.9)	
Quit <12 months	5732 (7.2)	5351 (7.2)	381 (7.1)	
Current smoker	10,785 (13.5)	10,193 (13.7)	592 (11.0)	
Comorbidities				
Hypertension	46,519 (40.1)	42,883 (39.7)	3636 (46.4)	<0.001
Diabetes	14,767 (12.7)	13,881 (12.8)	886 (11.3)	<0.001
Dyslipidemia	34,200 (29.5)	32,369 (30.0)	1831 (23.4)	<0.001
Chronic kidney disease	997 (0.9)	913 (0.8)	84 (1.1)	0.041
Anemia	17,715 (15.3)	15,715 (14.6)	2000 (25.6)	<0.001
Hyperthyroidism	2462 (2.1)	2341 (2.2)	121 (1.5)	<0.001
Hypothyroidism	2725 (2.4)	2583 (2.4)	142 (1.8)	0.001
COPD	6960 (6.0)	6262 (5.8)	698 (8.9)	<0.001
Liver disease	23,559 (20.3)	22,335 (20.7)	1224 (15.6)	<0.001
HCMP	156 (0.1)	149 (0.1)	7 (0.1)	0.331
Osteoporosis	33,139 (28.6)	30,569 (28.3)	2570 (32.8)	<0.001
Medications				
Aspirin	19,315 (16.7)	17,957 (16.6)	1358 (17.3)	0.102
P2Y12 inhibitor	872 (0.8)	816 (0.8)	56 (0.7)	0.742
ACE-inhibitor/ARB	18,425 (15.9)	17,110 (15.8)	1315 (16.8)	0.027
Beta blocker	18,115 (15.6)	16,815 (15.6)	1300 (16.6)	0.015
Calcium channel blocker	30,370 (26.2)	27,945 (25.9)	2425 (31.0)	<0.001
Statin	11,918 (10.3)	11,333 (10.5)	585 (7.5)	<0.001
Diuretics	23,665 (20.4)	21,728 (20.1)	1937 (24.7)	<0.001
MRA	1677 (1.4)	1533 (1.4)	144 (1.8)	0.003

BP, blood pressure; COPD, chronic obstructive pulmonary disease; HCMP, hypertrophic cardiomyopathy; ACE, angiotensin converting enzyme; ARB, angiotensin II receptor blocker; MRA, mineralocorticoid receptor antagonist. * Several parameters including diastolic BP, economic state showed exactly the same median values. However, still significant (admittedly $p < 0.05$) statistical differences because significantly different quartile values. † Male: >112 g/week or >42 g/day, Female: >56 g/week or >28 g/day. (14g per a glass). Values are presented as median (Q1-Q3 quartiles (25th and 75th percentiles)) or %.

3.2. BP and Incident AF in Different Age Groups

During 6.4 ± 2.1 years of follow-up and a total of 768,314 person-years, 4393, 3946, and 447 incident AF cases occurred in the overall, non-octogenarian, and octogenarian populations, respectively. The spline curves of the SBP and DBP and risk of AF in different age groups are presented in Figure 2. A U-shaped relationship between SBP or DBP and risk of AF was evident; however, the U-shaped relationship for SBP was not observed in the octogenarian population. There is the larger uncertainty in the older group because it is numerically small. The optimal SBP level associated with the lowest the risks of AF was 120–129 mm Hg in the overall population and the non-octogenarian population. The optimal DBP level with the lowest risk of AF was 70–79 mm Hg.

After multivariable adjustment for potentially confounding clinical covariates, in non-octogenarians, the risk of AF was higher in patients with BP levels of <120/<80 and ≥140/90 mm Hg with adjusted hazard ratios (HR) of 1.15 (95% CI, 1.03–1.28, $p < 0.001$) and 1.14 (95% CI, 1.04–1.26, $p < 0.001$), respectively, compared to BP levels of 120–129/<80 mm Hg. Amongst octogenarians, the risk of AF was significantly higher in patients with BP levels of ≥140/90 mm Hg with an HR of 1.26 (95% CI, 1.01–1.58, $p < 0.001$) compared with the optimal BP level (130–139/80–90 mm Hg; Table 2, Figure 3).

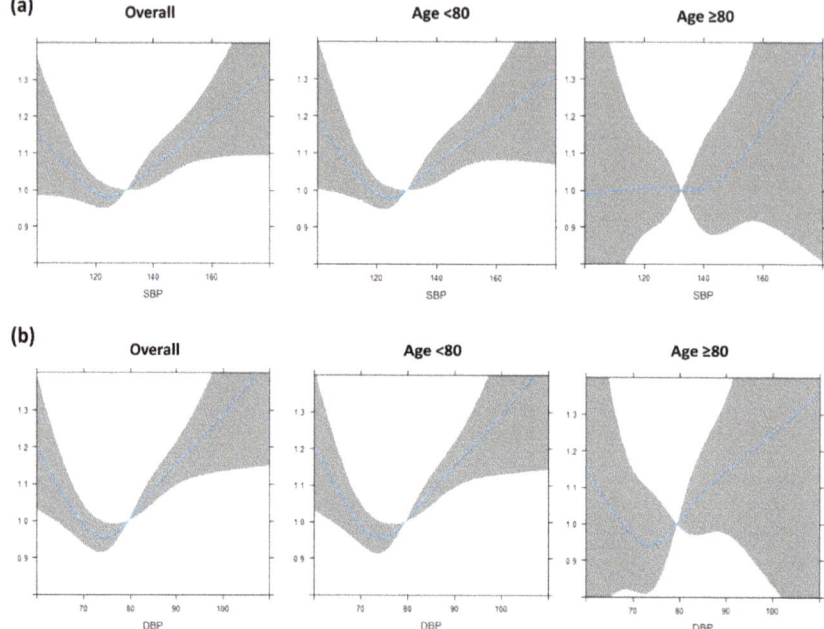

Figure 2. Systolic and diastolic blood pressure status of repeated measurement and risk of atrial fibrillation among elderly populations: (**a**) systolic blood pressure and (**b**) diastolic blood pressure. SBP, systolic blood pressure; DBP, diastolic blood pressure. The blue line shows relationship between hazard ratio of new-onset AF and blood pressure, and the gray area indicates the degree of confidence.

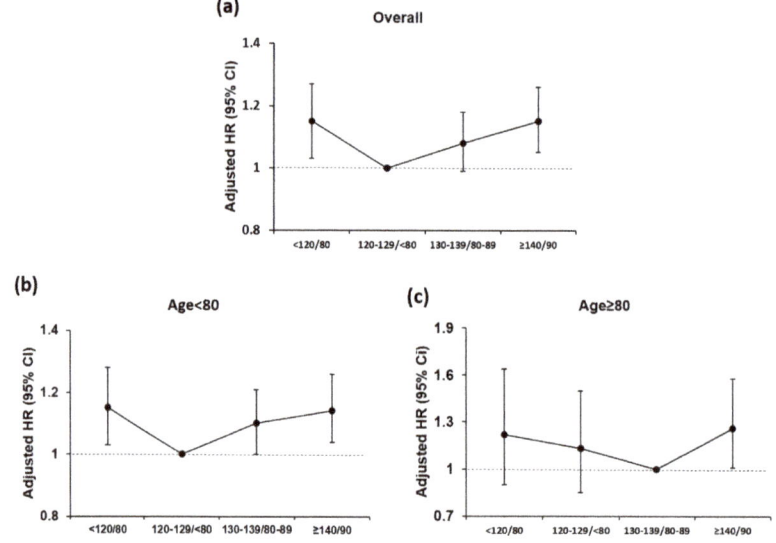

Figure 3. Blood pressure status of repeated measurement and risk of atrial fibrillation among elderly populations: (**a**) overall population, (**b**) age < 80 years, and (**c**) age ≥ 80 years. HR, hazard ratio.

Table 2. Incidence Rate of Atrial Fibrillation According to Blood Pressure.

Group	All Population			Age < 80 Years			Age ≥ 80 Years		
	No. /Total No. 4393 /115,866	Incidence Rate per 1000 Person-Years (95 CI)	Hazard Ratio (95 CI)	No. /Total No. 3946 /108,035	Incidence Rate Per 1000 Person-Years (95 CI)	Hazard Ratio (95 CI)	No. /Total No. 447 /7831	Incidence Rate Per 1000 Person-Years (95 CI)	Hazard Ratio (95 CI)
<120 /<80	713 /19,712	5.47 (5.07–5.88)	1.15 (1.03–1.27)	649 /18,556	5.24 (4.84–5.66)	1.15 (1.03–1.28)	64 /1156	9.78 (7.53–12.49)	1.22 (0.90–1.64)
120–129 /<80	721 /21,463	5.13 (4.76–5.52)	1 (reference)	647 /20,104	4.88 (4.51–5.27)	1 (reference)	74 /1359	9.37 (7.35–11.76)	1.13 (0.85–1.50)
130–139 /80–89	1526 /40,667	5.67 (5.39–5.96)	1.08 (0.99–1.18)	1386 /37,949	5.47 (5.19–5.77)	1.10 (1.00–1.21)	140 /2718	8.65 (7.28–10.21)	1 (reference)
≥140 /≥90	1433 /34,024	6.28 (5.96–6.62)	1.15 (1.05–1.26)	1264 /31,426	5.95 (5.63–6.29)	1.14 (1.04–1.26)	169 /2598	10.76 (9.20–12.52)	1.26 (1.01–1.58)

CI, confidence interval.

3.3. BP and Incident AF in Patients with Treated Hypertension

With a total of 298,087 person-years follow-up of patients with treated hypertension, there were 2069, 1846, and 3636 incident AF cases occurring in the overall, non-octogenarian, and octogenarian populations, respectively. The spline curves of the SBP and DBP and risk of AF in different age groups are presented in Figure 4 and had a similar pattern as the spline curve for the general populations (Figure 2).

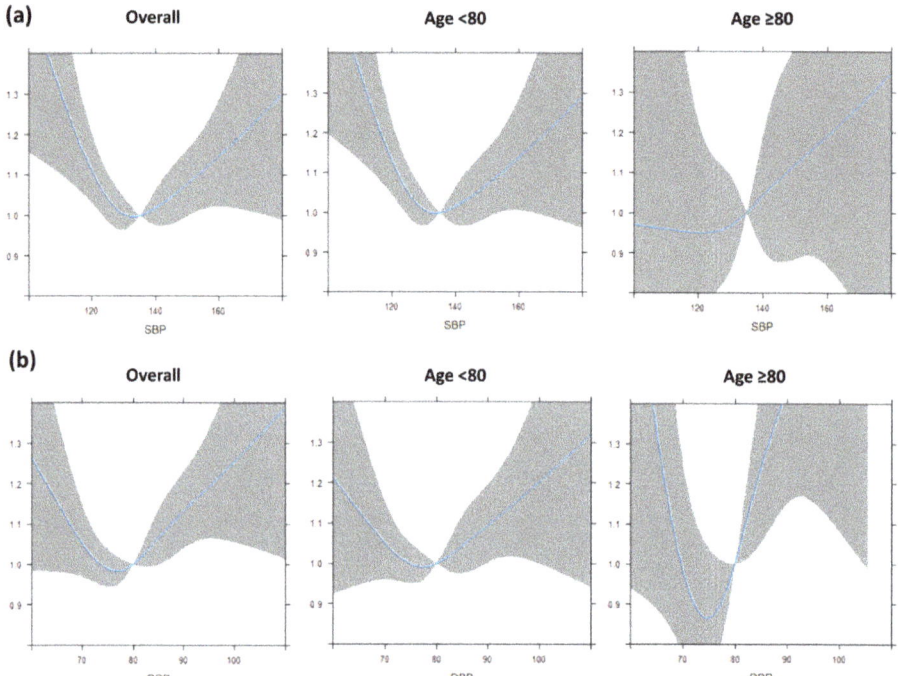

Figure 4. Systolic and diastolic blood pressure status of repeated measurement and risk of atrial fibrillation among elderly populations with antihypertensive medications: (**a**) systolic blood pressure and (**b**) diastolic blood pressure. SBP, systolic blood pressure; DBP, diastolic blood pressure. The blue line shows relationship between hazard ratio of new-onset AF and blood pressure, and the gray area indicates the degree of confidence.

After multivariable adjustment for potentially confounding clinical covariates in the non-octogenarian population, the risk of AF was higher in patients with intensive BP control (<120/<80 mm Hg) and poor (≥140/90 mm Hg) BP control with adjusted HRs of 1.37 (95% CI, 1.13–1.65, $p < 0.001$) and 1.16 (95% CI, 1.0–1.33, $p < 0.001$), respectively, compared to those with optimal BP control (120–129/<80 mm Hg). In octogenarians, the risk of AF was significantly higher in patients with a BP levels of ≥140/90 mm Hg with an HR of 1.42 (95% CI, 1.04–1.93, $p <0.001$) compared to those with optimal BP level (130–139/80–90 mm Hg; Table 3, Figure 5).

Table 3. Incidence Rate of Atrial Fibrillation According to Blood Pressure in Patients with Treated Hypertension.

Group	All Population			Age <80 Years			Age ≥ 80 Years		
	No./Total No. 2069/46,519	Incidence Rate per 1000 Person-Years (95 CI)	Hazard Ratio (95 CI)	No./Total No. 1846/42,883	Incidence Rate per 1000 Person-Years (95 CI)	Hazard Ratio (95 CI)	No./Total No. 223/3636	Incidence Rate Per 1000 Person-Years (95 CI)	Hazard Ratio (95 CI)
Intensive control (<120/80)	210/4159	8.22 (7.14–9.41)	1.34 (1.13–1.61)	189/3814	7.96 (6.87–9.18)	1.37 (1.13–1.65)	21/345	11.56 (7.16–17.67)	1.37 (0.83–2.24)
Optimal control (120–129/<80)	290/7466	6.22 (5.52–6.97)	1 (reference)	257/6893	5.91 (5.21–6.68)	1 (reference)	33/573	10.36 (7.13–14.55)	1.17 (0.77–1.79)
Suboptimal control (130–139/80–89)	735/17,268	6.66 (6.19–7.16)	1.09 (0.95–1.25)	667/15,934	6.49 (6.01–7.01)	1.12 (0.97–1.29)	68/1334	8.90 (6.91–11.29)	1 (reference)
Poor control (≥140/90)	834/17,626	7.22 (6.74–7.73)	1.16 (1.02–1.33)	733/16,242	6.83 (6.34–7.34)	1.16 (1.00–1.33)	101/1384	12.46 (10.15–15.14)	1.42 (1.04–1.93)

CI, confidence interval.

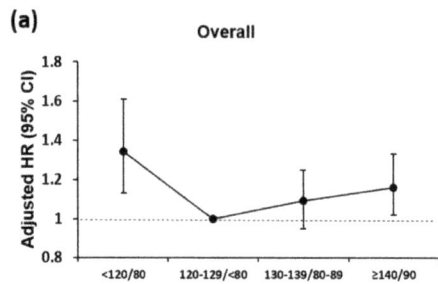

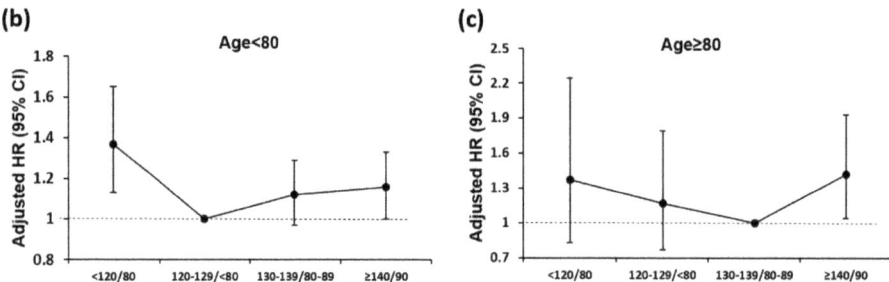

Figure 5. Blood pressure status of repeated measurement and risk of atrial fibrillation among elderly populations with antihypertensive medications: (**a**) overall population, (**b**) age < 80 years, and (**c**) age ≥ 80 years.

3.4. Serious Adverse Events according to BP Status in Different Age Groups

The incidence rate and HR of serious adverse events according to BP status in patients with hypertension treatment are presented in Table 4. In octogenarians, patients with intensive BP control (<120/<80 mm Hg) showed more hypotension requiring hospitalization than those with a BP levels of 130–139/80–90 mm Hg with an adjusted HR of 2.06 (95% CI, 1.12–3.81, $p < 0.001$). The composite adverse events (including hypotension requiring hospitalization, syncope, bradycardia, electrolyte abnormality, injurious falls, and acute kidney injury) were numerically more frequent but non-statistically significant in patients with intensive and optimal BP control compared to those with a BP level of 130–139/80–89 mm Hg.

Table 4. Incidence Rate and Hazard Ratio of Serious Adverse Events According to Blood Pressure Status in Patients with Hypertension Treatment.

		Blood Pressure Status			
		<120/80 mmHg	120–129/<80 mmHg	130–139/80–89 mmHg	≥140/90 mmHg
Overall	No. of total	4159	7466	17,268	17,626
Composite event	No. of events, HR (95 CI)	341 1.08 (0.94–1.23)	580 1 (reference)	1269 0.95 (0.86–1.04)	1437 1.01 (0.92–1.11)
Hypotension requiring hospitalization	No. of events, HR (95 CI)	95, 1.15 (0.89–1.48)	151, 1 (reference)	348, 0.99 (0.82–1.20)	366, 0.98 (0.81–1.19)
Syncope	No. of events HR (95 CI)	33, 1.08 (0.70–1.67)	55, 1 (reference)	155, 1.23 (0.90–1.67)	157, 1.18 (0.86–1.60)
Bradycardia	No. of events HR (95 CI)	22 0.99 (0.59–1.67)	41 1 (reference)	96 1.01 (0.70–1.45)	97 0.96 (0.67–1.39)
Electrolyte abnormality	No. of events HR (95 CI)	142 0.99 (0.80–1.21)	263 1 (reference)	523 0.86 (0.75–1.00)	646 1.01 (0.88–1.17)
Injurious falls	No. of events HR (95 CI)	11 1.11 (0.52–2.37)	17 1 (reference)	46 1.18 (0.67–2.06)	41 0.97 (0.55–1.71)
Acute kidney injury	No. of events HR (95 CI)	106 1.18 (0.93–1.50)	172 1 (reference)	364 0.90 (0.75–1.08)	433 0.96 (0.80–1.14)
Age < 80 Years	No. of total	3814	6893	15,934	16,242
Composite event	No. of events HR (95 CI)	298 1.08 (0.94–1.25)	506 1 (reference)	1124 0.96 (0.87–1.07)	1279 1.03 (0.93–1.15)
Hypotension requiring hospitalization	No. of events HR (95 CI)	80 1.13 (0.85–1.49)	129 1 (reference)	313 1.05 (0.85–1.28)	327 1.03 (0.84–1.27)
Syncope	No. of events HR (95 CI)	31 1.28 (0.81–2.02)	44 1 (reference)	141 1.39 (0.99–1.96)	143 1.33 (0.95–1.87)
Bradycardia	No. of events HR (95 CI)	18 0.88 (0.50–1.55)	38 1 (reference)	91 1.03 (0.71–1.51)	87 0.9. (0.63–1.36)
Electrolyte abnormality	No. of events HR (95 CI)	122 0.98 (0.79–1.22)	228 1 (reference)	453 0.87 (0.74–1.02)	573 1.04 (0.8–1.22)

Table 4. Cont.

		Blood Pressure Status			
		<120/80 mmHg	120–129/<80 mmHg	130–139/80–89 mmHg	≥140/90 mmHg
Injurious falls	No. of events HR (95 CI)	10 1.02 (0.45–2.24)	17 1 (reference)	40 1.04 (0.59–1.84)	38 0.91 (0.51–1.61)
Acute kidney injury	No. of events HR (95 CI)	96 1.25 (0.96–1.61)	148 1 (reference)	317 0.91 (0.75–1.11)	378 0.98 (0.81–1.18)
Age ≥ 80 Years	No of total	345	573	1334	1384
Composite event	No. of events HR (95 CI)	43 1.32 (0.94–1.86)	74 1.25 (0.94–1.66)	145 1 (reference)	158 1.03 (0.82–1.29)
Hypotension requiring hospitalization	No. of events HR (95 CI)	15 2.06 (1.12–3.81)	22 1.64 (0.96–2.81)	35 1 (reference)	39 1.08 (0.68–1.72)
Syncope	No. of events HR (95 CI)	2 0.57 (0.13–2.51)	11 1.69 (0.74–3.85)	14 1 (reference)	14 1.69 (0.74–3.85)
Bradycardia	No. of events HR (95 CI)	4 3.73 (0.97–14.32)	3 0.98 (0.19–5.14)	5 1 (reference)	10 2.02 (0.68–6.01)
Electrolyte abnormality	No. of events HR (95 CI)	20 1.21 (0.73–1.99)	35 1.18 (0.78–1.79)	70 1 (reference)	73 0.98 (0.70–1.36)
Injurious falls	No. of events HR (95 CI)	1 0.75 (0.09–5.90)	0	6 1 (reference)	3 0.44 (0.11–1.72)
Acute kidney Injury	No. of events HR (95 CI)	10 1.06 (0.53–2.11)	24 1.27 (0.77–2.11)	47 1 (reference)	55 1.02 (0.69–1.52)

CI, confidence interval.

4. Discussion

In this large nationwide study on the impact of hypertension on incident AF, our principal findings are that BP levels of 120–129/<80 mm Hg were associated with a lower risk of incident AF in non-octogenarians. Amongst octogenarians, an average 10 mm Hg higher BP level of 130–139/80–89 mm Hg was more optimal to prevent AF. Second, octogenarians with intensive BP control (<120/<80 mm Hg) showed more hypotension requiring hospitalization compared with BP level of 130–139/80–90 mm Hg. Hence, a less strict BP level may be better to prevent AF and adverse effects amongst octogenarians.

The relationship between high BP and high incidence of AF supports the importance of BP control to prevent AF in patients with hypertension. Hypertension is the most common and important modifiable AF risk factor [2,3,22,23]. In a SPRINT sub-analysis, intensive BP control targeting SBP < 120 mm Hg was related with a lower risk of new-onset AF [13]. In contrast, the present study found a U-shaped relationship was observed between BP and incident AF in both non-octogenarians and octogenarians. This U-shaped relationship could be related to several unique aspects of our study cohort.

The present study recruited participants aged over 60 years, with the median age of our population being 71.7 years, much older than previous studies [11–13], and 6.8% of overall population were individuals of age over 80 years. The elderly population had more comorbidities, and these factors may influence the U-shaped relationship. Since the incidence of AF increases with age, we evaluated the relationship between the optimal BP and AF risk for BP management in older individuals. When comparing the relationship between AF and DBP, a U-shaped pattern was also observed in the overall population and patients with hypertension.

4.1. Optimal BP Levels and Incident AF in Octogenarians

Amongst octogenarians, an average 10 mm Hg higher BP level of 130–139/80–89 mm Hg was more optimal to prevent AF; this compares to non-octogenarians where the optimal BP level was 120–129/<80 mm Hg. However, the management of hypertension in octogenarians offers more challenges than in non-octogenarians. Elderly patients (age > 80 years) have more comorbidities and higher risks other organ damage than patients aged under 80 years. In old patients, physicians should consider the risks and benefits when controlling BP due to aggravation of postural hypotension and reduction of renal function [16]. Also, intensive BP control has been related to increased serious adverse events such as hypotension, syncope, electrolyte abnormalities, and acute kidney injury [14]. Our results show an increased risk of hypotension requiring hospitalization in the intensive BP control group (BP < 120/80 mm Hg) compared with BPs 130–139/80–89 mm Hg. Even though other adverse events did not show significant differences, the composite outcome of adverse events showed a trend towards an increased risk in patients with intensive control (BP < 120/80 mm Hg) and optimal BP control (120–129/<80 mm Hg) compared to patients with BP levels of 130–139/80–89 mm Hg.

4.2. Limitations

The study has several limitations. First, in such studies using administrative databases, coding inaccuracies can lead to errors. Hence, we applied the definition that we had already validated in previous studies to minimize the problem [21,24–28]. Second, since the health examination of individuals was conducted in different hospitals and clinics, a uniformity of BP measurement could not be achieved. Third, the arbitrary cut-offs across continuous distributions (e.g., age, BP) were used to compare groups using simple binary statistical tests in this study. While the simplification can illustrate possible trends, it does automatically lead to a loss of detail in data analysis. Fourth, those who survive into their ninth decade are already a positively selected group and presumably with useful healthy characteristics. Fifth, since data about the types of AF and differential diagnosis between AF and atrial flutter (AFL) were not available, we could not investigate about the difference of optimal BP level according to the types of AF or AFL. Finally, hypertension and AF are associated with renal dysfunction. In our study, CKD was defined using the medical record with ICD-10 codes. There was no data on proteinuria. The lack of data on proteinuria, which is one of the criteria for CKD, may lead to low accuracy in defining CKD. This is one of the limitations of the study. Despite these limitations, the study is the first assessment to investigate the association between BP levels and incidental AF in a nationwide elderly population.

5. Conclusions

A U-shaped relationship for the development of incident AF was evident in non-octogenarians, and BP levels of 120–130/<80 mm Hg were associated the lowest risk of incident AF. Compared to non-octogenarians, the lowest risk of AF was associated with higher BP levels of 130–139/80–89 mm Hg amongst octogenarians.

Supplementary Materials: The following are available online at http://www.mdpi.com/2077-0383/9/9/2988/s1; Supplementary Table S1: Definitions and International Classification of Disease-10th Revision (ICD-10) codes used for defining the comorbidities and clinical outcomes; Supplementary Table S2: Comparison of baseline characteristics in patients with different blood pressure levels in overall population.

Author Contributions: Conceptualization, B.J. and G.Y.H.L.; methodology, P.-S.Y.; software, Y.J.P.; validation, E.J., H.T.Y., and T.-H.K.; formal analysis, J.-S.U.; investigation, Y.J.P.; resources, P.-S.Y.; data curation, H.-N.P.; writing—original draft preparation, Y.J.P.; writing—review and editing, G.Y.H.L.; visualization, M.-H.L.; supervision, M.-H.L.; project administration, B.J.; funding acquisition, B.J. All authors have read and agreed to the published version of the manuscript.

Funding: This research was funded by a research grant from the Korean Healthcare Technology R&D project funded by the Ministry of Health and Welfare (HI15C1200, HC19C0130) and a CMB-Yuhan research grant of Yonsei University College of Medicine (6-2019-0124).

Acknowledgments: The National Health Information Database was provided by the National Health Insurance Service of Korea. We thank the National Health Insurance Service for its cooperation.

Conflicts of Interest: G.Y.H.L.: Consultant for Bayer/Janssen, BMS/Pfizer, Biotronik, Medtronic, Boehringer Ingelheim, Microlife, and Daiichi-Sankyo. Speaker for Bayer, BMS/Pfizer, Medtronic, Boehringer Ingelheim, Microlife, Roche, and Daiichi-Sankyo. No fees were received personally. B.J.: Speaker for Bayer, BMS/Pfizer, Medtronic, and Daiichi-Sankyo and research funds from Medtronic and Abbott. No fees were directly received personally. None of the other authors have anything to disclose.

References

1. Kearney, P.M.; Whelton, M.; Reynolds, K.; Muntner, P.; Whelton, P.K.; He, J. Global burden of hypertension: Analysis of worldwide data. *Lancet* **2005**, *365*, 217–223. [CrossRef]
2. Huxley, R.R.; Lopez, F.L.; Folsom, A.R.; Agarwal, S.K.; Loehr, L.R.; Soliman, E.Z.; Maclehose, R.; Konety, S.; Alonso, A. Absolute and attributable risks of atrial fibrillation in relation to optimal and borderline risk factors: The Atherosclerosis Risk in Communities (ARIC) study. *Circulation* **2011**, *123*, 1501–1508. [CrossRef] [PubMed]
3. Emdin, C.A.; Anderson, S.G.; Salimi-Khorshidi, G.; Woodward, M.; MacMahon, S.; Dwyer, T.; Rahimi, K. Usual blood pressure, atrial fibrillation and vascular risk: Evidence from 4.3 million adults. *Int. J. Epidemiol.* **2017**, *46*, 162–172. [CrossRef]
4. Dzeshka, M.S.; Shantsila, A.; Shantsila, E.; Lip, G.Y.H. Atrial Fibrillation and Hypertension. *Hypertension* **2017**, *70*, 854–861. [CrossRef] [PubMed]
5. Gumprecht, J.; Domek, M.; Lip, G.Y.H.; Shantsila, A. Invited review: Hypertension and atrial fibrillation: Epidemiology, pathophysiology, and implications for management. *J. Hum. Hypertens.* **2019**, *33*, 824–836. [CrossRef] [PubMed]
6. Lip, G.Y.H.; Coca, A.; Kahan, T.; Boriani, G.; Manolis, A.S.; Olsen, M.H.; Oto, A.; Potpara, T.S.; Steffel, J.; Marin, F.; et al. Hypertension and cardiac arrhythmias: A consensus document from the European Heart Rhythm Association (EHRA) and ESC Council on Hypertension, endorsed by the Heart Rhythm Society (HRS), Asia-Pacific Heart Rhythm Society (APHRS) and Sociedad Latinoamericana de Estimulacion Cardiaca y Electrofisiologia (SOLEACE). *Europace* **2017**, *19*, 891–911. [CrossRef] [PubMed]
7. O'Neal, W.T.; Soliman, E.Z.; Qureshi, W.; Alonso, A.; Heckbert, S.R.; Herrington, D. Sustained pre-hypertensive blood pressure and incident atrial fibrillation: The Multi-Ethnic Study of Atherosclerosis. *J. Am. Soc Hypertens.* **2015**, *9*, 191–196. [CrossRef]

8. Conen, D.; Tedrow, U.B.; Koplan, B.A.; Glynn, R.J.; Buring, J.E.; Albert, C.M. Influence of systolic and diastolic blood pressure on the risk of incident atrial fibrillation in women. *Circulation* **2009**, *119*, 2146–2152. [CrossRef]
9. Grundvold, I.; Skretteberg, P.T.; Liestol, K.; Erikssen, G.; Kjeldsen, S.E.; Arnesen, H.; Erikssen, J.; Bodegard, J. Upper normal blood pressures predict incident atrial fibrillation in healthy middle-aged men: A 35-year follow-up study. *Hypertension* **2012**, *59*, 198–204. [CrossRef]
10. Thomas, M.C.; Dublin, S.; Kaplan, R.C.; Glazer, N.L.; Lumley, T.; Longstreth, W.T., Jr.; Smith, N.L.; Psaty, B.M.; Siscovick, D.S.; Heckbert, S.R. Blood pressure control and risk of incident atrial fibrillation. *Am. J. Hypertens.* **2008**, *21*, 1111–1116. [CrossRef]
11. Verdecchia, P.; Staessen, J.A.; Angeli, F.; de Simone, G.; Achilli, A.; Ganau, A.; Mureddu, G.; Pede, S.; Maggioni, A.P.; Lucci, D.; et al. Usual versus tight control of systolic blood pressure in non-diabetic patients with hypertension (Cardio-Sis): An open-label randomised trial. *Lancet* **2009**, *374*, 525–533. [CrossRef]
12. Chen, L.Y.; Bigger, J.T.; Hickey, K.T.; Chen, H.; Lopez-Jimenez, C.; Banerji, M.A.; Evans, G.; Fleg, J.L.; Papademetriou, V.; Thomas, A.; et al. Effect of Intensive Blood Pressure Lowering on Incident Atrial Fibrillation and P-Wave Indices in the ACCORD Blood Pressure Trial. *Am. J. Hypertens.* **2016**, *29*, 1276–1282. [CrossRef] [PubMed]
13. Soliman, E.Z.; Rahman, A.F.; Zhang, Z.M.; Rodriguez, C.J.; Chang, T.I.; Bates, J.T.; Ghazi, L.; Blackshear, J.L.; Chonchol, M.; Fine, L.J.; et al. Effect of Intensive Blood Pressure Lowering on the Risk of Atrial Fibrillation. *Hypertension* **2020**, *75*, 1491–1496. [CrossRef] [PubMed]
14. Group, S.R.; Wright, J.T., Jr.; Williamson, J.D.; Whelton, P.K.; Snyder, J.K.; Sink, K.M.; Rocco, M.V.; Reboussin, D.M.; Rahman, M.; Oparil, S.; et al. A Randomized Trial of Intensive versus Standard Blood-Pressure Control. *N. Engl. J. Med.* **2015**, *373*, 2103–2116. [CrossRef]
15. Williams, B.; Mancia, G.; Spiering, W.; Agabiti Rosei, E.; Azizi, M.; Burnier, M.; Clement, D.L.; Coca, A.; de Simone, G.; Dominiczak, A.; et al. 2018 ESC/ESH Guidelines for the management of arterial hypertension. *Eur. Heart J.* **2018**, *39*, 3021–3104. [CrossRef]
16. Kjeldsen, S.E.; Stenehjem, A.; Os, I.; Van de Borne, P.; Burnier, M.; Narkiewicz, K.; Redon, J.; Agabiti Rosei, E.; Mancia, G. Treatment of high blood pressure in elderly and octogenarians: European Society of Hypertension statement on blood pressure targets. *Blood Press.* **2016**, *25*, 333–336. [CrossRef]
17. Phillips, R.A.; Xu, J.; Peterson, L.E.; Arnold, R.M.; Diamond, J.A.; Schussheim, A.E. Impact of Cardiovascular Risk on the Relative Benefit and Harm of Intensive Treatment of Hypertension. *J. Am. Coll. Cardiol.* **2018**, *71*, 1601–1610. [CrossRef]
18. Lee, J.H.; Choi, J.K.; Jeong, S.N.; Choi, S.H. Charlson comorbidity index as a predictor of periodontal disease in elderly participants. *J. Periodontal Implant. Sci.* **2018**, *48*, 92–102. [CrossRef]
19. Lee, S.S.; Ae Kong, K.; Kim, D.; Lim, Y.M.; Yang, P.S.; Yi, J.E.; Kim, M.; Kwon, K.; Bum Pyun, W.; Joung, B.; et al. Clinical implication of an impaired fasting glucose and prehypertension related to new onset atrial fibrillation in a healthy Asian population without underlying disease: A nationwide cohort study in Korea. *Eur. Heart J.* **2017**, *38*, 2599–2607. [CrossRef]
20. Kim, D.; Yang, P.S.; Jang, E.; Yu, H.T.; Kim, T.H.; Uhm, J.S.; Kim, J.Y.; Pak, H.N.; Lee, M.H.; Joung, B.; et al. Increasing trends in hospital care burden of atrial fibrillation in Korea, 2006 through 2015. *Heart* **2018**, *104*, 2010–2017. [CrossRef]
21. Lee, H.Y.; Yang, P.S.; Kim, T.H.; Uhm, J.S.; Pak, H.N.; Lee, M.H.; Joung, B. Atrial fibrillation and the risk of myocardial infarction: A nation-wide propensity-matched study. *Sci. Rep.* **2017**, *7*, 12716. [CrossRef] [PubMed]
22. Verdecchia, P.; Angeli, F.; Reboldi, G. Hypertension and Atrial Fibrillation: Doubts and Certainties From Basic and Clinical Studies. *Circ. Res.* **2018**, *122*, 352–368. [CrossRef] [PubMed]
23. Dzeshka, M.S.; Shahid, F.; Shantsila, A.; Lip, G.Y.H. Hypertension and Atrial Fibrillation: An Intimate Association of Epidemiology, Pathophysiology, and Outcomes. *Am. J. Hypertens.* **2017**, *30*, 733–755. [CrossRef] [PubMed]
24. Kim, D.; Yang, P.S.; Yu, H.T.; Kim, T.H.; Jang, E.; Sung, J.H.; Pak, H.N.; Lee, M.Y.; Lee, M.H.; Lip, G.Y.H.; et al. Risk of dementia in stroke-free patients diagnosed with atrial fibrillation: Data from a population-based cohort. *Eur. Heart. J.* **2019**, *40*, 2313–2323. [CrossRef]

25. Kim, T.H.; Yang, P.S.; Uhm, J.S.; Kim, J.Y.; Pak, H.N.; Lee, M.H.; Joung, B.; Lip, G.Y.H. CHA2DS2-VASc Score (Congestive Heart Failure, Hypertension, Age >/=75 [Doubled], Diabetes Mellitus, Prior Stroke or Transient Ischemic Attack [Doubled], Vascular Disease, Age 65-74, Female) for Stroke in Asian Patients With Atrial Fibrillation: A Korean Nationwide Sample Cohort Study. *Stroke* **2017**, *48*, 1524–1530. [CrossRef]
26. Lee, H.; Kim, T.H.; Baek, Y.S.; Uhm, J.S.; Pak, H.N.; Lee, M.H.; Joung, B. The Trends of Atrial Fibrillation-Related Hospital Visit and Cost, Treatment Pattern and Mortality in Korea: 10-Year Nationwide Sample Cohort Data. *Korean Circ. J.* **2017**, *47*, 56–64. [CrossRef]
27. Baek, Y.S.; Yang, P.S.; Kim, T.H.; Uhm, J.S.; Park, J.; Pak, H.N.; Lee, M.H.; Joung, B. Associations of Abdominal Obesity and New-Onset Atrial Fibrillation in the General Population. *J. Am. Heart Assoc.* **2017**, *6*, e004705. [CrossRef]
28. Song, S.; Yang, P.S.; Kim, T.H.; Uhm, J.S.; Pak, H.N.; Lee, M.H.; Joung, B. Relation of Chronic Obstructive Pulmonary Disease to Cardiovascular Disease in the General Population. *Am. J. Cardiol.* **2017**, *120*, 1399–1404. [CrossRef]

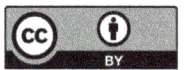

© 2020 by the authors. Licensee MDPI, Basel, Switzerland. This article is an open access article distributed under the terms and conditions of the Creative Commons Attribution (CC BY) license (http://creativecommons.org/licenses/by/4.0/).

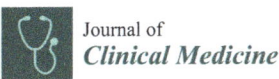

Journal of Clinical Medicine

Article

Ischemic Stroke Risk Factors in Patients with Atrial Fibrillation Treated with New Oral Anticoagulants

Paweł Wańkowicz [1,*], Jacek Staszewski [2], Aleksander Dębiec [2], Marta Nowakowska-Kotas [3], Aleksandra Szylińska [1] and Iwona Rotter [1]

1. Department of Medical Rehabilitation and Clinical Physiotherapy, Pomeranian Medical University in Szczecin, Żołnierska 48, 71-210 Szczecin, Poland; aleksandra.szylinska@gmail.com (A.S.); iwrot@wp.pl (I.R.)
2. Department of Neurology, Military Medical Institute, Warszawa, Szaserów 128, 04-141 Warszawa, Poland; jacekstaszewski@wp.pl (J.S.); adebiec@wim.mil.pl (A.D.)
3. Department of Neurology, Medical University of Wrocław, Borowska 213, 50-566 Wrocław, Poland; marnow64@interia.pl
* Correspondence: pawel.wankowicz@pum.edu.pl; Tel.: +48-91-48-00-914

Abstract: The most commonly used therapeutic option for the prevention of ischemic stroke in patients with atrial fibrillation is new- or old-generation oral anticoagulants. New oral anticoagulants are at least as effective as old-generation oral anticoagulants in the prevention of ischemic stroke, with a reduced risk of life-threatening hemorrhage. Moreover, the constant monitoring of these drugs in the patient's blood is not required during routine use. However, ischemic stroke can still occur in these patients. Therefore, the aim of this study was to investigate the pattern of risk factors for ischemic stroke in patients with atrial fibrillation treated with new oral anticoagulants. Our multicenter retrospective study involved 2032 patients with acute ischemic stroke. The experimental group consisted of 256 patients with acute ischemic stroke and nonvalvular atrial fibrillation, who were treated with new oral anticoagulants. The control group consisted of 1776 ischemic stroke patients without coexisting atrial fibrillation. The results of our study show that patients with atrial fibrillation treated with new oral anticoagulants are more likely to display thrombotic, proatherogenic, and proinflammatory factors in addition to the embolic factors associated with atrial fibrillation. Therefore, solely taking new oral anticoagulants is insufficient in protecting this group of patients from ischemic stroke.

Keywords: ischemic stroke; risk factor; atrial fibrillation; new oral anticoagulants

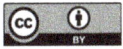

1. Introduction

Atrial fibrillation (AF) is the most common cardiac arrhythmia found in everyday clinical practice. Currently, the prevalence of AF in the global population ranges from 4 to 15 percent depending on the age of the patient [1–3]. This number is expected to double in the coming years due to the increasing life span of the general population, as well as the development of new techniques allowing faster detection of previously undiagnosed cases of AF [4,5].

The late detection or inadequate treatment of AF may result in serious complications, such as ischemic stroke. AF may account for up to 30% of cerebral ischemic strokes [6–8]. The most commonly used therapeutic option for the prevention of embolic complications in patients with AF is oral anticoagulants.

New oral anticoagulants (NOACs) are at least as effective as vitamin K antagonists (VKA) in the primary and secondary prevention of ischemic stroke, with a reduced risk of life-threatening hemorrhages—especially intracranial—as is confirmed in numerous studies [9–12]. Moreover, the constant monitoring of these drugs in the patient's blood is not required during routine use. However, data suggest that although the use of NOACs may be effective in preventing ischemic stroke associated with AF, a considerable number of patients still suffer from strokes [13,14].

Over the years, a number of factors have been identified as predisposing to the development of AF. Some of these are non-modifiable factors such as age, gender, genetic predisposition, or ethnicity. Others are modifiable—hypertension, coronary artery disease, heart failure, diabetes, or atherosclerosis [15–19]. Importantly, these AF risk factors are also risk factors for ischemic stroke [20]. Therefore, the aim of this study was to investigate the pattern of non-modifiable and modifiable risk factors for ischemic stroke in patients with nonvalvular atrial fibrillation (NVAF) treated with NOACs.

2. Materials and Methods

This was a multicenter retrospective study conducted between 2014 and 2020 at the Department of Neurology of the Pomeranian Medical University in Szczecin, the Department of Neurology of the Military Medical Institute in Warsaw, and the Department of Neurology of the Medical University of Wrocław in Poland.

The study included 2032 consecutive patients with acute ischemic stroke. Patients were divided into two groups. The experimental group consisted of 256 patients with acute ischemic stroke and nonvalvular atrial fibrillation. These patients had been treated with NOACs for the prevention of ischemic stroke. Because of the size of the study group, specific types of NOAC were not distinguished. The control group consisted of 1776 ischemic stroke patients without coexisting atrial fibrillation.

In accordance with international guidelines, all patients with ischemic stroke underwent neurological examination, electrocardiogram (ECG), diagnostic neuroimaging (computed tomography or magnetic resonance imaging of the brain), and vascular examination (Doppler ultrasound/angio-computed tomography/angio-magnetic resonance imaging of the carotid and vertebral arteries) [21]. All types of ischemic stroke were included in the study.

Data on the most common risk factors for ischemic stroke were collected by interview and through the analysis of medical records. These risk factors included baseline demographics such as sex, age, and comorbidities—for example, AF treated with NOACs, hypertension, diabetes mellitus, dyslipidemia, coronary artery disease, hemodynamically significant internal carotid artery (ICA) stenosis or ICA occlusion, peripheral arterial disease, previous stroke, and cigarette smoking. The Bioethics Committee of the Pomeranian Medical University issued consent to conduct the study (KB-0012/49/07/2020/Z).

The diagnosis of AF was based on the absence of P waves with the isoelectric line replaced by irregular high-frequency oscillations (f waves) in an ECG, either taken on admission to the neurology department or from the patient's medical records, which included information on the intake of NOACs. We also took into account patients who reported the presence of AF during the interview [22]. The diagnosis of hypertension was based on medical history and intake of hypotensive medications. Hypertension was defined by systolic blood pressure ≥ 140 mm Hg and/or diastolic blood pressure ≥ 90 mm Hg in repeated tests [23].

The diagnosis of diabetes mellitus was based on the patient's history, analysis of medical records, and intake of glucose-lowering medications. Diabetes mellitus was defined as a level of fasting blood glucose ≥ 126 mg/dL after a minimum of two tests, or a glucose level of ≥ 200 mg/dL measured at any time during the day [24].

The diagnosis of dyslipidemia was based on the interview, analysis of patient medical records, and intake of lipid-lowering medications. Dyslipidemia was defined as a serum cholesterol concentration of >190 mg/dL, low-density lipoprotein cholesterol >115 mg/dL, serum triglyceride concentration >150 mg/dL, and high-density lipoprotein cholesterol <40 mg/dL in males and <45 mg/dL in females [25].

The diagnosis of coronary heart disease was based on the interview, analysis of the patient's medical records, or intake of cardiovascular medications.

The diagnosis of ICA hemodynamically significant stenosis was based on medical records and/or vascular examination (Doppler ultrasound/angio-computed tomography/angio-magnetic resonance imaging) where the degree of stenosis was 50% or greater [26,27].

The diagnosis of peripheral arterial disease was based on the interview and an analysis of medical records.

The determination of cigarette smoking was based on the interview and medical records. Smoking was defined as current smoking of any number of cigarettes.

The diagnosis of recurrent stroke was based on patient history according to medical records or if the patient, caregiver, or relative reported this diagnosis.

Statistical Analysis

The null hypothesis was that there would be no differences in risk factors between ischemic stroke patients with NVAF who took NOACs and ischemic stroke patients without AF. The alternative hypothesis was that there would be significant differences in risk factors between ischemic stroke patients with NVAF who took NOACs and ischemic stroke patients without AF. In order to compare the characteristics of both groups, the Mann–Whitney U test was used for quantitative data. Fisher's exact test was used for qualitative data. Multiple logistic regression was calculated in order to assess the odds ratio of independent risk factors for both groups. Differences were considered significant at $p < 0.05$. All computations were performed using licensed Statistica 13.0 software (StatSoft, Tulsa, OK, USA).

3. Results

In total, 256 (12.6%) patients of the 2032 acute ischemic stroke cohort included in this study had a diagnosis of NVAF and were taking NOACs. The median age of all patients was 71 years (69.9 ± 8.7 years). In total, 958 patients (47.15%) were male. Hypertension was present in 1543 patients (75.94%), diabetes mellitus in 685 (33.71%), dyslipidemia in 876 (43.11%), ICA significant stenosis/occlusion in 298 (14.67%), coronary heart disease in 873 (42.96%), peripheral arterial disease in 262 (12.89%), previous stroke in 954 (46.95%), and cigarette smoking in 1041 (51.23%).

3.1. Comparison of Risk Factors for Ischemic Stroke in Patients with Nonvalvular Atrial Fibrillation Treated with New-Generation Oral Anticoagulants versus Patients without Atrial Fibrillation

A comparison of both groups is shown in Table 1.

Table 1. Baseline characteristics of patients with ischemic stroke with nonvalvular atrial fibrillation treated with new oral anticoagulants and patients without atrial fibrillation.

Parameter	AF NOAC (n = 256)	No-AF (n = 1776)	p-Value
Age, mean ± SD; Me	78.23 ± 7.32; 79.0	68.66 ± 8.41; 69.0	<0.001
Female, n (%)	181 (70)	893 (50)	<0.001
Comorbidities, n (%)			
Diabetes mellitus	134 (52)	551 (31)	<0.001
Dyslipidemia	152 (59)	724 (40)	<0.001
Hypertension	237 (92)	1306 (73)	<0.001
ICA significant stenosis/occlusion	43 (16)	255 (14)	0.302
Coronary heart disease	166 (64)	707 (39)	<0.001
Peripheral arterial disease	51 (19)	211 (11)	<0.001
Smoking	151 (58)	890 (50)	0.008
Previous stroke	161 (62)	793 (44)	<0.001

Legend: n—number of patients, SD—standard deviation, Me—median, AF—atrial fibrillation, ICA—internal carotid artery, NOAC—nonvalvular atrial fibrillation treated with new oral anticoagulants.

3.2. Analysis of Risk Factors for Ischemic Stroke in Patients with Nonvalvular Atrial Fibrillation Treated with a New Oral Anticoagulant and Patients without Atrial Fibrillation

A univariate and multivariate logistic regression model is shown in Table 2.

Table 2. Analysis of risk factors of ischemic stroke in patients with atrial fibrillation, who suffered a stroke despite NOAC therapy, compared to patients without AF (multivariate logistic regression).

Factors		Univariable Logistic Regression Models				Multivariable Logistic Regression Model *			
		OR	CI 95%	CI 95%	p	OR	CI 95%	CI 95%	p
Age		1.16	1.14	1.18	<0001	1.22	1.18	1.25	<0.001
Gender	Female	2.38	1.79	3.17	<0.001	1.93	1.37	2.70	<0.001
	Male	1.00				1.00			
Diabetes mellitus	Yes	2.44	1.87	3.18	<0.001	1.90	1.38	2.63	<0.001
	No	1.00				1.00			
Dyslipidemia	Yes	2.12	162	2.77	<0.001	2.48	1.80	3.42	<0.001
	No	1.00				1.00			
Hypertension	Yes	4.48	2.78	7.24	<0.001	4.20	2.48	7.10	<0.001
	No	1.000				1.00			
Coronary heart disease	Yes	2.78	2.12	3.66	<0.001	1.79	1.27	2.51	0.001
	No	1.00				1.00			
Peripheral arterial disease	Yes	1.84	1.31	2.58	<0.001	1.11	0.72	1.71	0.634
	No	1.00				1.00			
Smoking	Yes	1.43	1.09	1.86	0.008	2.67	1.91	3.74	<0.001
	No	1.00				1.00			
Previous stroke	Yes	2.10	1.60	2.75	<0.001	0.39	0.26	0.60	<0.001
	No	100				1.00			

Legend: OR—odds ratio, CI—confidence interval. * Note: Model was adjusted for the following variables: age, sex, diabetes mellitus, dyslipidemia, hypertension, coronary heart disease, peripheral arterial disease, smoking, previous stroke.

4. Discussion

The most common therapeutic option for the prevention of ischemic stroke in patients with AF is treatment with VKA or NOACs. Chronic use of oral anticoagulants reduces the risk of ischemic stroke by 64% [28]. Nevertheless, this does not completely prevent the risk of ischemic stroke in these patients. In VKA treatment, one popular explanation for this is that the patient did not follow the physician's recommendations regarding the frequency of administration, resulting in nontherapeutic international normalized ratio (INR). However, this cannot be the case for NOACs, which do not require constant monitoring of blood levels.

The results of some reports suggest that the sole use of anticoagulants for AF patients is insufficient in significantly reducing the risk of stroke, due to the presence of other factors that often accompany AF. In a study by Tokunaga et al. on AF patients, prior use of warfarin, an old-generation oral anticoagulant, was associated with a higher risk of ischemic events in the two years following therapy when compared with no such treatment [29]. Evans et al. observed that, among AF patients who had an ischemic stroke, there was a higher rate of recurrent lacunar stroke than cardioembolic stroke, which suggests that, although the incidence of one type of stroke associated with AF may be reduced, the presence of other factors in the patient may result in a different type of stroke [30]. Many studies have also considered genetic variability as an expression of increased susceptibility to stroke in AF patients taking old-generation anticoagulants. It is apparent that the majority of patients, despite switching to a NOAC, developed ischemic stroke nonetheless [31–34].

The results of our study showed that, in addition to the embolic factor linked directly to AF, patients with this condition who were taking NOACs and suffered ischemic stroke had higher odds of developing hypertension, diabetes mellitus, dyslipidemia, and cigarette smoking compared to patients without AF—factors that favor thrombogenic, proatherogenic, and proinflammatory mechanisms.

Although it is well known that hypertension is a major risk factor for ischemic stroke, the complexity of cerebrovascular problems associated with hypertension is generally underestimated. Hypertension causes structural vascular changes that increase peripheral resistance, even with a relaxed vascular bed, which predisposes patients to distal ischemia resulting from stenosis or occlusion.

Hypertension also causes degenerative changes in the small intracerebral arteries, which can lead to extravasation and the development of focal cerebral edema, as well as lacunar infarcts. The last classic atherosclerotic mechanism leads to transient cerebral ischemic attacks or cerebral ischemic stroke via embolism or hemodynamic perfusion abnormalities [35].

Diabetes mellitus is a model of chronic vascular disease. It induces changes in microcirculation through the synthesis of extracellular matrix proteins and a thickening of the capillary basement membrane. These changes, in combination with advanced glycation end-products, oxidative stress, and inflammation, can lead to macroangiopathy. The risk for ischemic stroke in patients with diabetes is closely correlated with the severity and type of diabetes [36].

Cigarette smoking is an extremely important and independent risk factor for ischemic stroke, as confirmed by numerous studies. Probable mechanisms increasing the risk of ischemic stroke in smokers are numerous and include increased platelet aggregation, increased fibrinogen levels, and the direct effects of 1,3-Butadiene in tobacco smoke. These mechanisms accelerate atherosclerotic processes. Interestingly, it has been suggested that the risk of ischemic stroke in the smoking population is related to a chronic inflammation that leads to advanced atherosclerosis of the intracerebral and cerebral vessels [37,38].

The role of dyslipidemia in the pathogenesis of ischemic stroke, although initially unclear, is now given more credence. Dyslipidemia is a modifiable risk factor for vasculopathy [39].

Our study also showed that patients taking NOACs were significantly more likely to have non-modifiable factors—namely older age and female gender—than patients without AF.

Aging is associated with a multitude of changes in the hemostatic system. Increased procoagulant activity and a prothrombotic state are inherent in aging, through increased concentrations of procoagulant factors, thrombin formation, and platelet activation. Aging is also associated with increased levels of fibrin and fibrinogen degradation products [40,41]. All of these changes can be considered aspects of physiological aging or are provoked by other abnormalities such as chronic inflammation, malnutrition, and decreased physical activity.

Our study had several limitations. First, it was a retrospective study. Second, reference to specific types of NOAC was not possible because of the limited number of cases. Third, the time of the last administration of a NOAC was unknown in many cases. Fourth, we were unable to determine whether patients previously treated with a NOAC had their dose adjusted according to their age, weight, and creatinine levels. Fifth, only the most common risk factors for ischemic stroke were considered. Sixth, we had no information about therapy, especially those that might affect AF, such as angiotensin-converting-enzyme inhibitors, beta-blockers, and statins. Seventh, we had no information about data regarding some critical risk factors of ischemic stroke: diet (high in sodium, high in red meat, low in fruits, low in vegetables, low in fiber, and low in whole grains), alcohol consumption (any dosage), low physical activity, high BMI, high fasting plasma glucose, high systolic blood pressure, high low-density lipoprotein cholesterol, and kidney dysfunction, as measured by low glomerular filtration rate (GFR).

However, our study had some strengths. We analyzed a large group of patients with ischemic stroke that occurred during NOAC treatment. To the best of our knowledge, the risk factor profile of patients with ischemic stroke with NVAF who take NOAC has not been previously studied or reported on. Our study showed that in addition to the embolic factor linked directly to AF, patients with this condition who were taking NOACs were significantly more likely to have factors that favor thrombogenic, proatherogenic, and proinflammatory mechanisms than patients without AF. NOAC treatment is insufficient in protecting this group of patients against ischemic stroke. We presume that combination strategies, adding antiplatelet therapy or left atrial appendage occlusion to oral anticoagulation, might be helpful for this group of patients, but this requires further investigation in controlled trials.

5. Conclusions

The results of our study show that patients with NVAF treated with NOACs are more likely to display thrombotic, proatherogenic, and proinflammatory factors in addition to the embolic factors associated with AF. Therefore, solely ingesting NOAC is insufficient in protecting this group of patients from ischemic stroke. In light of the aforementioned data, primary or secondary prevention of ischemic stroke in this group of patients requires a modification of lifestyle, better health education, increased attention to therapeutic recommendations, and regular exercise, even at minimal intensity.

Author Contributions: Conceptualization, P.W.; Formal analysis, P.W., J.S., A.D., M.N.-K., A.S. and I.R.; Investigation, P.W., J.S., A.D., M.N.-K., A.S. and I.R.; Methodology, P.W.; Supervision, I.R.; Writing—original draft, P.W., J.S., A.D., M.N.-K., A.S. and I.R.; Writing—review and editing, P.W., J.S., A.D., M.N.-K., A.S. and I.R. All authors have read and agreed to the published version of the manuscript.

Funding: This research received no external funding.

Institutional Review Board Statement: The study was conducted according to the guidelines of the Declaration of Helsinki, and approved by the Bioethics Committee of the Pomeranian Medical University in Szczecin was received (KB-0012/49/07/2020/Z; 29 July 2020).

Informed Consent Statement: Informed consent was obtained from all subjects involved in the study.

Data Availability Statement: All data that support the findings of this study are available upon request from the corresponding author.

Conflicts of Interest: The authors have declared that no competing interest exist.

References

1. Zoni-Berisso, M.; Lercari, F.; Carazza, T.; Domenicucci, S. Epidemiology of atrial fibrillation: European perspective. *Clin. Epidemiol.* **2014**, *6*, 213–220. [CrossRef] [PubMed]
2. Wolowacz, S.E.; Samuel, M.; Brennan, V.K.; Jasso-Mosqueda, J.G.; Van Gelder, I.C. The cost of illness of atrial fibrillation: A systematic review of the recent literature. *Europace* **2011**, *13*, 1375–1385. [CrossRef]
3. Friberg, L.; Bergfeldt, L. Atrial fibrillation prevalence revisited. *J. Intern. Med.* **2013**, *274*, 461–468. [CrossRef] [PubMed]
4. Go, A.S.; Hylek, E.M.; Phillips, K.A.; Chang, Y.; Henault, L.E.; Selby, J.V.; Singer, D.E. Prevalence of diagnosed atrial fibrillation in adults: National implications for rhythm management and stroke prevention: The AnTicoagulation and Risk Factors in Atrial Fibrillation (ATRIA) Study. *JAMA* **2001**, *285*, 2370–2375. [CrossRef]
5. Krijthe, B.P.; Kunst, A.; Benjamin, E.J.; Lip, G.Y.; Franco, O.H.; Hofman, A.; Witteman, J.C.; Stricker, B.H.; Heeringa, J. Projections on the number of individuals with atrial fibrillation in the European Union, from 2000 to 2060. *Eur. Hear J.* **2013**, *34*, 2746–2751. [CrossRef]
6. Becker, E.I.; Jung, A.; Völler, H.; Wegscheider, K.; Vogel, H.P.; Landgraf, H. Cardiogenic embolism as the main cause of ischemic stroke in a city hospital: An interdisciplinary study. *Vasa* **2001**, *30*, 43–52. [CrossRef]
7. Johnson, W.D.; Ganjoo, A.; Stone, C.D.; Srivyas, R.C.; Howard, M. The left atrial appendage: Our most lethal human attachment! Surgical implications. *Eur. J. Cardio-Thorac. Surg.* **2000**, *17*, 718–722. [CrossRef]
8. Olsson, S.B.; Halperin, J.L. Prevention of stroke in patients with atrial fibrillation. *Semin. Vasc. Med.* **2005**, *5*, 285–292. [CrossRef]
9. Connolly, S.J.; Ezekowitz, M.D.; Yusuf, S.; Eikelboom, J.; Oldgren, J.; Parekh, A.; Pogue, J.; Reilly, P.A.; Themeles, E.; Varrone, J.; et al. Dabigatran versus warfarin in patients with atrial fibrillation. *N. Engl. J. Med.* **2009**, *361*, 1139–1151. [CrossRef]
10. Patel, M.R.; Mahaffey, K.W.; Garg, J.; Pan, G.; Singer, D.E.; Hacke, W.; Breithardt, G.; Halperin, J.L.; Hankey, G.J.; Piccini, J.P.; et al. Investigators. Rivaroxaban versus warfarin in nonvalvular atrial fibrillation. *N. Engl. J. Med.* **2011**, *365*, 883–891. [CrossRef]
11. Granger, C.B.; Alexander, J.H.; McMurray, J.J.; Lopes, R.D.; Hylek, E.M.; Hanna, M.; Al-Khalidi, H.R.; Ansell, J.; Atar, D.; Avezum, A.; et al. Apixaban versus warfarin in patients with atrial fibrillation. *N. Engl. J. Med.* **2011**, *365*, 981–992. [CrossRef] [PubMed]
12. Giugliano, R.P.; Ruff, C.T.; Braunwald, E.; Murphy, S.A.; Wiviott, S.D.; Halperin, J.L.; Waldo, A.L.; Ezekowitz, M.D.; Weitz, J.I.; Špinar, J.; et al. Edoxaban versus warfarin in patients with atrial fibrillation. *N. Engl. J. Med.* **2013**, *369*, 2093–2104. [CrossRef]

13. Diener, H.-C.; Connolly, S.J.; Ezekowitz, M.D.; Wallentin, L.; Reilly, P.A.; Yang, S.; Xavier, D.; Di Pasquale, G.; Yusuf, S.; RE-LY Study Group. Dabigatran compared with warfarin in patients with atrial fibrillation and previous transient ischaemic attack or stroke: A subgroup analysis of the RE-LY trial. *Lancet Neurol.* **2010**, *9*, 1157–1163. [CrossRef]
14. Rost, N.S.; Giugliano, R.P.; Ruff, C.T.; Murphy, S.A.; Crompton, A.E.; Norden, A.D.; Silverman, S.; Singhal, A.B.; Nicolau, J.C.; SomaRaju, B.; et al. Outcomes With Edoxaban Versus Warfarin in Patients With Previous Cerebrovascular Events: Findings From ENGAGE AF-TIMI 48 (Effective Anticoagulation With Factor Xa Next Generation in Atrial Fibrillation-Thrombolysis in Myocardial Infarction 48). *Stroke* **2016**, *47*, 2075–2082. [CrossRef] [PubMed]
15. Benjamin, E.J.; Levy, D.; Vaziri, S.M.; D'Agostino, R.B.; Belanger, A.J.; Wolf, P.A. Independent risk factors for atrial fibrillation in a population-based cohort. The Framingham Heart Study. *JAMA* **1994**, *271*, 840–844. [CrossRef] [PubMed]
16. Psaty, B.M.; Manolio, T.A.; Kuller, L.H.; Kronmal, R.A.; Cushman, M.; Fried, L.P.; White, R.; Furberg, C.D.; Rautaharju, P.M. Incidence of and risk factors for atrial fibrillation in older adults. *Circulation* **1997**, *96*, 2455–2461. [CrossRef] [PubMed]
17. Conen, D.; Tedrow, U.B.; Koplan, B.A.; Glynn, R.J.; Buring, J.E.; Albert, C.M. Influence of systolic and diastolic blood pressure on the risk of incident atrial fibrillation in women. *Circulation* **2009**, *119*, 2146–2152. [CrossRef]
18. Huxley, R.R.; Lopez, F.L.; Folsom, A.R.; Agarwal, S.K.; Loehr, L.R.; Soliman, E.Z.; Maclehose, R.; Konety, S.; Alonso, A. Absolute and attributable risks of atrial fibrillation in relation to optimal and borderline risk factors: The Atherosclerosis Risk in Communities (ARIC) study. *Circulation* **2011**, *123*, 1501–1508. [CrossRef]
19. Nalliah, C.J.; Sanders, P.; Kottkamp, H.; Kalman, J.M. The role of obesity in atrial fibrillation. *Eur. Hear J.* **2016**, *37*, 1565–1572. [CrossRef]
20. Wańkowicz, P.; Nowacki, P.; Gołąb-Janowska, M. Atrial fibrillation risk factors in patients with ischemic stroke. *Arch. Med. Sci.* **2021**, *17*, 19–24. [CrossRef]
21. Powers, W.J.; Rabinstein, A.A.; Ackerson, T.; Adeoye, O.M.; Bambakidis, N.C.; Becker, K.; Biller, J.; Brown, M.; Demaerschalk, B.M.; Hoh, B. Guidelines for the Early Management of Patients With Acute Ischemic Stroke: 2019 Update to the 2018 Guidelines for the Early Management of Acute Ischemic Stroke: A Guideline for Healthcare Professionals From the American Heart Association/American Stroke Association. *Stroke* **2019**, *50*, e344–e418. [PubMed]
22. Steinberg, J.S.; O'Connell, H.; Li, S.; Ziegler, P.D. Thirty-Second Gold Standard Definition of Atrial Fibrillation and Its Relationship With Subsequent Arrhythmia Patterns: Analysis of a Large Prospective Device Database. *Circ. Arrhythm. Electrophysiol.* **2018**, *11*, e006274. [CrossRef] [PubMed]
23. Mancia, G.; De Backer, G.; Dominiczak, A.; Cifkova, R.; Fagard, R.; Germano, G.; Grassi, G.; Heagerty, A.M.; Kjeldsen, S.E.; Laurent, S.; et al. 2007 Guidelines for the Management of Arterial Hypertension: The Task Force for the Management of Arterial Hypertension of the European Society of Hypertension (ESH) and of the European Society of Cardiology (ESC). *J. Hypertens.* **2007**, *25*, 1105–1187. [CrossRef]
24. Tahrani, A.A.; Bailey, C.J.; Del Prato, S.; Barnett, A.H. Management of type 2 diabetes: New and future developments in treatment. *Lancet* **2011**, *378*, 182–197. [CrossRef]
25. Grundy, S.M.; Cleeman, J.I.; Merz, C.N.B.; Brewer, H.B.; Clark, L.T.; Hunninghake, D.B.; Pasternak, R.C.; Smith, S.C.; Stone, N.J. Implications of recent clinical trials for the National Cholesterol Education Program Adult Treatment Panel III guidelines. *Circulation* **2004**, *110*, 227–239. [CrossRef]
26. Inzitari, D.; Eliasziw, M.; Gates, P.; Sharpe, B.L.; Chan, R.K.; Meldrum, H.E.; Barnett, H.J. The causes and risk of stroke in patients with asymptomatic internal-carotid-artery stenosis. North American Symptomatic Carotid Endarterectomy Trial Collaborators. *N. Engl. J. Med.* **2000**, *342*, 1693–1700. [CrossRef]
27. Halliday, A.; Harrison, M.; Hayter, E.; Kong, X.; Mansfield, A.; Marro, J.; Pan, H.; Peto, R.; Potter, J.; Rahimi, K.; et al. 10-year stroke prevention after successful carotid endarterectomy for asymptomatic stenosis (ACST-1): A multicentre randomised trial. *Lancet* **2010**, *376*, 1074–1084. [CrossRef]
28. Hart, R.G.; Pearce, L.A.; Aguilar, M.I. Meta-analysis: Antithrombotic therapy to prevent stroke in patients who have nonvalvular atrial fibrillation. *Ann. Intern. Med.* **2007**, *146*, 857–867. [CrossRef]
29. Tokunaga, K.; Koga, M.; Itabashi, R.; Yamagami, H.; Todo, K.; Yoshimura, S.; Kimura, K.; Sato, S.; Terasaki, T.; Inoue, M.; et al. Prior Anticoagulation and Short- or Long-Term Clinical Outcomes in Ischemic Stroke or Transient Ischemic Attack Patients With Nonvalvular Atrial Fibrillation. *J. Am. Heart Assoc.* **2019**, *8*. [CrossRef] [PubMed]
30. Evans, A.; Perez, I.; Yu, G.; Kalra, L. Should stroke subtype influence anticoagulation decisions to prevent recurrence in stroke patients with atrial fibrillation? *Stroke* **2001**, *32*, 2828–2832. [CrossRef] [PubMed]
31. D'Andrea, G.; D'Ambrosio, R.L.; Di Perna, P.; Chetta, M.; Santacroce, R.; Brancaccio, V.; Grandone, E.; Margaglione, M. A polymorphism in the VKORC1 gene is associated with an interindividual variability in the dose-anticoagulant effect of warfarin. *Blood* **2005**, *105*, 645–649. [CrossRef]
32. Wadelius, M.; Chen, L.Y.; Downes, K.; Ghori, J.; Hunt, S.; Eriksson, N.; Wallerman, O.; Melhus, H.; Bentley, D.; Deloukas, P.; et al. Common VKORC1 and GGCX polymorphisms associated with warfarin dose. *Pharm. J.* **2005**, *5*, 262–270. [CrossRef]
33. Anderson, J.L.; Horne, B.D.; Stevens, S.M.; Grove, A.S.; Barton, S.; Nicholas, Z.P.; Kahn, S.F.; May, H.T.; Samuelson, K.M.; Muhlestein, J.B.; et al. Randomized trial of genotype-guided versus standard warfarin dosing in patients initiating oral anticoagulation. *Circulation* **2007**, *116*, 2563–2570. [CrossRef]
34. International Warfarin Pharmacogenetics Consortium; Klein, T.E.; Altman, R.B.; Eriksson, N.; Gage, B.F.; Kimmel, S.E.; Lee, M.-T.M.; Limdi, N.A.; Page, D.; Roden, D.M.; et al. Estimation of the warfarin dose with clinical and pharmacogenetic data. *N. Engl. J. Med.* **2009**, *360*, 753–764. [PubMed]

35. Johansson, B.B. Hypertension mechanisms causing stroke. *Clin. Exp. Pharmacol. Physiol.* **1999**, *26*, 563–565. [CrossRef] [PubMed]
36. Chawla, A.; Chawla, R.; Jaggi, S. Microvascular and macrovascular complications in diabetes mellitus: Distinct or continuum? *Indian J. Endocrinol. Metab.* **2016**, *20*, 546–551. [CrossRef] [PubMed]
37. Shah, R.S.; Cole, J.W. Smoking and stroke: The more you smoke the more you stroke. *Expert Rev. Cardiovasc. Ther.* **2010**, *8*, 917–932. [CrossRef]
38. Mannami, T.; Iso, H.; Baba, S.; Sasaki, S.; Okada, K.; Konishi, M.; Tsugane, S. Cigarette smoking and risk of stroke and its subtypes among middle-aged Japanese men and women: The JPHC Study Cohort I. *Stroke* **2004**, *35*, 1248–1253. [CrossRef]
39. Heart Protection Study Collaborative Group. Effects on 11-year mortality and morbidity of lowering LDL cholesterol with simvastatin for about 5 years in 20,536 high-risk individuals: A randomised controlled trial. *Lancet* **2011**, *378*, 2013–2020. [CrossRef]
40. Aw, D.; Silva, A.B.; Palmer, D.B. Immunosenescence: Emerging challenges for an ageing population. *Immunology* **2007**, *120*, 435–446. [CrossRef] [PubMed]
41. Sanada, F.; Taniyama, Y.; Muratsu, J.; Otsu, R.; Shimizu, H.; Rakugi, H.; Morishita, R. Source of Chronic Inflammation in Aging. *Front. Cardiovasc. Med.* **2018**, *5*, 12. [CrossRef] [PubMed]

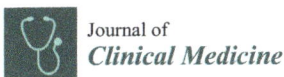 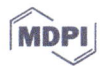

Article

Atrial Fibrillation Increases the Risk of Early-Onset Dementia in the General Population: Data from a Population-Based Cohort

Dongmin Kim [1,2,†], Pil-Sung Yang [3,†], Gregory Y.H. Lip [4,*] and Boyoung Joung [5]

1. Division of Cardiology, Department of Internal Medicine, College of Medicine, Dankook University, Cheonan-si, Chungnam 31116, Korea; kdongmin@dkuh.co.kr
2. Department of Medicine, The Graduate School, Yonsei University, Seoul 03722, Korea
3. Department of Cardiology, CHA Bundang Medical Centre, CHA University, Seongnam 13496, Korea; psyang01@cha.ac.kr
4. Liverpool Centre for Cardiovascular Science, University of Liverpool and Liverpool Heart & Chest Hospital, Liverpool L14 3PE, UK
5. Division of Cardiology, Department of Internal Medicine, Severance Cardiovascular Hospital, Yonsei University College of Medicine, Seoul 03722, Korea; cby6908@yuhs.ac
* Correspondence: gregory.lip@liverpool.ac.uk; Tel.: +82-2-2228-846
† The first two authors contributed equally to this work.

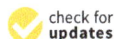

Received: 22 October 2020; Accepted: 9 November 2020; Published: 14 November 2020

Abstract: Atrial fibrillation (AF) is considered a risk factor for dementia, especially in the elderly. However, the association between the two diseases is not well identified in different age subgroups. The association of incident AF with the development of dementia was assessed from 1 January 2005, to 31 December 2013, in 428,262 participants from a longitudinal cohort (the Korea National Health Insurance Service-Health Screening cohort). In total, 10,983 participants were diagnosed with incident AF during the follow-up period. The incidence of dementia was 11.3 and 3.0 per 1000 person-years in the incident-AF and without-AF groups, respectively. After adjustment for clinical variables, the risk of dementia was significantly elevated by incident AF, with a hazard ratio (HR) of 1.98 (95% confidence interval [CI]: 1.80–2.17, $p < 0.001$), even after censoring for stroke (HR: 1.74, 95% CI: 1.55–1.94, $p < 0.001$). The HRs of incident AF for dementia onset before the age of 65 (early-onset dementia) and for onset after the age of 65 (late-onset dementia) were 2.91 (95% CI: 1.93–4.41) and 1.67 (95% CI: 1.49–1.87), respectively. Younger participants with AF were more prone to dementia development than older participants with AF (p for trend < 0.001). AF was associated with an increased risk of both early- and late-onset dementia, independent of clinical stroke.

Keywords: atrial fibrillation; dementia; early-onset; prognosis; age

1. Introduction

With the aging of the population, atrial fibrillation (AF) and dementia have become important health-care problems worldwide. AF is the most common sustained cardiac arrhythmia and is widespread in the older age group, leading to substantial public health and economic burdens [1,2]. Patients with AF have an increased risk of mortality and morbidity due to stroke, congestive heart failure, and hospitalization, in association with an increase in comorbid chronic diseases [3].

Approximately 40 million people worldwide have dementia, and this number is projected to increase owing to population aging [4]. Although the exact mechanism of the pathophysiology of dementia has not been well elucidated, a growing body of evidence suggests that AF might contribute to the development of cognitive dysfunction and dementia [5–8]. Oral anticoagulant therapy was associated with a reduced risk of developing dementia in an elderly AF population [8].

In contrast to the aged population, there is little evidence on the association of AF and early-onset dementia (EOD), with onset at age < 65 years. EOD can be a more devastating condition affecting patients who still have an active socioeconomic involvement.

In this study, we investigated the association between incident AF and the risk of EOD and late-onset dementia (LOD) in a general population cohort including middle-aged groups, using the nationwide population-based database of the Korea National Health Insurance Service-Health Screening (NHIS-HEALS) [9].

2. Experimental Section

2.1. Source of Study Data

This study was based on Korea NHIS-HEALS data released in 2015 [9]. The dataset included 514,866 Koreans comprising a 10% random sample of all health-screened participants aged 40–79 years as an initial 2002–2003 cohort, who were followed-up through 2013 with data related to lifestyle and behavior from a questionnaire survey and the major results of health examinations. The NHIS-HEALS database incorporates sociodemographic information of the beneficiaries, a medical claims dataset including information on diagnosis based on the 10th revision of the International Classification of Disease (ICD-10) codes, medical bill details, medical treatments, disease histories, prescription drug use, and personal information of inpatients and outpatients in the National Health Information Database. The national health screening program is conducted biennially and includes regular blood tests, chest radiographic examinations, physical examination, and questionnaire survey on medical history. The date and cause of death of individual participants were extracted from the death registration database of the Korea National Statistical office and were linked to the NHIS-HEALS database. The Korean social security numbers linked every individual in the cohort, and all social security numbers were deleted after constructing the cohort by assigning serial numbers to prevent leakage of personal information. This study was approved by the Institutional Review Board of the Yonsei University Health System (Seoul, Republic of Korea, IRB No, 4-2020-0827), and the need for informed consent was waived.

2.2. Study Population

From the Korean NHIS-HEALS database, a total of 457,510 individuals who underwent a health check-up between 2005 and 2010 were enrolled. Follow-up data were reviewed until December 2013. Participants with the following conditions were excluded: (i) valvular heart disease (presence of prosthetic heart valves, diagnosis of mitral stenosis, or insurance claims for valve replacement or valvuloplasty) (n = 1606), (ii) a history of ischemic stroke or transient ischemic attack before enrollment (n = 22,515), (iii) a history of hemorrhagic stroke before enrollment (n = 1130), (iv) a diagnosis of dementia before enrollment (n = 506), and (v) a diagnosis of AF before enrollment (n = 3491). Finally, we included 428,262 participants, among whom 10,983 had incident AF during the follow-up period (Figure 1).

The definition of AF was based on ICD-10 code I48. To ensure diagnostic accuracy, participants were considered to have AF only when AF was a discharge diagnosis or had been confirmed at least twice in the outpatient department. The positive predictive value of this definition of AF was 94.1% and was previously validated in the NHIS database [1,2,8].

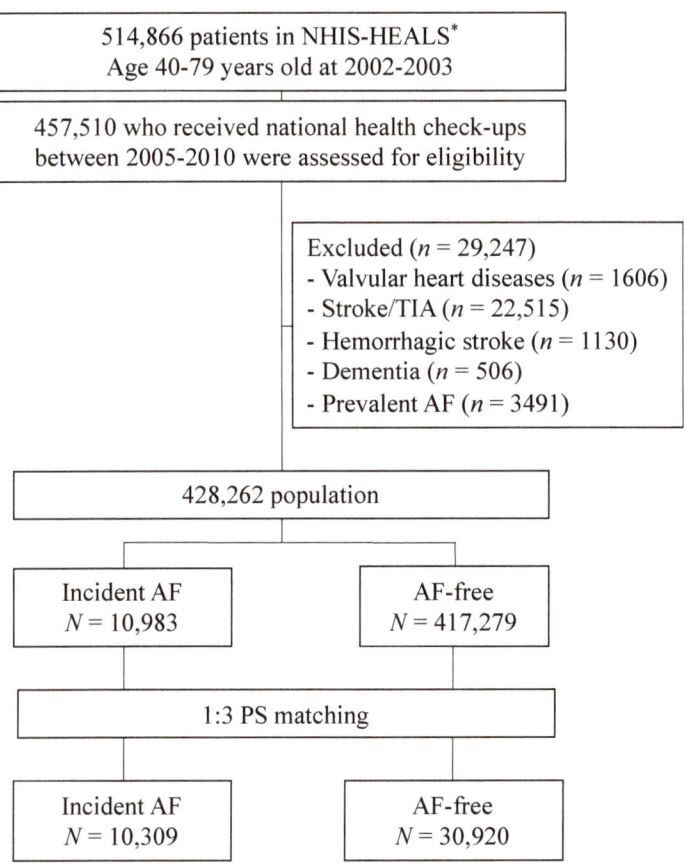

Figure 1. Flowchart of the enrollment procedure of the study population and analyses. TIA, transient ischemic attack; AF, atrial fibrillation. * The National Health Insurance Service-Health Screening Cohort (NHIS-HEALS) in Korea.

2.3. Assessment of Dementia

Patients with dementia are registered in the national registry for severe disease and can receive medical expense reductions from the Korean government. Therefore, the assignment of the dementia diagnostic code is well controlled. The diagnosis of dementia was defined using the ICD-10 codes for dementia (F00 or G30 for Alzheimer's dementia, F01 for vascular dementia, F02 for dementia with other diseases classified elsewhere, and F03 or G31 for unspecified dementia) with prescription of dementia drugs (rivastigmine, galantamine, memantine, or donepezil). To evaluate the accuracy of our definition of dementia, a validation study was conducted at two teaching hospitals with a total of 972 patients, using the medical records of the patients and the results of cognitive function tests. The positive predictive value was 94.7%.

2.4. Covariates

The medical claims and information on prescribed medication prior to the index date were used to define baseline comorbidities. When the condition was a discharge diagnosis or had been confirmed at least twice in an outpatient department, then the participants were considered to have comorbidities, as in previous studies with the NHIS (Table S1) [1,2,8,10]. Baseline income status was estimated by the total amount of national health insurance premiums paid by the individual in the index year, proportional to the individual's income.

2.5. Statistical Analysis

The baseline characteristics of the participants with and without incident AF were compared using logistic regression models, adjusting for age and sex where appropriate. The association between incident AF and incident dementia was assessed by Cox proportional hazard regression models. Incident AF was entered into the models as a time-varying variable. Follow-up began on the date of enrollment into the study and ended on the date of dementia diagnosis, date of death, or end of the study period (31 December 2013; defined as the last date of follow-up), whichever came first. In model I, we adjusted for age and sex. In model II, we adjusted for additional covariates, including hypertension, diabetes mellitus, dyslipidemia, previous myocardial infarction, peripheral artery disease, heart failure, chronic kidney disease, osteoporosis, chronic obstructive lung disease, liver disease, history of a malignant neoplasm, economic status, cardiovascular medications (aspirin, P2Y12 inhibitor, statin, anticoagulation agents, beta-blockers, angiotensin-converting enzyme inhibitors or angiotensin receptor blockers, calcium channel blockers, digoxin, diuretics), body mass index, blood glucose level, total cholesterol, and alcohol and smoking habits. Missing values were excluded case-wise.

Stroke censoring was done for the sensitivity analyses. Participants were censored on the date of the stroke, if it developed before the end of the follow-up period. Any potential effect of age was assessed by stratifying the analysis at each decade of age and by using an interaction. Furthermore, propensity score matching was used to minimize potential systematic differences between the AF and the without-AF groups. The propensity scores for the incident AF of each study participant were calculated and adjusted for the above-mentioned variables in a logistic regression analysis. All tests were two-tailed, and $p < 0.05$ was considered significant. Statistical analyses were conducted with SAS version 9.4 (SAS Institute, Cary, NC, USA).

3. Results

3.1. Baseline Characteristics

Over a follow-up period of 310,6109 person-years, incident AF was diagnosed in 10,983 participants (3.5/1000 person-years). Participants with incident AF were older (age 61.7 ± 9.9 vs. 55.5 ± 9.1 years, $p < 0.001$), showed a male predominance, had more comorbidities, and were taking more cardiovascular medications. The follow-up duration was longer in the AF group (96 months, interquartile range (IQR) 86–101 months) than in the group without AF (93 months, IQR 84–100 months) ($p < 0.001$) (Table 1). At baseline, 0.44% of participants in the AF group received anticoagulation therapy. After diagnosis of AF, anticoagulation therapy was performed in 16.9% of participants in the AF group.

Table 1. Baseline characteristics.

	No AF	Incident AF	p-Value
	(N = 417,279)	(N = 10,983)	
Age, mean (SD), years	55.5 ± 9.1	61.7 ± 9.9	<0.001
Age > 65 No. (%)	74,143 (17.8)	4531 (41.3)	<0.001
Female, No. (%)	191,431 (45.9)	4318 (39.3)	0.002
BMI, mean (SD), kg/m^2	24.0 ± 2.9	24.3 ± 3.1	<0.001
SBP, mean (SD), mmHg	125.8 ± 16.6	130.2 ± 17.6	0.072
DBP, mean (SD), mmHg	78.4 ± 10.7	80.1 ± 11.0	0.038
Blood glucose, mean (SD), mg/dL	98.4 ± 26.8	101.9 ± 32.5	0.008
Total cholesterol, mean (SD), mg/dL	198.9 ± 36.9	195.4 ± 38.0	<0.001
Serum creatinine, mean (SD), mg/dL	0.99 ± 0.97	1.08 ± 1.02	0.75

Table 1. Cont.

	No AF	Incident AF	p-Value
	(N = 417,279)	(N = 10,983)	
Blood hemoglobin, mean (SD), mg/dL	13.9 ± 1.5	13.9 ± 1.5	0.012
Hypertension, No. (%)	94,332 (22.6)	4450 (40.5)	<0.001
Diabetes, No. (%)	31,483 (7.5)	1359 (12.4)	0.003
Dyslipidemia, No. (%)	95,735 (22.9)	3571 (32.5)	<0.001
Heart failure, No. (%)	10,191 (2.4)	977 (8.9)	<0.001
History of MI, No. (%)	3423 (0.8)	273 (2.5)	0.207
PAOD, No. (%)	7150 (1.7)	356 (3.2)	0.809
CKD or ESRD, No. (%)	2764 (0.7)	142 (1.3)	0.032
Osteoporosis, No. (%)	56,584 (13.6)	2042 (18.6)	<0.001
COPD, No. (%)	10,609 (2.5)	708 (6.5)	<0.001
History of liver disease, No. (%)	84,708 (20.3)	2828 (25.8)	<0.001
History of malignancy, No. (%)	27,063 (6.5)	1118 (10.2)	<0.001
CHA_2DS_2-VASc score	1.0 ± 1.0	1.6 ± 1.3	<0.001
Income level			0.095
Low, No. (%)	120,422 (28.9)	3354 (30.5)	
Middle, No. (%)	151,912 (36.4)	3868 (35.2)	
High, No. (%)	144,945 (34.7)	3761 (34.2)	
Smoking			0.571
No, No. (%)	283,087 (71.7)	7384 (71.4)	
Former, No. (%)	36,450 (9.2)	1060 (10.3)	
Current, No. (%)	75,477 (19.1)	1894 (18.3)	
Alcohol consumption			0.004
Low, No. (%)	308,731 (74.0)	8000 (72.8)	
Moderate, No. (%)	67,780 (16.2)	1610 (14.7)	
Heavy, No. (%)	40,768 (9.8)	1373 (12.5)	
Exercise			<0.001
None, No. (%)	7882 (1.9)	153 (1.4)	
Seldom, No. (%)	10,850 (2.6)	158 (1.4)	
Regular, No. (%)	398,547 (95.5)	10,672 (97.2)	
ACE inhibitor or ARB, No. (%)	39,615 (9.5)	1982 (18.1)	0.313
Beta-Blocker, No. (%)	37,528 (9.0)	2015 (18.4)	<0.001
Diuretics, No. (%)	44,803 (10.4)	2294 (20.9)	0.073
Potassium-sparing diuretics, No. (%)	3791 (0.9)	305 (2.8)	0.361
NDHP-CCB, No. (%)	3744 (0.9)	340 (3.1)	<0.001
DHP-CCB, No. (%)	53,735 (12.9)	2478 (22.6)	0.16
Digoxin, No. (%)	889 (0.2)	249 (2.3)	<0.001
Alpha-blocker, No. (%)	8574 (2.1)	490 (4.5)	0.805
Statin, No. (%)	25,263 (6.1)	1018 (9.3)	<0.001
Antiarrhythmic agents, No. (%)	139 (0.03)	46 (0.42)	<0.001
Aspirin, No. (%)	36,385 (8.7)	2034 (18.5)	<0.001
P_2Y_{12} inhibitor, No. (%)	2020 (0.5)	140 (1.3)	0.577
Anticoagulation, No. (%)	179 (0.04)	48 (0.44)	<0.001
F/U duration, median (IQR), months	93 (84, 100)	96 (86, 101)	<0.001

Values are expressed in No. (%), mean ± standard deviation (SD), or median (interquartile range; IQR). Abbreviation: BMI, body mass index; SBP, systolic blood pressure; DBP, diastolic blood pressure; MI, myocardial infarction; PAOD, peripheral artery occlusive disease; CKD, chronic kidney disease; ESRD, end-stage renal disease; COPD, chronic obstructive pulmonary disease; ACE, angiotensin-converting enzyme; ARB, angiotensin type II receptor blocker; NDHP, non-dihydropyridine; CCB, calcium channel blocker; DHP, dihydropyridine; F/U, follow-up; CHA2DS2-VASc score (congestive heart failure, blood pressure consistently above 140/90 mm Hg or treated hypertension on medication, age ≥ 75 years, diabetes mellitus, prior stroke, transient ischemic attack, or thromboembolism)–(vascular disease (e.g., peripheral artery disease, myocardial infarction, aortic plaque), age 65–74 years, female sex).

3.2. Risk of Dementia in the Overall Population

Compared to the group without AF, the cumulative incidence of dementia was higher in the incident-AF group (log-rank $p < 0.001$, Figure 2A). Among patients with incident AF, 880 (8.0%) participants developed dementia during 77,851 person-years of follow-up, compared with 9172 participants (2.2%) who developed dementia among patients without AF during 3,033,519 person-years. The incidence of dementia was 11.3 and 3.0 per 1000 person-years in the incident-AF and without-AF groups, respectively.

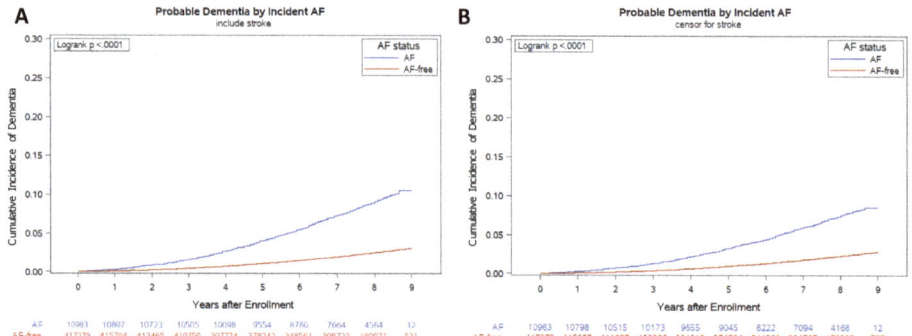

Figure 2. Cumulative incidence of dementia before (**A**) and after (**B**) censoring for stroke.

As quantified using the age- and sex-adjusted hazard ratios (HRs) with 95% confidence intervals (CIs), the risk of dementia was increased in participants with incident AF (HR: 2.06, 95% CI: 1.88–2.25). After additional adjustments for clinical variables, the risk of dementia was still significantly elevated by incident AF, with an HR of 1.98 (95% CI: 1.80–2.17) (Table 2, Figure 2A). Incident AF increased the risk of dementia in all decades of age. The risk of dementia due to AF was greater in young participants than in old participants (p for trend < 0.001) (Figure 3A).

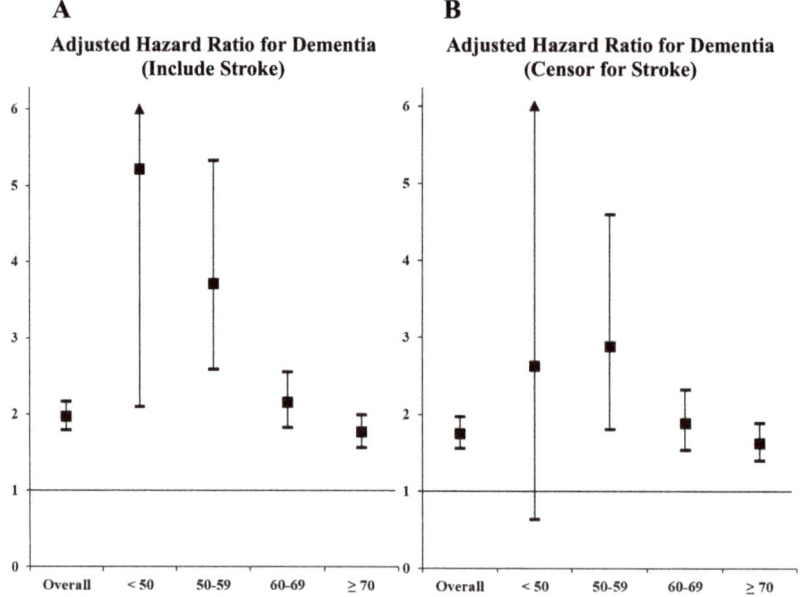

Figure 3. Hazard ratios for dementia per decade of age in the presence of AF. (**A**) Including stroke during the follow-up; (**B**) excluding stroke during the follow-up. The hazard ratios are expressed as boxes, the 95% confidence intervals are expressed as limit lines, and the horizontal line (at hazard ratio 1) indicates no difference in hazard ratios between the AF and the without-AF groups.

During the follow-up period, 12.7% and 2.0% of participants in the AF and without-AF groups developed stroke, respectively. After censoring for stroke, a higher cumulative incidence of dementia was observed in the incident-AF group than in the without-AF group (log-rank $p < 0.001$; Figure 2B). The incidence of dementia after censoring for stroke was 9.1 and 2.7 per 1000 person-years in the incident-AF and without-AF groups, respectively. Incident AF increased the risk of dementia, with an age- and sex-adjusted HR of 1.81 (95% CI: 1.63–2.02) and clinical variable-adjusted HR of 1.74 (95% CI: 1.55–1.94) (Table 2). After censoring for stroke, the trend of a greater risk of dementia due to AF in younger participants was still significant (p for trend < 0.001) (Figure 3B).

Table 2. Incidence of dementia during follow-up periods according to the AF status.

Dementia	Cases, No. (%)	Incidence *	Adjusted HR (95% CI)	
			Model I †	Model II ‡
Including Stroke				
Overall dementia				
No AF (n = 417,279)	9172 (2.2)	3.0	1.00 (Reference)	1.00 (Reference)
AF (n = 10,983)	880 (8.0)	11.3	2.06 (1.88–2.25)	1.98 (1.80–2.17)
Early-onset dementia				
No AF (n = 409,145)	1038 (0.3)	0.3	1.00	1.00
AF (n = 10,177)	74 (0.7)	1.0	3.93 (2.88–5.38)	3.81 (2.75–5.29)
Late-onset dementia				
No AF (n = 416,241)	8134 (2.0)	2.7	1.00	1.00
AF (n = 10,909)	806 (7.4)	10.4	1.95 (1.78–2.15)	1.88 (1.70–2.07)
Alzheimer Dementia				
No AF (n = 417,253)	6797 (1.6)	2.2	1.00	1.00
AF (n = 10,981)	611 (5.6)	7.8	1.76 (1.58–1.97)	1.69 (1.51–1.90)
Vascular Dementia				
No AF (n = 417,253)	1159 (0.3)	0.4	1.00	1.00
AF (n = 10,981)	151 (1.4)	1.9	3.45 (2.81–4.24)	3.22 (2.61–3.99)
Censored for Stroke				
Overall dementia				
No AF (n = 417,279)	8246 (2.0)	2.7	1.00	1.00
AF (n = 10,983)	680 (6.2)	9.1	1.81 (1.63–2.02)	1.74 (1.55–1.94)
Early-onset dementia				
No AF (n = 409,145)	902 (0.2)	0.3	1.00	1.00
AF (n = 10,177)	53 (0.5)	0.7	2.92 (1.95–4.36)	2.91 (1.93–4.41)
Late-onset dementia				
No AF (n = 416,241)	7344 (1.8)	2.4	1.00	1.00
AF (n = 10,909)	627 (5.7)	8.4	1.75 (1.57–1.95)	1.67 (1.49–1.87)
Alzheimer Dementia				
No AF (n = 417,253)	6246 (1.5)	2.1	1.00	1.00
AF (n = 10,981)	493 (4.5)	6.6	1.61 (1.41–1.82)	1.54 (1.35–1.76)
Vascular Dementia				
No AF (n = 417,253)	911 (0.2)	0.3	1.00	1.00
AF (n = 10,981)	91 (0.8)	1.2	2.82 (2.16–3.67)	2.57 (1.95–3.38)

HR, hazard ratio. * Incidence: per 1000 person-year † Model I was adjusted for age and sex. ‡ Model II was additionally adjusted for hypertension, diabetes mellitus, dyslipidemia, heart failure, previous myocardial infarction, peripheral artery disease, osteoporosis, chronic kidney disease, chronic obstructive pulmonary disease, malignant neoplasm, liver disease, CHA2DS2-VASc score, cardiovascular medications (e.g., ACE inhibitors or ARB, beta-blockers, diuretics, statin, alpha-blockers, K-sparing diuretics, digoxin, calcium channel blockers, antiarrhythmic drugs, aspirin, P2Y12 inhibitors, oral anticoagulants), economic status, alcohol consumption, smoking status, exercise habits, follow-up duration, body mass index, systolic and diastolic blood pressure, blood glucose, total cholesterol, and blood hemoglobin level.

3.3. Risk of EOD and LOD

During the follow-up, EOD developed at a rate of 1.0 case per 1000 person-years and 0.3 cases per 1000 person-years in the AF and without-AF groups, respectively. Among EOD cases, Alzheimer's dementia regarded 65.4% of the patients, whereas vascular and other types of dementia regarded 20.0% and 14.7% of the patients, respectively. AF showed a significantly higher association with EOD (clinical variable-adjusted HR: 3.81, 95% CI: 2.75–5.29) than with LOD (clinical variable-adjusted HR: 1.88, 95% CI: 1.70–2.07).

After censoring for stroke, incident AF increased the risk of both EOD and LOD, with clinical variable-adjusted HRs of 2.91 (95% CI: 1.93–4.41) and 1.67 (95% CI: 1.49–1.87), respectively (Table 2).

3.4. Risk of Dementia According to the Type of Dementia

Of all dementia cases, 73.7%, 13.0%, and 13.3% were classified as Alzheimer's dementia, vascular dementia, and other dementia, respectively. In the AF group, Alzheimer's dementia developed in 5.6% of participants, whereas 1.5% of patients in the without-AF group had Alzheimer's dementia. The clinical variable-adjusted HRs for Alzheimer's dementia were 1.69 (95% CI: 1.51–1.90) and 1.54 (95% CI: 1.35–1.76), including and censoring for stroke events during the observational period, respectively. The risk of vascular dementia was significantly high in the AF group (HR: 3.22, 95% CI: 2.61–3.99). After censoring for stroke, the HR for vascular dementia was still higher in the AF group than in the without-AF group (HR: 2.57, 95% CI: 1.95–3.38) (Table 2).

3.5. Subgroup Analyses

The risk of dementia was significantly increased in all subgroups of the incident-AF group compared to the without-AF group, except in patients with chronic kidney disease and previous myocardial infarction (Figure 4).

3.6. Sensitivity Analysis with a Propensity Score-Matched Population

With propensity score matching, the baseline characteristics of the incident-AF and without-AF groups became similar (Table S2). As quantified by age- and sex-adjusted HRs (95% CI), patients with incident AF had an elevated risk for dementia (HR: 1.90, 95% CI: 1.72–2.11). After additional clinical variable adjustments, the risk of dementia was still significantly elevated by incident AF, with an HR of 1.89 (95% CI: 1.70–2.09) (Tables S3 and S4, Figure S1A). The increased risk for dementia of younger participants with incident AF was still significant (Figure S2A).

The cumulative incidence of stroke-censored dementia was higher in the incident-AF group than the without-AF group (log-rank $p < 0.001$; Figure S1B). The incidence of stroke-censored dementia per 1000 person-years was 9.1 and 6.4 in the incident-AF and without-AF groups, respectively. Incident AF increased the risk of dementia, with an age- and sex-adjusted HR of 1.68 (95% CI: 1.49–1.89) and a clinical variable-adjusted HR of 1.65 (95% CI: 1.46–1.86) (Tables S3 and S4). After censoring for stroke, incident AF elevated the risk of dementia in those older than 50 years (Figure S2B). Both EOD and LOD were associated with AF. The greater risk of EOD than LOD due to AF was also observed in the propensity score-matched population (Table S3).

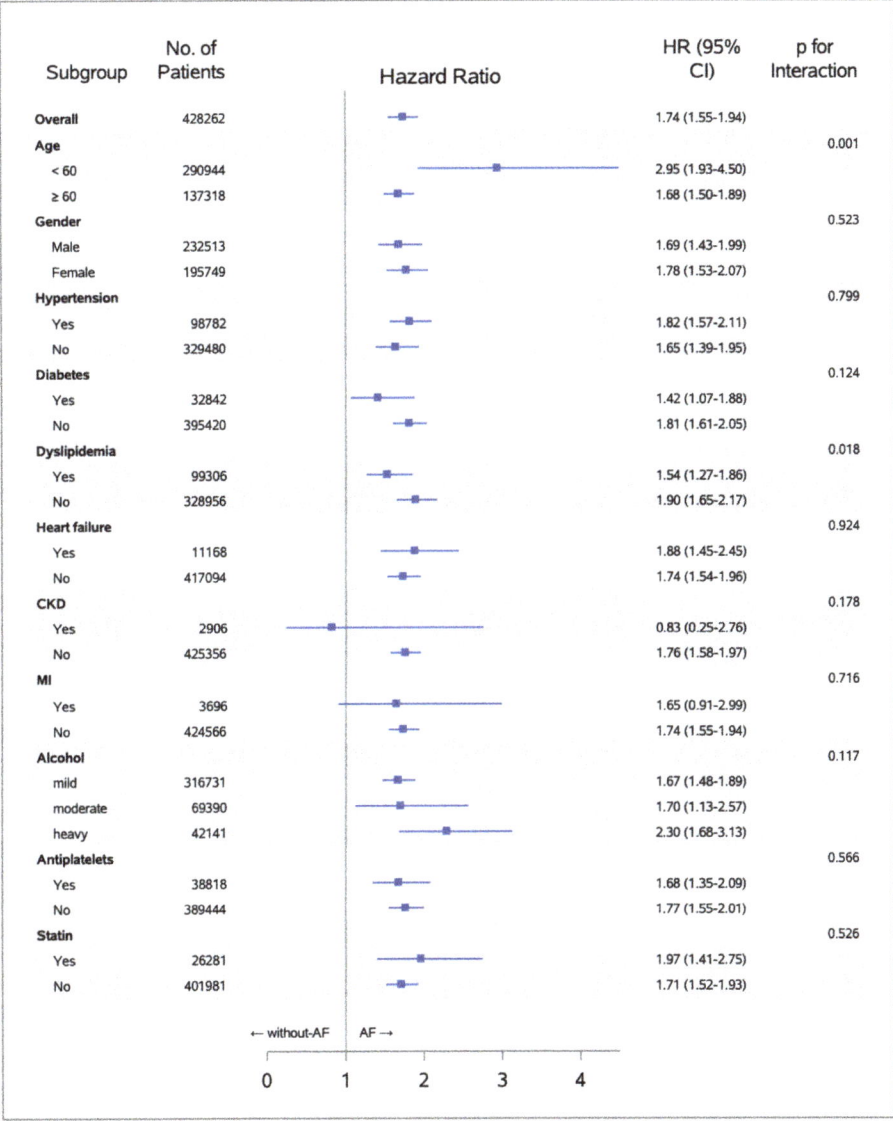

Figure 4. Subgroup analysis for the risk of dementia according to the AF status. The hazard ratios and the 95% confidence intervals are expressed as boxes and limit lines, respectively. The vertical line (at hazard ratio 1) indicates no difference in hazard ratios between AF and without-AF groups.

4. Discussion

Our findings from this population-based study are consistent with those of previous studies, indicating that incident AF is associated with an elevated risk of dementia. In addition, we found this relationship was independent of clinical stroke and was significant in different age subgroups. AF was also associated with an elevated risk of EOD, and the risk of dementia due to AF was greater in younger participants. These results suggest a strong association between AF and dementia in various age groups.

Previous studies have shown that the risk of dementia is associated with AF. However, various associations according to age were observed in different studies. In one study, AF increased the risk of dementia only in the younger age group [11]. In contrast, another study showed that only late-life AF was associated with dementia [12]. Previously, we reported similar results showing that AF increased the risk of dementia in an elderly population aged over 60 years from the Korean NIHS cohort [8]. In that study, AF was associated with all age groups. In the present study, we showed that the association was significant for middle- and late-life AF. The risk of dementia was higher in the younger age group.

Various mechanisms are suggested for the relationship between AF and dementia [13–15], including vascular mechanisms closely related to both Alzheimer's disease and vascular dementia [16, 17]. Stroke might also be a main mechanism of this association. The association between AF and dementia was stronger in individuals with both AF and stroke at baseline than in those without stroke at baseline. These findings support a possible interaction of stroke with AF and dementia. Although the association remained significant after censoring for stroke in our study, subclinical cerebral infarctions are known to be related to both AF and dementia [18].

Stroke is also known as a risk factor for EOD [19]. Various etiologies can result in presenile dementia, including genetic factors. Although genetic factors are considered strong risk factors for EOD in affected patients, familial dementia is extremely rare, and a very small proportion of EOD was attributable to familial dementia. Previous studies indicated that vascular risk factors including stroke might be more potent risk factors than genetic causes [19]. One study showed that stroke increased the risk of EOD by about three times. Another cross-sectional study showed a high prevalence of stroke or transient ischemic attack in the EOD group. In that study, other vascular risk factors, such as chronic kidney disease, ischemic heart disease, diabetes, hypertension, and peripheral vascular disease, were associated with EOD [20].

However, the effect of AF on EOD has not been well identified. In this study, incident AF was associated with an increased risk of dementia, even after censoring for stroke during follow-up and adjusting for vascular risk factors. Interestingly, while AF increased the risk of EOD by 3.88 times, it increased the risk of LOD by 1.88 times. Although we cannot provide the exact reason for this discrepancy, it might be explained by the causes of cerebrovascular events at a young age. Cardio-embolic stroke accounted for a significant proportion of the etiologies of stroke in the young-age group [21].

In terms of long-term effects of AF, a study proposed that the reason for the strong association between AF and dementia in the young-age group is the latent effect of AF, similar to those of other dementia risk factors, which also seems to differ with age [11]. Although the direct latent effect of AF on dementia could not be elucidated in this study, the vulnerability to dementia development was high in the young-age group, which supports the latent effect of AF.

Limitations of the present study were as follows. First, this study was based on administrative databases, and ICD-10 codes were used to define diseases. This type of study has potential vulnerabilities linked to inaccurate coding and definition. Appropriate validation of the definition is required to address these issues, and we have used the validated definition in previous studies based on a Korean NHIS cohort [1,2,8]. Dementia diagnosis was defined as in a previous study [22], and internal validation was performed for accuracy. Although we analyzed after censoring stroke, a significant proportion of participants with EOD and AF might already had subclinic or overt cerebral events, as stroke was defined by ICD-10 codes rather than brain imaging. Second, the type (paroxysmal vs. persistent) of AF could not be defined. As asymptomatic AF is not an uncommon condition, we may have misclassified some participants with this condition. Third, owing to the observational nature of this study, there might be residual unidentified confounders. Sleep apnea is an emerging risk factor for dementia and is also strongly associated with AF [23,24]. Unfortunately, we could not exclude possibilities that the relationship between AF and dementia was mediated by sleep apnea. To reduce those biases, we performed a sensitivity analysis with propensity score matching.

5. Conclusions

Incident AF was associated with an increased risk of both EOD and LOD, independent of clinical stroke. Younger participants with AF were more prone to dementia development than older participants with AF.

Supplementary Materials: The following are available online at http://www.mdpi.com/2077-0383/9/11/3665/s1, Table S1: Definitions and ICD-10 codes used for defining the comorbidities and clinical outcomes, Table S2: Baseline characteristics of overall population and propensity score (PS)-matched population, Table S3: Incidence of dementia during follow-up periods according to the AF status in the propensity score-matched population, Table S4: Types of dementia during follow-up periods according to the AF status in the propensity score-matched population, Figure S1: Cumulative incidence of dementia before (A) and after (B) censoring for stroke in the propensity score-matched population, Figure S2: Hazard ratios for dementia per decade of age with atrial fibrillation in the propensity score-matched population.

Author Contributions: Conceptualization, B.J. and G.Y.H.L.; methodology, D.K. and P.-S.Y.; software, D.K.; validation, P.-S.Y.; formal analysis, D.K.; investigation, P.-S.Y.; resources, D.K.; data curation, P.-S.Y.; writing—original draft preparation, D.K.; writing—review and editing, G.Y.H.L.; visualization, D.K.; supervision, B.J.; project administration, B.J.; funding acquisition, B.J. All authors have read and agreed to the published version of the manuscript.

Funding: This study was supported by a research grant from the Korean Healthcare Technology R&D project funded by the Ministry of Health and Welfare (HI15C1200, HC19C0130) and a CMB-Yuhan research grant of Yonsei University College of Medicine (6-2019-0124).

Acknowledgments: The National Health Information Database was provided by the National Health Insurance Service of Korea. We thank the National Health Insurance Service for its cooperation.

Conflicts of Interest: GYHL: Consultant for Bayer/Janssen, BMS/Pfizer, Biotronik, Medtronic, Boehringer Ingelheim, Microlife, and Daiichi-Sankyo. Speaker for Bayer, BMS/Pfizer, Medtronic, Boehringer Ingelheim, Microlife, Roche, and Daiichi-Sankyo. No fees were received personally. JB: Speaker for Bayer, BMS/Pfizer, Medtronic, and Daiichi-Sankyo and research funds from Medtronic and Abbott. No fees were directly received personally. None of the other authors have any disclosures to make.

References

1. Lee, H.; Kim, T.H.; Baek, Y.S.; Uhm, J.S.; Pak, H.N.; Lee, M.H.; Joung, B. The Trends of Atrial Fibrillation-Related Hospital Visit and Cost, Treatment Pattern and Mortality in Korea: 10-Year Nationwide Sample Cohort Data. *Korean Circ. J.* **2017**, *47*, 56–64. [CrossRef]
2. Kim, D.; Yang, P.S.; Jang, E.; Yu, H.T.; Kim, T.H.; Uhm, J.S.; Kim, J.Y.; Pak, H.N.; Lee, M.H.; Joung, B.; et al. 10-year nationwide trends of the incidence, prevalence, and adverse outcomes of non-valvular atrial fibrillation nationwide health insurance data covering the entire Korean population. *Am. Heart J.* **2018**, *202*, 20–26. [CrossRef] [PubMed]
3. Stewart, S.; Hart, C.L.; Hole, D.J.; McMurray, J.J. A population-based study of the long-term risks associated with atrial fibrillation: 20-year follow-up of the Renfrew/Paisley study. *Am. J. Med.* **2002**, *113*, 359–364. [CrossRef]
4. Wortmann, M. Dementia: A global health priority—Highlights from an ADI and World Health Organization report. *Alzheimer's Res. Ther.* **2012**, *4*, 40. [CrossRef] [PubMed]
5. Ott, A.; Breteler, M.M.; de Bruyne, M.C.; van Harskamp, F.; Grobbee, D.E.; Hofman, A. Atrial fibrillation and dementia in a population-based study. The Rotterdam Study. *Stroke* **1997**, *28*, 316–321. [CrossRef]
6. Rastas, S.; Verkkoniemi, A.; Polvikoski, T.; Juva, K.; Niinisto, L.; Mattila, K.; Lansimies, E.; Pirttila, T.; Sulkava, R. Atrial fibrillation, stroke, and cognition: A longitudinal population-based study of people aged 85 and older. *Stroke* **2007**, *38*, 1454–1460. [CrossRef]
7. Bunch, T.J.; Weiss, J.P.; Crandall, B.G.; May, H.T.; Bair, T.L.; Osborn, J.S.; Anderson, J.L.; Muhlestein, J.B.; Horne, B.D.; Lappe, D.L.; et al. Atrial fibrillation is independently associated with senile, vascular, and Alzheimer's dementia. *Heart Rhythm* **2010**, *7*, 433–437. [CrossRef]
8. Kim, D.; Yang, P.S.; Yu, H.T.; Kim, T.H.; Jang, E.; Sung, J.H.; Pak, H.N.; Lee, M.Y.; Lee, M.H.; Lip, G.Y.H.; et al. Risk of dementia in stroke-free patients diagnosed with atrial fibrillation: Data from a population-based cohort. *Eur. Heart J.* **2019**, *40*, 2313–2323. [CrossRef]

9. Seong, S.C.; Kim, Y.Y.; Park, S.K.; Khang, Y.H.; Kim, H.C.; Park, J.H.; Kang, H.J.; Do, C.H.; Song, J.S.; Lee, E.J.; et al. Cohort profile: The National Health Insurance Service-National Health Screening Cohort (NHIS-HEALS) in Korea. *BMJ Open* **2017**, *7*, e016640. [CrossRef]
10. Kim, T.H.; Yang, P.S.; Uhm, J.S.; Kim, J.Y.; Pak, H.N.; Lee, M.H.; Joung, B.; Lip, G.Y.H. CHA2DS2-VASc Score (Congestive Heart Failure, Hypertension, Age >/=75 [Doubled], Diabetes Mellitus, Prior Stroke or Transient Ischemic Attack [Doubled], Vascular Disease, Age 65–74, Female) for Stroke in Asian Patients With Atrial Fibrillation: A Korean Nationwide Sample Cohort Study. *Stroke* **2017**, *48*, 1524–1530. [CrossRef]
11. De Bruijn, R.F.; Heeringa, J.; Wolters, F.J.; Franco, O.H.; Stricker, B.H.; Hofman, A.; Koudstaal, P.J.; Ikram, M.A. Association Between Atrial Fibrillation and Dementia in the General Population. *JAMA Neurol.* **2015**, *72*, 1288–1294. [CrossRef] [PubMed]
12. Rusanen, M.; Kivipelto, M.; Levalahti, E.; Laatikainen, T.; Tuomilehto, J.; Soininen, H.; Ngandu, T. Heart diseases and long-term risk of dementia and Alzheimer's disease: A population-based CAIDE study. *J. Alzheimers Dis.* **2014**, *42*, 183–191. [CrossRef] [PubMed]
13. Wardlaw, J.M.; Smith, C.; Dichgans, M. Mechanisms of sporadic cerebral small vessel disease: Insights from neuroimaging. *Lancet Neurol.* **2013**, *12*, 483–497. [CrossRef]
14. Goette, A.; Kalman, J.M.; Aguinaga, L.; Akar, J.; Cabrera, J.A.; Chen, S.A.; Chugh, S.S.; Corradi, D.; D'avila, A.; Dobrev, D.; et al. EHRA/HRS/APHRS/SOLAECE expert consensus on Atrial cardiomyopathies: Definition, characterisation, and clinical implication. *J. Arrhythm.* **2016**, *32*, 247–278. [CrossRef]
15. Poggesi, A.; Pasi, M.; Pescini, F.; Pantoni, L.; Inzitari, D. Circulating biologic markers of endothelial dysfunction in cerebral small vessel disease: A review. *J. Cereb. Blood Flow Metab. Off. J. Int. Soc. Cereb. Blood Flow Metab.* **2016**, *36*, 72–94. [CrossRef]
16. Viticchi, G.; Falsetti, L.; Buratti, L.; Sajeva, G.; Luzzi, S.; Bartolini, M.; Provinciali, L.; Silvestrini, M. Framingham Risk Score and the Risk of Progression from Mild Cognitive Impairment to Dementia. *J. Alzheimers Dis.* **2017**, *59*, 67–75. [CrossRef]
17. Falsetti, L.; Viticchi, G.; Buratti, L.; Grigioni, F.; Capucci, A.; Silvestrini, M. Interactions between Atrial Fibrillation, Cardiovascular Risk Factors, and ApoE Genotype in Promoting Cognitive Decline in Patients with Alzheimer's Disease: A Prospective Cohort Study. *J. Alzheimers Dis.* **2018**, *62*, 713–725. [CrossRef]
18. Vermeer, S.E.; Prins, N.D.; den Heijer, T.; Hofman, A.; Koudstaal, P.J.; Breteler, M.M. Silent brain infarcts and the risk of dementia and cognitive decline. *N. Engl. J. Med.* **2003**, *348*, 1215–1222. [CrossRef]
19. Nordstrom, P.; Nordstrom, A.; Eriksson, M.; Wahlund, L.O.; Gustafson, Y. Risk factors in late adolescence for young-onset dementia in men: A nationwide cohort study. *JAMA Intern. Med.* **2013**, *173*, 1612–1618. [CrossRef]
20. Heath, C.A.; Mercer, S.W.; Guthrie, B. Vascular comorbidities in younger people with dementia: A cross-sectional population-based study of 616,245 middle-aged people in Scotland. *J. Neurol. Neurosurg. Psychiatry* **2015**, *86*, 959–964. [CrossRef]
21. Smajlovic, D. Strokes in young adults: Epidemiology and prevention. *Vasc. Health Risk. Manag.* **2015**, *11*, 157–164. [CrossRef] [PubMed]
22. Lee, S.-H.; Han, K.; Cho, H.; Park, Y.-M.; Kwon, H.-S.; Kang, G.; Yoon, K.-H.; Kim, M.K. Variability in metabolic parameters and risk of dementia: A nationwide population-based study. *Alzheimer's Res. Ther.* **2018**, *10*, 110. [CrossRef] [PubMed]
23. Buratti, L.; Viticchi, G.; Baldinelli, S.; Falsetti, L.; Luzzi, S.; Pulcini, A.; Petrelli, C.; Provinciali, L.; Silvestrini, M. Sleep Apnea, Cognitive Profile, and Vascular Changes: An Intriguing Relationship. *J. Alzheimers Dis.* **2017**, *60*, 1195–1203. [CrossRef]
24. Cadby, G.; McArdle, N.; Briffa, T.; Hillman, D.R.; Simpson, L.; Knuiman, M.; Hung, J. Severity of OSA is an independent predictor of incident atrial fibrillation hospitalization in a large sleep-clinic cohort. *Chest* **2015**, *148*, 945–952. [CrossRef] [PubMed]

Publisher's Note: MDPI stays neutral with regard to jurisdictional claims in published maps and institutional affiliations.

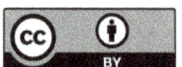

© 2020 by the authors. Licensee MDPI, Basel, Switzerland. This article is an open access article distributed under the terms and conditions of the Creative Commons Attribution (CC BY) license (http://creativecommons.org/licenses/by/4.0/).

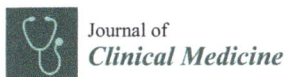

Article

Involvement of Autonomic Nervous System in New-Onset Atrial Fibrillation during Acute Myocardial Infarction

Audrey Sagnard [1,†], Charles Guenancia [1,2,*,†], Basile Mouhat [1,2], Maud Maza [1,2], Marie Fichot [1], Daniel Moreau [1], Fabien Garnier [1], Luc Lorgis [1,2], Yves Cottin [1,2] and Marianne Zeller [1,2]

1. Cardiology Department, University Hospital, 21000 Dijon, France; audrey.sagnard@chu-dijon.fr (A.S.); basile.mouhat@gmail.com (B.M.); maud.maza@chu-dijon.fr (M.M.); marie.fichot@chu-dijon.fr (M.F.); daniel.moreau@u-bourgogne.fr (D.M.); fabien.garnier@chu-dijon.fr (F.G.); luc.lorgis@chu-dijon.fr (L.L.); yves.cottin@chu-dijon.fr (Y.C.); marianne.zeller@u-bourgogne.fr (M.Z.)
2. PEC 2 EA 7460, University of Burgundy and Franche-Comté, 21000 Dijon, France
* Correspondence: charles.guenancia@gmail.com; Tel.: +33-380-293-536; Fax: +33-380-293-879
† These authors contributed equally to this work.

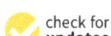

Received: 14 April 2020; Accepted: 5 May 2020; Published: 14 May 2020

Abstract: Background: Atrial fibrillation (AF) is common after acute myocardial infarction (AMI) and associated with in-hospital and long-term mortality. However, the pathophysiology of AF in AMI is poorly understood. Heart rate variability (HRV), measured by Holter-ECG, reflects cardiovascular response to the autonomic nervous system and altered (reduced or enhanced) HRV may have a major role in the onset of AF in AMI patients. **Objective:** We investigated the relationship between autonomic dysregulation and new-onset AF during AMI. **Methods:** As part of the RICO survey, all consecutive patients hospitalized for AMI at Dijon (France) university hospital between June 2001 and November 2014 were analyzed by Holter-ECG <24 h following admission. HRV was measured using temporal and spectral analysis. **Results:** Among the 2040 included patients, 168 (8.2%) developed AF during AMI. Compared to the sinus-rhythm (SR) group, AF patients were older, had more frequent hypertension and lower left ventricular ejection fraction LVEF. On the Holter parameters, AF patients had higher pNN50 values (11% vs. 4%, p < 0.001) and median LH/HF ratio, a reflection of sympathovagal balance, was significantly lower in the AF group (0.88 vs 2.75 p < 0.001). The optimal LF/HF cut-off for AF prediction was 1.735. In multivariate analyses, low LF/HF <1.735 (OR(95%CI) = 3.377 (2.047–5.572)) was strongly associated with AF, ahead of age (OR(95%CI) = 1.04(1.01–1.06)), mean sinus-rhythm rate (OR(95%CI) = 1.03(1.02–1.05)) and log NT-proBNP (OR(95%CI) = 1.38(1.01–1.90)). **Conclusion:** Our study strongly suggests that new-onset AF in AMI mainly occurs in a dysregulated autonomic nervous system, as suggested by low LF/HF, and higher PNN50 and RMSSD values.

Keywords: acute myocardial infarction; atrial fibrillation; heart rate variability; autonomic nervous system

1. Introduction

Atrial fibrillation (AF) is one of the most common cardiovascular (CV) diseases worldwide, with an increasing global burden associated with the ageing of the population. AF frequently occurs in patients with acute myocardial infarction (AMI), with an incidence ranging from 6% to 21% [1], and is associated with an increased risk of death and rehospitalisation for heart failure, which in turn have major economic consequences [2]. AF leads to atrial remodeling through an alteration of the electrical and structural properties of the atria, thus facilitating the maintenance and recurrence of AF [3]. Several risk factors for AF have already been identified in various populations, but the predictive power of individual risk factors is still far from accurate. Heart rate variability (HRV), measured by Holter-ECG, reflects cardiovascular response to the autonomic nervous system (ANS) and altered (reduced or enhanced) HRV may have a major role in the onset of AF in AMI patients with coronary artery disease (CAD) [4]. However, in the setting of AMI, the role of the ANS is uncertain and data are scarce [5]. The aim of this retrospective analysis of a large database of patients was to evaluate whether autonomic dysfunction (measured by HRV) could be associated with new-onset AF in AMI: is it an epiphenomenon related to sympathetic activation linked to the severity of the infarction, or is it related to parasympathetic dependence which would suggest chronic electrical and anatomical atrial remodeling and therefore risk of recurrence?

2. Experimental Section

2.1. Patients

The participants were recruited from the RICO (obseRvatoire des Infarctus de Côte-d'Or) database, a regional registry for cases of acute myocardial infarction (MI). Briefly, RICO collects data from all patients hospitalized for acute MI in all public or privately funded hospitals of one department in the east of France [6]. The present study included all consecutive patients admitted between 20th June 2001 and 2nd November 2014 (>18 years old) who underwent a 24-h Holter ECG recording during their coronary care unit stay. Patients with a history of AF (n = 94) were excluded, we checked for each patient admission his/her previous medical history, baseline treatments and medical recording in the hospital files. In case of suspicion of previous AF that cannot be confirmed by the patient (anticoagulant therapy, antiarrhythmic drug) we systematically called the general practitioner or the cardiologist of the patient to explain this drug prescriptions. A flow chart reporting the inclusion and exclusion criteria is shown in Figure 1. The present study complied with the Declaration of Helsinki and was approved by the ethics committee of the University Hospital of Dijon. Each patient provided written consent before participation.

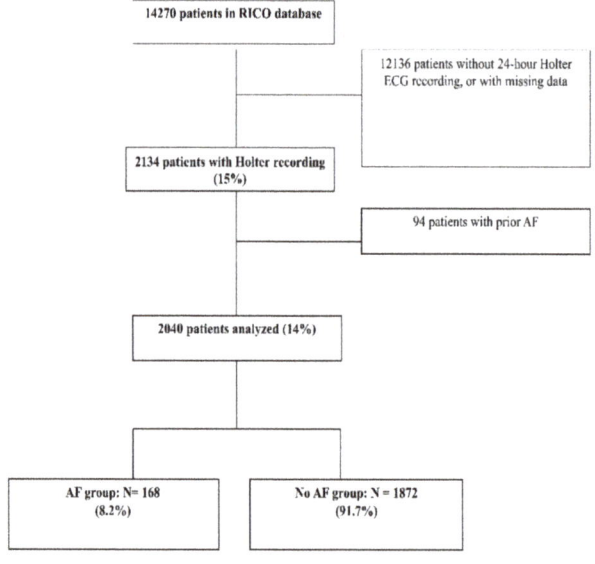

Figure 1. Study Flow Chart.

2.2. Data Collection

Patient data were collected from the RICO database: continuous electrocardiographic monitoring (CEM) data (rhythm status during AMI), cardiovascular risk factors, clinical data, type of AMI, acute management, acute and discharge medications, biological data, echocardiography data including LVEF (with a cut-off at 40% using Simpson's method for more clinical relevance) and left atrial dimensions as previously described [7].

2.3. AF Definition

AF was diagnosed in accordance with the current European Society of Cardiology Guidelines as absolutely irregular RR intervals and no discernible, distinct P waves and an episode duration of at least 30 s. Flutter episodes were included as AF episodes [8].

2.4. Biological Data

Blood samples were drawn on admission. Plasma creatinine levels were measured on a Vitros 950 analyzer (Ortho Clinical Diagnostics, Rochester, New York, USA). Glomerular filtration rate was calculated with the Chronic Kidney Disease Epidemiology Collaboration (CKD-EPI) formula. C-reactive protein (CRP) was determined on a dimension Xpand (Dade Behring, Deerfield, Illinois, USA) using enzymatic methods. CRP level was dichotomized into high and low categories at 3 mg/L for more clinical relevance.

2.5. Holter ECG Data

If the patient consented to undergo a 24-h (Holter) ECG, it was done in the coronary care unit within the 24 h following admission. Holter monitoring was based on device availability [6], patient consent and expected hospital stay >48 h within our cardiology department to be able to obtain Holter results before hospital discharge. Long ECG tracing was recorded and analyzed by two experienced observers using a Syneflash digital recorder Holter (Ela medical and Spieder Viers, le Plessis Robinson, France), with seven surface electrode signals (acquisition sampling rate: 1000 Hz). After classifying the QRS morphology, the RR intervals (longest and shortest) were confirmed manually until no QRS sequences were incorrectly labelled. Only sequences with normal QRS characteristics during 24 h (sinus rhythm) were analysed for HRV study. HRV was addressed from the time or frequency domain in accordance with the 1996 guidelines of the ESC Task Force [9]: Time domain variables: (1) rMSSD: root mean square of successive differences in NN intervals is considered an estimate of the short-term components of HRV, which correspond to parasympathetic activity. (2) pNN50: proportion derived by dividing NN50 (the number of interval differences of successive NN intervals greater than 50 ms) by the total number of NN intervals. This is a measure of parasympathetic activity. (3) SDNN: the standard deviation of all intervals between adjacent QRS complexes resulting from sinus node depolarization (NN), i.e., the square root of variance, reflects the cyclic components responsible for variability in the period of recording and is considered as an estimate of overall HRV, encompassing vagal and sympathetic influences [10,11].

Frequency domain variables: Fast Fourier transform was used to convert the different successive RR intervals in the frequency domain. Low frequencies (LF), between 0.04 and 0.15 Hz, are affected by both vagal and sympathetic activity, whereas high frequencies (HF), between 0.15 and 0.4 Hz, are affected by vagal tone. The LF/HF ratio is therefore considered an indicator of sympathovagal balance; oscillations in very low frequencies VLF (range 0.00 to 0.04 Hz) reflect peripheral vasomotor regulation. Total power (TP), combining the sum of all the frequencies, is a global measure of ANS activity [10,11].

2.6. Statistical Analyses

Results were expressed as medians [IQR] for continuous variables and as percentages for dichotomized variables. Normality was tested with the Kolmogorov-Smirnov test. For continuous data, we used the Mann-Whitney test. Categorical variables were compared with the χ^2 or Fisher exact test. A p value of less than 0.05 was considered statistically significant. Since the NT-proBNP values do not follow a normal distribution, a logarithmic transformation was performed. To assess discrimination for AF recurrences, we examined the area under the receiver-operating characteristic (ROC) curve (plot of sensitivity versus 1—specificity for all possible cut-off values to classify predictions) for the LF-HF with the best sensitivity, specificity, positive predictive value and negative predictive value according to the Youden index. Multivariate logistic regression models were built to estimate the odds ratio (OR) of in-hospital AF and of a LF/HF ratio cut-off value. Variables that met the statistical significance threshold of 5% in univariable analysis were included in the multivariate models. LVEF was not included in the final model because of collinearity with NT-proBNP. To improve the robustness of results, the AF patients were matched 1:1 with the SR patients using nearest neighbor matching on the linear propensity score with a tolerance of 0.02. The same logistic regression model was used to compare AF with SR patients. The statistical tests were performed with SPSS software version 26 (IBM Corp., Armonk, NY, USA).

3. Results

3.1. Patient Characteristics

Of the 14,270 patients in the RICO database, 2040 (14.3%) met the main inclusion criteria of having a 24-h Holter ECG recording and no prior AF (Figure 1).

AF was identified in 168 (8.2%) of the included patients. Tables 1–4 summarize the characteristics of the study population.

Patients from the AF group were almost 10 y older (77 vs. 64 y; $p < 0.001$), more frequently hypertensive (68% vs 49%; $p < 0.001$) and less likely to smoke (15% vs. 35%; $p < 0.001$) then the rest of the study population. The pNN50 values of the AF group were almost thrice higher (11% vs. 4%; $p < 0.001$), their rMSSD values were higher (45 vs. 27 ms; $p < 0.001$) and the HR by Holter ECG was faster (73 vs. 66 beats/min; $p < 0.001$). More AF patients had a LF/HF ratio < 1.735% (75% vs. 30%; $p < 0.001$). High creatinine (98 vs. 87 µmol/L; $p < 0.001$), glycaemia (7.92 vs. 7.00 mmol/L; $p < 0.001$) and NT-proBNP levels (2450 vs. 542 pg/mL; $p < 0.001$) were observed in AF patients. They were also more likely to have a history of cardiovascular disease, including CAD, stroke, and renal failure. Accordingly, they were more likely to be taking chronic CV medications such as beta blockers and amiodarone (medication used for a history of ventricular arrhythmia (no atrial fibrillation ECG traces in their medical records)). The other admission parameters (including diabetes, time to admission, and troponin Ic peak) were not significantly different except for multivessel disease.

Table 1. Patient Baseline Characteristics (n (%) or median (interquartile range)).

	No AF N = 1872	AF N = 168	p
Risk factors			
Age. years	64 (53–76)	77 (70–83)	<0.001
Female	519 (28%)	63 (38%)	0.007
BMI. kg/m^2	26 (24–29)	26 (23–28)	0.067
Hypertension	924 (49%)	114 (68%)	<0.001
Hypercholesterolemia	832 (44%)	73 (44%)	0.804
Family history of CAD	503 (27%)	41 (24%)	0.489
Diabetes	388 (21%)	36 (21%)	0.830
Smoking	649 (35%)	25 (15%)	<0.001

Table 1. Cont.

	No AF N = 1872	AF N = 168	p
	CV history		
CAD	350 (19%)	40 (24%)	0.106
Stroke	99 (5%)	16 (10%)	0.023
Chronic renal failure	67 (4%)	8 (5%)	0.435
	Clinical data on admission		
HR. beats/min	76 (65–89)	89 (70–108)	<0.001
SBP	140 (121–160)	130 (116–150)	<0.001
DBP	80 (70–92)	80 (64–90)	0.019
Heart failure (Killip >1)	315 (17%)	59 (35%)	<0.001
Anterior wall location	677 (36%)	58 (35%)	0.671
STEMI	1075 (57%)	107 (64%)	0.115
LVEF. %	55 (45–61)	47 (40–56)	<0.001
LVEF <40%	224 (13%)	33 (21%)	0.004
GRACE risk score	138 (115–163)	179 (150–202)	<0.001
Time to admission. min	192 (105–450)	180 (106–373)	0.818
ICU stay. days	4 (3–5)	5 (3–8)	<0.001
	Biological data on admission		
Creatinine, μmol/l	87 (74–105)	98 (79–117)	<0.001
eGFR CKD, mL/min	76.3 (58.8–91.6)	60.9 (45.6–74.8)	<0.001
Glycaemia. mmol/L	7.00 (5.92–8.77)	7.92 (6.45–10.41)	<0.001
CRP ≥ 3 mg/L	1064 (63%)	111 (76%)	0.003
Troponin Ic peak, μg/L	18.5 (3.8–41.0)	20.5 (6.5–41.0)	0.204
NT-proBNP, pg/mL	542 (138–2177)	2450 (735–6915)	<0.001
Log NT-proBNP, pg/mL	2.73 (2.14–3.34)	3.39 (2.87–3.84)	<0.001
	Chronic medication on admission		
Amiodarone	10 (1%)	5 (3%)	0.005
ARB/ACE inhibitors	633 (34%)	76 (45%)	0.002
Beta blockers	463 (25%)	63 (38%)	<0.001
Diuretic	408 (22%)	64 (38%)	<0.001
Antiplatelet	206 (11%)	25 (15%)	0.129
Aspirin	360 (19%)	51 (30%)	0.001
VKA	28 (2%)	5 (3%)	0.187
Statin	463 (25%)	46 (27%)	0.447
	Acute medications <48 h		
Amiodarone	72 (4%)	58 (35%)	<0.001
ARB/ACE inhibitors	1413 (75%)	103 (61%)	<0.001
Beta blockers	1508 (81%)	109 (65%)	<0.001
Statin	1533 (82%)	121 (72%)	0.002

ACE: angiotensin conversion enzyme; ARB: angiotensin receptor blockers; AF: atrial fibrillation; BMI: body mass index; CAD: Coronary artery disease; CRP: C–reactive protein; CK: creatine kinase; CKD: chronic kidney disease; COPD: chronic obstructive pulmonary disease; DBP: diastolic blood pressure; eGFR: estimated glomerular filtration rate; HR: heart rate; ICU: Intensive Care Unit; LVEF: left ventricular ejection fraction; LWM: low molecular weight; NT-proBNP: N-terminal pro brain natriuretic peptide. PAD: peripheral artery disease; SBP: systolic blood pressure; STEMI: ST segment elevation myocardial infarction; VKA: vitamin K antagonist.

Table 2. Acute myocardial infarction management (n (%)).

	No AF N = 1872	AF N = 168	p
Invasive treatment			
Coronary angiography	1782 (95%)	154 (92%)	0.047
TIMI class on culprit artery	N = 1716	N = 150	0.308
0	789 (46%)	76 (51%)	
1	93 (5%)	7 (5%)	
2	179 (11%)	20 (13%)	
3	655 (38%)	47 (31%)	
TIMI class on culprit artery <2	882 (51%)	83 (55%)	0.355
CABG	71 (4%)	8 (5%)	0.533
Medical treatment			
Thrombolysis	274 (15%)	24 (14%)	0.902
Antiplatelet	1632 (87%)	135 (80%)	0.013
Aspirin	1811 (97%)	155 (92%)	0.003
Low molecular weight heparin	1238 (66%)	62 (37%)	<0.001
Unfractionated heparin	850 (45%)	116 (69%)	<0.001
Glycoprotein IIbIIIa inhibitors	798 (43%)	53 (32%)	0.005

AF: atrial fibrillation; CABG: coronary artery byass graft surgery; PCI: percutaneous coronary intervention.

Table 3. Holter parameters according to the onset of new AF during AMI, n (%), median (interquartile range) or mean (± standard deviation).

	No AF N = 1872	AF N = 168	p
Heart rate. beats/min	66 (60–73)	73 (60–84)	<0.001
Premature Ventricular Contractions (/24 h)	11 (2–92)	70 (7–378)	<0.001
VT episode (/24 h)	0 (0–0)/1 ± 22	0 (0–0)/4 ± 44	0.011
pNN50. %	4 (1–11)	11 (2–36)	<0.001
rMSSD. ms	27 (19–41)	45 (24–108)	<0.001
SDNN. ms	83 (64–107)	90 (61–119)	0.123
Power. ms^2	1850 (925–3507)	2007 (1036–5171)	0.044
LF/HF	2.75 (1.46–4.58)	0.88 (0.57–2.00)	<0.001
LF/HF < 1.735	532 (30%)	111 (75%)	<0.001

AF: atrial fibrillation; VT: ventricular tachycardia; pNN50: proportion derived by dividing NN50 (the number of interval differences of successive NN intervals greater than 50 ms) by the total number of NN intervals; rMSSD: root mean square of successive differences in NN intervals; SDNN: standard deviation of all intervals between adjacent QRS complexes resulting from sinus node depolarization; LF: low frequencies; HF: high frequencies.

Table 4. In-hospital outcomes according to the onset of new AF during AMI n (%).

	No AF N = 1872	AF N = 168	p
Death	21 (1.1%)	8 (4.8%)	0.002
CV death	17 (0.9%)	6 (3.6%)	0.009
Recurrent MI	89 (4.8%)	10 (6.0%)	0.489
Heart Failure	417 (22%)	93 (55%)	<0.001
Stroke	19 (1.0%)	5 (3.0%)	0.042
VT or VF	130 (6.9%)	29 (17.3%)	<0.001

AF: atrial fibrillation; CV: cardio vascular; MI: myocardial infarction; VT: ventricular tachycardia; VF: ventricular fibrillation.

3.2. ROC Curve

The optimal cut-offs for continuous test variables were determined from the ROC curve, which was used to estimate the optimal threshold value of LF-HF. The best LF/HF value to characterize our population according to AF occurrence was a LF/HF ratio <1.735, with an AUC of 0.73 (95% CI (0.69–0.78); $p < 0.001$), sensitivity of 69% and specificity of 70% (Figure 2).

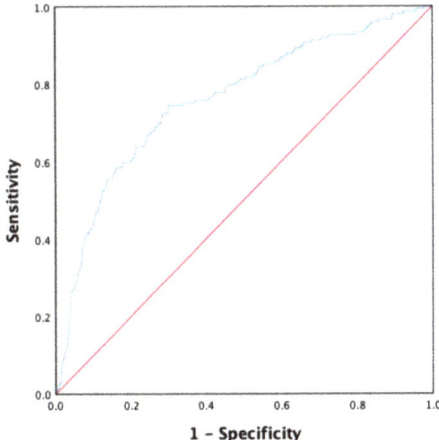

Figure 2. ROC curve demonstrating the predictive performance of LF/HF ratio for the onset of new AF during AMI: AUC = 0.73 (0.69–0.78); $p < 0.001$); optimal threshold: 1.735; sensitivity = 0.698; specificity = 0.707.

3.3. LF/HF Determinants: Multivariate Analysis

In multivariate analysis, only age, female sex and diabetes were associated with low LF/HF, therefore excluding the influence of treatments such as beta blockers or the severity of AMI on this ANS parameter.

3.4. AF Determinants in Acute Myocardial Infarction

In univariate analysis (Table 5) the risk factors for developing AF in the acute phase of infarction were: female sex, age, hypertension, smoking HR on Holter, CRP > 3 mg/L, eGFR, log-NTproBNP, chronic use of ARB/ACE inhibitors and chronic use of beta-blockers.

In multivariate analysis, the independent risk factors for developing AF were age (OR 1.05 (1.03–1.07); $p < 0.001$), HR (OR 1.04 (1.02–1.05); $p < 0.001$) and log NT-proBNP (OR: 1.48(1.10–1.99, $p = 0.010$)) with a good predictive performance.

The addition of the LF/HF < 1.735 variable significantly improved our ability to predict in-hospital AF (OR 3.38 (2.05–5.57); $p < 0.001$).

Moreover, after 1:1 propensity score matching (on age, sex, previous hypertension, previous stroke, BMI, LVEF), LF/HF ratio <1.735 (OR 3.49 (2.03–5.99), $p < 0.001$) remained independently associated with the new-onset of AF during AMI.

Table 5. Logistic regression analysis for the prediction of in-hospital AF.

Characteristic	Univariate OR (95% CI)	p	Multivariable 1 OR (95% CI)	p	Multivariable 2 OR (95% CI)	p
Female	1.564 (1.126–2.172)	0.008	0.756 (0.501–1.140)	0.182	0.671 (0.434–1.038)	0.073
Age, Years	1.063 (1.049–1.077)	<0.001	1.049 (1.028–1.071)	<0.001	1.036 (1.01–1.060)	0.002
Hypertension	2.166 (1.547–3.032)	<0.001	1.160 (0.734–1.834)	0.525	1.234 (0.756–2.014)	0.400
Smoker	0.329 (0.213–0.509)	<0.001	0.996 (0.561–1.766)	0.988	1.078 (0.586–1.980)	0.810
Previous Stroke	1.885 (1.084–3.279)	0.025	0.994 (0.513–1.926)	0.986	0.949 (0.484–1.862)	0.879
HR (holter), bpm	1.043 (1.031–1.055)	<0.001	1.039 (1.025–1.054)	<0.001	1.034 (1.019–1.048)	<0.001
CRP >3 mg/L	1.785 (1.210–2.633)	0.003	1.189 (0.741–1.910)	0.473	1.199 (0.722–1.992)	0.482
eGFR CKD, mL/min	0.975 (0.969–0.981)	<0.001	0.997 (0.987–1.008)	0.616	0.998 (0.987–1.008)	0.659
NT–proBNP (log)	2.687 (2.143–3.369)	<0.001	1.479 (1.100–1.990)	0.010	1.379 (1.001–1.899)	0.049
Glycemia, mmol/L	1.000 (0.995–1.005)	0.998	X		X	
Troponin I Peak, µg/L	1.001 (0.997–1.004)	0.699	X		X	
Beta Blockers (Chronic)	1.826 (1.313–2.539)	<0.001	1.067 (0.701–1.624)	0.763	0.950 (0.604–1.493)	0.823
ARB/ACE Inhibitors (Chronic)	1.680 (1.222–2.311)	0.001	0.921 (0.601–1.411)	0.704	0.866 (0.550–1.361)	0.532
LF/HF <1.735	6.748 (4.605–9.889)	<0.001	X		3.377 (2.047–5.572)	<0.001
Quality Indexes			PhI = 0.324; −2LL = 796.132; %class = 92.5		pHL = 0.106; −2LL = 706.701; %class = 92.8	

ACE: angiotensin conversion enzyme; ARB: angiotensin receptor blockers; CRP: C-reactive protein; CKD: chronic kidney disease; eGFR: estimated glomerular filtration rate; HR: heart rate.

3.5. Echocardiographic Parameters of Left Atrium

We performed a subgroup analysis using left atrial (LA) echocardiographic parameters in patients for whom these parameters were available (n = 121 for LA diameter, 117 for LA area and n = 100 for LA volume). We started by conducting a univariate analysis to identify the LA size variable that could most powerfully predict AF. Next, we added the variable to a bivariate model and observed whether LF/HF remained independently associated with AF after adjustment on left atrial size. In univariate analysis, the only LA size parameter that was a predictor of in-hospital AF was LA volume (OR 1.03 (1.00–1.05); $p < 0.001$). Among the patients included in the subgroup analysis, eight had a new-onset of AF during AMI. However, after bivariate analysis, neither LA volume nor LH/HF remained significantly associated with AF ($p = 0.062$ for both variables). Collinearity between the variables was not significant (variation inflation factor = 1.07).

4. Discussion

The results of our large, population-based study indicate that a low LF/HF (<1.735) ratio was strongly associated with new-onset AF during AMI. Indeed, investigation of the median LF/HF ratio revealed that the sinus rhythm group and the AF group had a marked difference in sympathovagal balance. In our population, 75% of AF patients had a LF/HF ratio < 1.735, compared to 30% of patients in the sinus rhythm group. Lower values of LF/HF ratio are thought to reflect decreased sympathetic activity and/or increased parasympathetic activity, i.e., above all, an imbalance of this sympathovagal tone.

4.1. AF in Acute Myocardial Infarction

It is still not known whether AF in AMI is promoted by acute activation of the sympathetic nervous system and is therefore a reversible arrhythmia, or if it occurs on a pre-existing atrial substrate that is prone to chronic dysregulation of ANS, indicating potential recurrence. This question is of particular interest considering the potential therapeutic consequences, particularly the initiation of oral anticoagulation therapy on top of the dual antiplatelet treatment prescribed to AMI patients. The role of autonomic tone in the genesis of atrial arrhythmia has been clinically recognized for many years, but autonomic modulation is extremely complex to characterize and quantify [4]. In clinical cardiology, the main tool to evaluate ANS activity is the analysis of HRV parameters on continuous ECG recordings [9]. The frequency-domain HRV parameters obtained by spectral analysis are considered the most useful parameters for addressing the sympathetic/parasympathetic balance. The HF components are thought to primarily reflect vagal tone, whereas the more complex LF components probably reflect sympathetic activity [4]. Both the parasympathetic and the sympathetic nervous systems have been shown to play a role in AF. Amar et al., showed that the onset of AF was preceded by a primary increase in the sympathetic drive, followed by marked modulation toward vagal predominance [12]. Our results suggest that there appears to be an ANS dysregulation prior to AMI, resulting in a paradoxical ANS response on the parasympathetic side where we would have expected an over-expression of the sympathetic system only.

4.2. LF/HF Ratio Findings

The ANS plays a central pathophysiological role in the initiation and progression of AF [13]. Power spectral analysis of the beat-to-beat variations of heart rate or the heart period (R–R interval) has become widely used to quantify cardiac autonomic regulation. This technique partitions the total variance (the "power") of a continuous series of beats into its frequency components, typically identifying two main peaks: low frequency (LF), 0.04–0.15 Hz, and high frequency (HF) 0.15–0.4 Hz [9]. The HF peak is widely believed to reflect cardiac parasympathetic nerve activity while the LF, although more complex, is often assumed to have a dominant sympathetic component. Based upon these assumptions, Pagani and colleagues suggested that the ratio of LF to HF (LF/HF) could be used to quantify the changing relationship between sympathetic and parasympathetic nerve activities (i.e., the sympathovagal balance) in both healthy and diseased organisms [14]. The clinical determinants influencing HRV values were evaluated from Framingham's study, which showed that age and HR were the two main determinants of HRV in healthy subjects, in addition to sex and smoking [15]. The LF/HF ratio has gained wide acceptance as a tool for assessing cardiovascular autonomic regulation where increases in LF/HF are assumed to reflect a shift towards "sympathetic dominance" and decreases indicate "parasympathetic dominance" [9]. Moreover, it has been proved that non-linearity of neural modulation of cycle length may result in an intrinsic rate-dependency of autonomic indexes, with the exception of normalized frequency-domain indexes (like LF/HF), which appear to be devoid of intrinsic rate-dependency [16]. Thus, LF/HF ratio is considered the more appropriate to assess ANS independently of heart rate and was also the most powerful predictor of AF in our results. The intrinsic rate-independency of LF/HF is very important: indeed, in our study, heart rate at admission was also associated with new-onset AF on top of LF/HF.

4.3. AF Determinants in Acute Myocardial Infarction

The present findings also confirm the significance of several known clinical risk factors, such as age, CAD, blood pressure and heart rate for the development of AF. We found that, after adjustment, only age, HR on Holter recording, and LF/HF ratio remained significant predictors of AF. Indeed, our results show that patients with low a LF/HF ratio are three times more likely to develop AF than patients with a higher LF/HF ratio (OR 3.65 (2.20–0.76; $p < 0.001$)). The addition of LF/HF ratio to the classical AF predictors improved the diagnostic performance of the model, indicating that the parameters of the ANS are not fully covered by the classical clinical and biological predictors of AF during AMI. It therefore seems important to include this variable in existing risk scores. ANS plays an independent role on top of the variables classically used to predict AF, particularly on the parasympathetic side with a decrease in the LF/HF ratio. In addition, the other Holter ECG parameters used to evaluate parasympathetic activity, such as PNN50 or rMSSD, were consistent with our main hypothesis [9]. In our population, the AF group had higher PNN50 and rMSSD values, stressing the importance of the parasympathetic component as an AF substrate. This result has led us to speculate that an underlying chronic disease may have preceded the onset of AMI. Indeed, some authors have shown that parasympathetic tone is increased by expansion and atrial fibrosis in experimental models of AF [17]. In heart failure models, there is also an increase in sympathetic, parasympathetic and lymph node fibers in the left atrium that promote the maintenance and upkeep of arrhythmia [18]. These results are strong evidence that parasympathetic activation is related to the electrical remodeling of the LA through myocyte remodeling, and that parasympathetic activation occurs before the AMI [19]. Non-invasive measures obtained from Holter monitoring could identify an increased risk of AF in patients hospitalized for AMI, and could justify prolonged rhythm monitoring in patients identified as at-risk [20]. Moreover, in addition to AF prediction, HRV data on scopes could improve the stratification of ventricular rhythmic risk, as previously shown [21]. Consequently, we suggest that systematic and automated analysis of HRV data be added to the management of patients in the acute phase of MI. The contribution of LF/HF ratio to the prediction of AF recurrence risk at distance from the acute episode remains to be determined, but it may prove to be a useful tool for differentiating between acute AF episodes resulting from AMI and AF linked to pre-existing conditions at a high risk of recurrence [7].

4.4. Limitations

Among the 14,270 patients included in the RICO registry, 12,136 (85.0%) were excluded due to a lack of Holter monitoring. This could lead to a selection bias, considering that only patients for whom the hospital stay was scheduled to be >48h within our cardiology department were eligible to receive a Holter monitor, and this was also according to device availability. However, the large sample size of our included population, as well as the baseline characteristics that are close to the usual data obtained from the whole registry population in terms of age, CV risk factors and AMI type, should reduce this bias [22].

We were not able to provide the dimensions of LA for all patients, which is unfortunate seeing as these parameters are known to be associated with the onset of AF. In the subgroup of patients for whom LA parameters were available, we found that LA volume and LF/HF ratio were not collinear variables. This result suggests that the predictive value of LF/HF ratio on new-onset AF in the whole population is not likely to be related to a statistical relationship between the ANS and LA dimensions' parameters.

Moreover, we can not exclude that new-onset AF patients had previous asymptomatic paroxysmal AF episodes (silent atrial fibrillation). However, we carefully checked patients medical history at admission to exclude previously known AF [3].

5. Conclusions

The results of our large HRV analysis indicate that autonomic dysregulation is strongly associated with new-onset AF in AMI. It would appear that AF in AMI is not related to an acute sympathetic activation, but rather on a parasympathetic one, suggesting the presence of chronically impaired cardiac autonomic regulation in patients who experience such events. However, in the absence of direct assessment of ANS activity, the causality between ANS dysfunction and increased risk of new-onset AF can only be inferred. Future studies are needed to test the clinical management of AMI patients guided by HRV [20].

Author Contributions: Conceptualization, C.G.; Data curation, A.S. and M.M.; Formal analysis, M.M.; Investigation, A.S. and F.G.; Methodology, B.M. and M.M.; Supervision, C.G., D.M., L.L., Y.C. and M.Z.; Validation, B.M. and M.F.; Writing—original draft, A.S.; Writing—review & editing, C.G., M.F. and M.Z. All authors have read and agreed to the published version of the manuscript.

Funding: This study was supported by the University Hospital of Dijon, the Association de Cardiologie de Bourgogne and by grants from the Agence Régionale de Santé (ARS) de Bourgogne Franche-Comté, French Ministry of Research, Institut National de la Santé et de la Recherche Médicale (INSERM), Fédération Française de Cardiologie, Société Française de Cardiologie and from the Conseil Regional de Bourgogne Franche-Comté.

Acknowledgments: The authors thank Theresa Daily and Suzanne Rankin for English revision of the paper, Florence Bichat, Morgane Laine and Aline Chagon for technical assistance.

Conflicts of Interest: The authors declare no conflict of interest.

References

1. Jabre, P.; Jouven, X.; Adnet, F.; Thabut, G.; Bielinski, S.J.; Weston, S.A.; Roger, V.L. Atrial fibrillation and death after myocardial infarction: A community study. *Circulation* **2011**, *123*, 2094–2100. [CrossRef] [PubMed]
2. Bengtson, L.G.S.; Chen, L.Y.; Chamberlain, A.M.; Michos, E.D.; Whitsel, E.A.; Lutsey, P.L.; Duval, S.; Rosamond, W.D.; Alonso, A. Temporal trends in the occurrence and outcomes of atrial fibrillation in patients with acute myocardial infarction (from the Atherosclerosis Risk in Communities Surveillance Study). *Am. J. Cardiol.* **2014**, *114*, 692–697. [CrossRef] [PubMed]
3. Guenancia, C.; Garnier, F.; Fichot, M.; Sagnard, A.; Laurent, G.; Lorgis, L. Silent atrial fibrillation: Clinical management and perspectives. *Future Cardiol.* **2020**, *16*, 133–142. [CrossRef]
4. Bettoni, M.; Zimmermann, M. Autonomic tone variations before the onset of paroxysmal atrial fibrillation. *Circulation* **2002**, *105*, 2753–2759. [CrossRef]
5. Nortamo, S.; Ukkola, O.; Kiviniemi, A.; Tulppo, M.; Huikuri, H.; Perkiömäki, J.S. Impaired cardiac autonomic regulation and long-term risk of atrial fibrillation in patients with coronary artery disease. *Heart Rhythm* **2018**, *15*, 334–340. [CrossRef] [PubMed]
6. Lorgis, L.; Moreau, D.; Mock, L.; Daumas, B.; Potard, D.; Touzery, C.; Cottin, Y.; Zeller, M. High N-Terminal Pro-B-Type Natriuretic Peptide Levels Are Associated with Reduced Heart Rate Variability in Acute Myocardial Infarction. *PLoS ONE* **2012**, *7*, e44677. [CrossRef]
7. Guenancia, C.; Toucas, C.; Fauchier, L.; Stamboul, K.; Garnier, F.; Mouhat, B.; Sagnard, A.; Lorgis, L.; Zeller, M.; Cottin, Y. High rate of recurrence at long-term follow-up after new-onset atrial fibrillation during acute myocardial infarction. *Eur. Eur. Pacing Arrhythm. Card. Electrophysiol. J. Work. Groups Card. Pacing Arrhythm. Card. Cell. Electrophysiol. Eur. Soc. Cardiol.* **2018**. [CrossRef]
8. Kirchhof, P.; Benussi, S.; Kotecha, D.; Ahlsson, A.; Atar, D.; Casadei, B.; Castella, M.; Diener, H.-C.; Heidbuchel, H.; Hendriks, J.; et al. 2016 ESC Guidelines for the management of atrial fibrillation developed in collaboration with EACTS. *Eur. J. Cardio-Thorac. Surg. Off. J. Eur. Assoc. Cardio-Thorac. Surg.* **2016**, *50*, e1–e88. [CrossRef]
9. Malik, M.; Bigger, J.T.; Camm, A.J.; Kleiger, R.E.; Malliani, A.; Moss, A.J.; Schwartz, P.J. Heart rate variability. Standards of measurement, physiological interpretation, and clinical use. Task Force of the European Society of Cardiology and the North American Society of Pacing and Electrophysiology. *Eur. Heart J.* **1996**, *17*, 354–381.
10. Billman, G.E. Heart Rate Variability—A Historical Perspective. *Front. Physiol.* **2011**, *2*. [CrossRef]
11. Rajendra Acharya, U.; Paul Joseph, K.; Kannathal, N.; Lim, C.M.; Suri, J.S. Heart rate variability: A review. *Med. Biol. Eng. Comput.* **2006**, *44*, 1031–1051. [CrossRef] [PubMed]
12. Amar, D.; Zhang, H.; Miodownik, S.; Kadish, A.H. Competing autonomic mechanisms precede the onset of postoperative atrial fibrillation. *J. Am. Coll. Cardiol.* **2003**, *42*, 1262–1268. [CrossRef]
13. Linz, D.; Elliott, A.D.; Hohl, M.; Malik, V.; Schotten, U.; Dobrev, D.; Nattel, S.; Böhm, M.; Floras, J.; Lau, D.H.; et al. Role of autonomic nervous system in atrial fibrillation. *Int. J. Cardiol.* **2018**. [CrossRef]
14. Pagani, M.; Lombardi, F.; Guzzetti, S.; Sandrone, G.; Rimoldi, O.; Malfatto, G.; Cerutti, S.; Malliani, A. Power spectral density of heart rate variability as an index of sympatho-vagal interaction in normal and hypertensive subjects. *J. Hypertens. Suppl. Off. J. Int. Soc. Hypertens.* **1984**, *2*, S383–S385.

15. Tsuji, H.; Larson, M.G.; Venditti, F.J.; Manders, E.S.; Evans, J.C.; Feldman, C.L.; Levy, D. Impact of reduced heart rate variability on risk for cardiac events. The Framingham Heart Study. *Circulation* **1996**, *94*, 2850–2855. [CrossRef] [PubMed]
16. Zaza, A.; Lombardi, F. Autonomic indexes based on the analysis of heart rate variability: A view from the sinus node. *Cardiovasc. Res.* **2001**, *50*, 434–442. [CrossRef]
17. Lau, D.H.; Schotten, U.; Mahajan, R.; Antic, N.A.; Hatem, S.N.; Pathak, R.K.; Hendriks, J.M.L.; Kalman, J.M.; Sanders, P. Novel mechanisms in the pathogenesis of atrial fibrillation: Practical applications. *Eur. Heart J.* **2016**, *37*, 1573–1581. [CrossRef]
18. Ng, J.; Villuendas, R.; Cokic, I.; Schliamser, J.E.; Gordon, D.; Koduri, H.; Benefield, B.; Simon, J.; Murthy, S.N.P.; Lomasney, J.W.; et al. Autonomic remodeling in the left atrium and pulmonary veins in heart failure: Creation of a dynamic substrate for atrial fibrillation. *Circ. Arrhythm. Electrophysiol.* **2011**, *4*, 388–396. [CrossRef]
19. Jayachandran, J.V.; Sih, H.J.; Winkle, W.; Zipes, D.P.; Hutchins, G.D.; Olgin, J.E. Atrial fibrillation produced by prolonged rapid atrial pacing is associated with heterogeneous changes in atrial sympathetic innervation. *Circulation* **2000**, *101*, 1185–1191. [CrossRef]
20. Jons, C.; Raatikainen, P.; Gang, U.J.; Huikuri, H.V.; Joergensen, R.M.; Johannesen, A.; Dixen, U.; Messier, M.; McNitt, S.; Thomsen, P.E.B.; et al. Autonomic dysfunction and new-onset atrial fibrillation in patients with left ventricular systolic dysfunction after acute myocardial infarction: A CARISMA substudy. *J. Cardiovasc. Electrophysiol.* **2010**, *21*, 983–990. [CrossRef]
21. Kalla, M.; Herring, N.; Paterson, D.J. Cardiac sympatho-vagal balance and ventricular arrhythmia. *Auton. Neurosci.* **2016**, *199*, 29–37. [CrossRef] [PubMed]
22. Farnier, M.; Salignon-Vernay, C.; Yao, H.; Chague, F.; Brunel, P.; Maza, M.; Brunet, D.; Bichat, F.; Beer, J.-C.; Cottin, Y.; et al. Prevalence, risk factor burden, and severity of coronary artery disease in patients with heterozygous familial hypercholesterolemia hospitalized for an acute myocardial infarction: Data from the French RICO survey. *J. Clin. Lipidol.* **2019**, *13*, 601–607. [CrossRef] [PubMed]

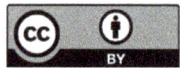

© 2020 by the authors. Licensee MDPI, Basel, Switzerland. This article is an open access article distributed under the terms and conditions of the Creative Commons Attribution (CC BY) license (http://creativecommons.org/licenses/by/4.0/).

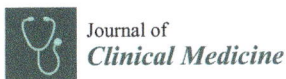 Journal of *Clinical Medicine*

Article

Real-Life Incident Atrial Fibrillation in Outpatients with Coronary Artery Disease

Sandro Ninni [1,2,*], Gilles Lemesle [1,2], Thibaud Meurice [3], Olivier Tricot [4], Nicolas Lamblin [1,5] and Christophe Bauters [1,5]

1. CHU Lille, Department of Cardiology, University of Lille, F-59000 Lille, France; gilles.lemesle@chru-lille.fr (G.L.); nicolas.lamblin@chru-lille.fr (N.L.); christophe.bauters@chru-lille.fr (C.B.)
2. Institut Pasteur de Lille, U1011, F-59000 Lille, France
3. Hôpital Privé Le Bois, 59003 Lille, France; tmeurice@me.com
4. Centre Hospitalier de Dunkerque, 59240 Dunkerque, France; oliviertricot@gmail.com
5. Institut Pasteur de Lille, U1167, F-59000 Lille, France
* Correspondence: sandro.ninni@chru-lille.fr; Tel.: +33-320-429373

Received: 1 July 2020; Accepted: 22 July 2020; Published: 24 July 2020

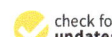

Abstract: Background: The risk, correlates, and consequences of incident atrial fibrillation (AF) in patients with chronic coronary artery disease (CAD) are largely unknown. **Methods and results:** We analyzed incident AF during a 3-year follow-up in 5031 CAD outpatients included in the prospective multicenter CARDIONOR registry and with no history of AF at baseline. Incident AF occurred in 266 patients (3-year cumulative incidence: 4.7% (95% confidence interval (CI): 4.1 to 5.3)). Incident AF was diagnosed during cardiology outpatient visits in 177 (66.5%) patients, 87 of whom were asymptomatic. Of note, 46 (17.3%) patients were diagnosed at time of hospitalization for heart failure, and a few patients ($n = 5$) at the time of ischemic stroke. Five variables were independently associated with incident AF: older age ($p < 0.0001$), heart failure ($p = 0.003$), lower left ventricle ejection fraction ($p = 0.008$), history of hypertension ($p = 0.010$), and diabetes mellitus ($p = 0.033$). Anticoagulant therapy was used in 245 (92%) patients and was associated with an antiplatelet drug in half ($n = 122$). Incident AF was a powerful predictor of all-cause (adjusted hazard ratio: 2.04; 95% CI: 1.47 to 2.83; $p < 0.0001$) and cardiovascular mortality (adjusted hazard ratio: 2.88; 95% CI: 1.88 to 4.43; $p < 0.0001$). **Conclusions:** In CAD outpatients, real-life incident AF occurs at a stable rate of 1.6% annually and is frequently diagnosed in asymptomatic patients during cardiology outpatient visits. Anticoagulation is used in most cases, often combined with antiplatelet therapy. Incident AF is associated with increased mortality.

Keywords: coronary artery disease; atrial fibrillation; prognosis; anticoagulation; antiplatelet therapy

1. Introduction

Atrial fibrillation (AF) is commonly observed in patients with coronary artery disease (CAD) [1–3]. Thanks to major therapeutic advances in recent decades [4,5], survival of patients with CAD has increased considerably, leaving more opportunity for the development of age-dependent diseases such as AF. The presence of concomitant AF in CAD patients is important in daily practice. Indeed, it may target higher risk patients for both ischemic and bleeding events and critically affect patient management, especially regarding antithrombotic strategies [1,3,6]. Although the risk, correlates, and consequences of incident AF have been extensively studied in the general population [7,8], and to the best of our knowledge, data are lacking in patients with chronic CAD. In addition, how antithrombotic drugs are managed in contemporary practice in such a setting is not known. The level of evidence of guidelines is indeed very low and practices may, therefore, widely differ between physicians. Given the specificities of the CAD population (routine follow-up by cardiologists, background secondary medical prevention therapy including antiplatelet drugs, prognostic implications of concomitant diseases), we sought to investigate these issues.

We analyzed data for 5031 CAD outpatients without prevalent AF included in a prospective registry. Here, we report the incidence, correlates, diagnostic circumstances, management, and prognostic impact of a first episode of AF occurring during the 3-year study follow-up.

2. Methods

2.1. Study Population

The CARDIONOR study is a multicenter registry that enrolled 10,517 consecutive outpatients with a diagnosis of CAD, AF, and/or heart failure (HF) between January 2013 and May 2015 [9]. The patients were included by 81 cardiologists from the French Region of Nord-Pas-de-Calais during outpatient visits. Documented CAD was defined as a history of myocardial infarction (MI), coronary revascularization, and/or the presence of coronary stenosis >50% on a coronary angiogram. Documented AF was defined as a history of AF, even if in sinus rhythm at inclusion. The sole exclusion criterion was age < 18 years. Patients with other cardiovascular or non-cardiovascular illnesses or co-morbidities were not excluded.

A case record form was completed at the initial visit with information regarding demographic and clinical details of the patients, including current medications. The treating cardiologists then followed up with the patients, with the number of outpatient visits at clinician discretion. Protocol-specified follow-up was performed at three years using a standardized case record form to report clinical events. In the case of missing information, a research technician contacted general practitioners and/or patients. The identification of patients with events for adjudication was based on interviews with patients/relatives during outpatient visits, discharge summaries for hospitalization during follow-up that were sent to treating cardiologists, and information obtained by the research technician. The events that patients reported were systematically confirmed from the medical reports.

This study was approved by the French medical data protection committee and authorized by the Commission Nationale de l'Informatique et des Libertés for the treatment of personal health data. All patients consented to the study after being informed in writing of the study's objectives and treatment of the data, as well as about their rights to object and about access and rectification.

2.2. Study Design and Definitions

Figure 1 shows the study flow chart. Among the 10517 outpatients included in the CARDIONOR registry, a total of 6313 had documented CAD. We excluded 1282 patients with prevalent AF, leaving 5031 CAD patients with no history of AF at registry inclusion. For the present analysis, we focused on the 5015 patients (99%) for whom follow-up was available. Two investigators adjudicated incident AF, with a third opinion sought in cases of disagreement.

The diagnostic circumstances of AF, as well as the antithrombotic strategy, were systematically assessed and adjudicated. No specific screening was performed for AF detection; documented AF episodes, therefore, represented daily practice. Data on therapeutic management represent the initial cardiologist recommendation, as described in the medical report associated with the AF diagnosis. Patients with implanted devices who had documented atrial high rate episodes and whose treating cardiologists had diagnosed them as having probable AF (as documented in the medical report) were adjudicated as incident AF. HF was defined as a history of hospitalization for HF and/or a history of symptoms and signs of HF associated with echocardiographic evidence of systolic dysfunction, left ventricular hypertrophy, left atrial enlargement, or diastolic dysfunction. Cause of death was determined after a detailed review of the circumstances of death and classified as cardiovascular or non-cardiovascular, as previously defined [10]. Death by an unknown cause was kept as a separate category.

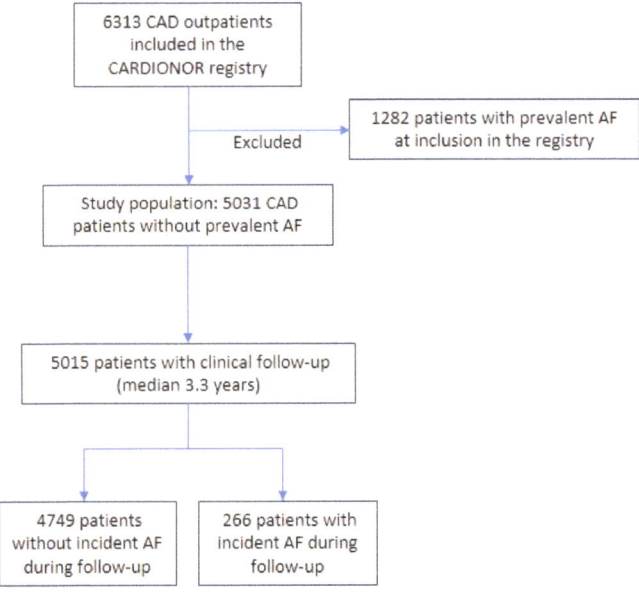

Figure 1. Study flow chart.

2.3. Statistical Analysis

Continuous variables are described as mean ± standard deviation (SD). Categorical variables are presented as absolute numbers and/or percentages. The incidence of AF was estimated with the cumulative incidence function, with death as the competing event. Univariable and multivariable assessments of baseline variables associated with incident AF were performed with the use of a cause-specific hazard model [11,12]. Hazard ratios (HRs) and 95% confidence intervals (CIs) were calculated. The proportional hazards assumption was tested visually using Kaplan–Meier curves and by examining plots of −ln [−ln (survival time)] against the ln (time). For continuous variables, the linearity assumption was assessed by plotting Schoenfeld residuals versus time. Collinearity was excluded by constructing a correlation matrix between candidate predictors. The comparison of baseline variables in patients with incident AF according to antithrombotic treatment was performed using the χ^2 test, the Fisher's exact test for categorical variables, and the Student's unpaired t test for continuous variables. The associations between incident AF and mortality were assessed with Cox analyses, and incident AF was modeled as a time-dependent variable. HRs and 95% CIs were calculated. All statistical analyses were performed using STATA 14.2 software (STATA Corporation, College Station, TX, USA). Significance was assumed at $p < 0.05$.

3. Results

3.1. Study Population

A clinical follow-up was obtained at a median of 3.3 (interquartile range: 3.0 to 3.6) years in 5015 (99%) of the 5031 CAD outpatients without prevalent AF. As shown in Table 1, most patients were male (77.8%), with a mean age of 66.1 ± 11.7 years. A history of MI was documented in 50.7% of the cases, with 72.7% of the patients having had previous percutaneous coronary intervention (PCI) and 19.5% with a previous coronary bypass (CABG). The mean left ventricular ejection fraction (LVEF) was 57 ± 11%, and 18.2% of the patients had LVEF <50%. Secondary prevention medications were widely prescribed (antiplatelet agents 98%, statins 92.5%, angiotensin-converting enzyme inhibitors or angiotensin receptor blockers 83.2%, beta-blockers 82.4%).

Table 1. Baseline characteristics of the study population and correlates of incident atrial fibrillation (AF) according to univariable analysis.

	All Patients with Follow-Up (n = 5015)	No Incident AF (n = 4749)	Incident AF (n = 266)	HR [95% CI]	p
Age, years	66.1 ± 11.7	65.8 ± 11.6	72.6 ± 10.4	1.06 [1.05–1.07]	<0.0001
Women	22.2	21.9	27.8	1.37 [1.05–1.79]	0.021
History of hypertension	59.2	58.4	73.2	1.95 [1.48–2.56]	<0.0001
History of diabetes mellitus	31.7	31.3	39.9	1.46 [1.14–1.86]	0.003
Previous MI	50.7	50.8	49.2	0.96 [0.75–1.22]	0.715
Previous PCI	72.7	73.1	65.8	0.69 [0.53–0.88]	0.004
Previous coronary bypass	19.5	19.3	22.9	1.25 [0.94–1.66]	0.127
Previous stroke	4.7	4.6	6.0	1.39 [0.84–2.30]	0.202
History of peripheral artery disease	23.5	23.3	27.1	1.25 [0.96–1.64]	0.104
Heart failure	14.5	13.8	27.8	2.67 [2.04–3.50]	<0.0001
LVEF, %	57 ± 11	57 ± 10	54 ± 13	0.97 [0.96–0.98]	<0.0001
LVEF < 50%	18.2	17.6	28.2	1.95 [1.49–2.54]	<0.0001
Medications at inclusion:					
Antiplatelet drug	98.0	97.9	98.9	1.80 [0.58–5.62]	0.311
Oral anticoagulant	4.1	4.1	3.4	0.81 [0.42–1.57]	0.533
At least 1 antithrombotic drug	99.3	99.3	99.6	1.82 [0.26–13.0]	0.550
Angiotensin-Converting enzyme inhibitor or angiotensin receptor blocker	83.2	82.9	88.4	1.53 [1.05–2.22]	0.027
Beta-Blocker	82.4	82.2	86.8	1.39 [0.98–1.99]	0.067
Statin	92.5	92.7	90.2	0.72 [0.48–1.07]	0.107

Data are presented as mean ± standard deviation (SD) or %. HR, hazard ratio; CI, confidence interval; MI, myocardial infarction; PCI, percutaneous coronary intervention; LVEF, left ventricular ejection fraction.

3.2. Incident AF

During the follow-up period, there were 495 deaths (cardiovascular deaths: $n = 200$) among the 5015 patients. During the same period, 266 patients experienced real-life incident AF. Risk of AF increased progressively, with cumulative incidences including death as the competing event of 1.6% (95% CI: 1.3 to 1.9), 2.9% (95% CI: 2.4 to 3.3), and 4.7% (95% CI: 4.1 to 5.3) at years 1–3, respectively. Figure 2A shows the cumulative incidence of AF over the time and Figure 2B according to age at inclusion.

We performed univariable and multivariable assessments of baseline variables that might be associated with incident AF (Tables 1 and 2). Five variables determined at registry inclusion were independently associated with incident AF: older age ($p < 0.0001$), heart failure ($p = 0.003$), lower LVEF ($p = 0.008$), history of hypertension ($p = 0.010$), and diabetes mellitus ($p = 0.033$). Of note, a history of MI was not associated with an increased risk for incident AF.

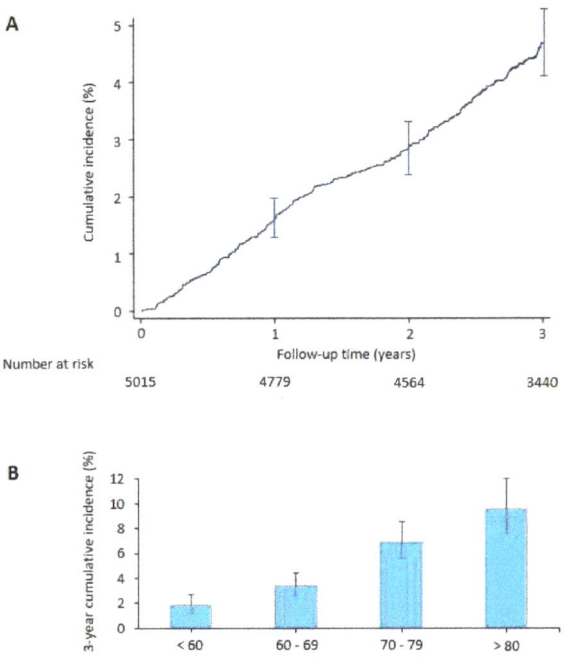

Figure 2. Incidence of a first episode of atrial fibrillation (AF). (**A**) Cumulative incidence of AF during the follow-up period (death as the competing event). (**B**) 3-year cumulative incidence of AF (death as the competing event) according to age at inclusion. Error bars are 95% CI.

Table 2. Independent correlates of incident atrial fibrillation (AF) by multivariable analysis.

	HR [95% CI]	p
Age (per year)	1.05 [1.04–1.07]	<0.0001
Heart failure	1.67 [1.19–2.35]	0.003
LVEF (per %)	0.98 [0.97–0.99]	0.008
History of hypertension	1.45 [1.09–1.93]	0.010
History of diabetes mellitus	1.31 [1.02–1.69]	0.033

HR, hazard ratio; CI, confidence interval; LVEF, left ventricular ejection fraction. The variables included in the model were age, sex, history of hypertension, history of diabetes mellitus, previous myocardial infarction, previous percutaneous coronary intervention, previous coronary bypass, previous stroke, history of peripheral artery disease, heart failure, and LVEF. A stepwise approach was used with forward selection (the p value for entering into the stepwise model was set at 0.05).

3.3. Diagnosis and Management of Incident AF

As shown in Figure 3A, the diagnosis of AF in the 266 patients took place in different settings. In two thirds of cases, incident AF was diagnosed during cardiology outpatient visits. Almost half of the patients in these situations had no evident symptoms of AF. Other relatively frequent diagnostic circumstances included hospitalization for heart failure ($n = 46$) and monitoring of implanted devices ($n = 15$). Of note, the number of patients who had AF diagnosed at the time of hospitalization for ischemic stroke was low ($n = 5$).

We assessed the antithrombotic strategy that was chosen in patients with incident AF. The mean CHA_2DS_2-VASc score in the 266 patients was 4.3 (±1.5). The proportion of women with a CHA_2DS_2-VASc score ≥ 3 was 97%, and the proportion of men with a CHA_2DS_2-VASc score ≥ 2 was 96%. As shown in Figure 3B, most patients were prescribed an anticoagulant (any anticoagulant:

$n = 245$ (92%); direct oral anticoagulant: $n = 127$; vitamin K antagonist: $n = 110$; low-molecular-weight heparin: $n = 8$). When anticoagulation was not used, 12 patients received single-antiplatelet therapy and 8 patients received dual-antiplatelet therapy; one patient had no antithrombotic therapy. When an anticoagulant was used, the antithrombotic regimen also included an antiplatelet drug in half of cases (anticoagulant alone: $n = 123$; anticoagulant + single-antiplatelet therapy: $n = 111$; anticoagulant + dual-antiplatelet therapy: $n = 11$). At time of incident AF, 26 of the 266 patients had a recent (<1 year) history of MI and/or PCI. When focusing on the 240 remaining patients who experienced incident AF in the context of chronic CAD (i.e., previous MI and/or PCI > 12 months) (Figure 3C), an anticoagulant was used in 225 (94%), still often combined with an antiplatelet drug (anticoagulant alone: $n = 121$; anticoagulant + single-antiplatelet therapy: $n = 102$; anticoagulant + dual-antiplatelet therapy: $n = 2$). Apart from higher proportions of previous PCI (75% vs. 54.6%, $p = 0.001$) and previous stroke (8.7% vs. 1.7%, $p = 0.026$), patients who received anticoagulant and antiplatelet therapy had similar characteristics to patients treated with anticoagulant alone (Table 3).

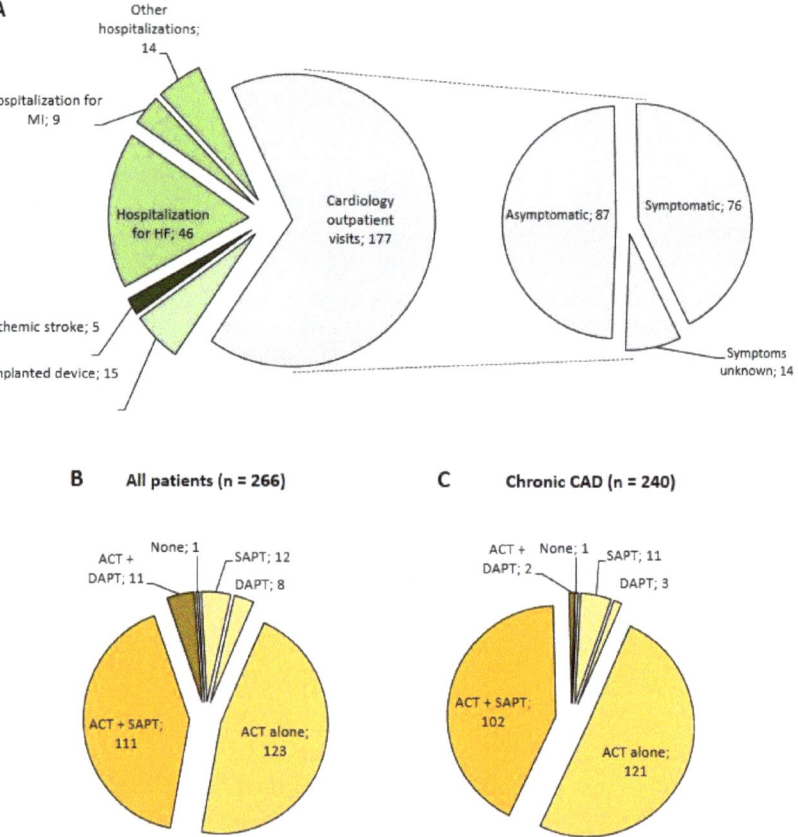

Figure 3. Diagnostic circumstances and antithrombotic management of incident atrial fibrillation (AF) in coronary artery disease (CAD) outpatients. (**A**) Diagnostic circumstances of incident atrial fibrillation (AF) in coronary artery disease (CAD) outpatients. HF, heart failure; MI, myocardial infarction (**B**) Antithrombotic strategy in all coronary artery disease (CAD) outpatients with incident atrial fibrillation (AF); ACT, anticoagulant therapy; DAPT, dual-antiplatelet therapy; SAPT, single-antiplatelet therapy. (**C**) Antithrombotic strategy in patients with incident AF in a context of chronic CAD (i.e., patients without recent (<1 year) history of myocardial infarction and/or percutaneous coronary intervention).

Table 3. Comparison of patients receiving anticoagulant therapy (ACT) alone vs. ACT and antiplatelet therapy (APT) ($n = 225$ patients with incident atrial fibrillation (AF) and without a recent (<1 year) history of myocardial infarction (MI) or percutaneous coronary intervention (PCI)).

	ACT Alone ($n = 121$)	ACT + APT ($n = 104$)	p
Baseline characteristics			
Age, years	73.5 ± 10.0	71.5 ± 10.8	0.137
Women	29.8	25.0	0.426
History of hypertension	69.4	74.8	0.376
History of diabetes mellitus	37.2	44.2	0.283
Previous MI	46.3	52.9	0.323
Previous PCI	54.6	75.0	0.001
Previous coronary bypass	30.6	20.2	0.076
Previous stroke	1.7	8.7	0.026
History of peripheral artery disease	28.9	22.1	0.244
Heart failure	24.8	32.7	0.190
LVEF, %	55 ± 12	53 ± 14	0.149
AF diagnosis			
Cardiology outpatient—asymptomatic	37.2	32.7	0.481
Cardiology outpatient—symptomatic	30.6	28.9	0.777
Hospitalization for heart failure	16.5	19.2	0.597
Implanted device	7.4	3.9	0.391
CHA_2DS_2-VASc score at AF diagnosis	4.3 ± 1.5	4.3 ± 1.3	0.700

Data are presented as mean ± SD or %. LVEF, left ventricular ejection fraction.

3.4. Outcome After Incident AF

For the 266 patients with incident AF, the median clinical follow-up after AF diagnosis was 1.2 (interquartile range: 0.5 to 2.2) years. A total of 42 deaths (cardiovascular deaths: $n = 26$) occurred during the post-AF period. Table 4 shows the impact of incident AF, analyzed as a time-dependent variable, on all-cause and cardiovascular mortality. In adjusted models, incident AF during follow-up was associated with significant increases in the risk of all-cause mortality (HR: 2.04; 95% CI: 1.47 to 2.83) and cardiovascular mortality (HR: 2.88; 95% CI: 1.88 to 4.43).

Table 4. Association of incident atrial fibrillation (AF) with mortality.

	HR [95% CI]	p
All-Cause Mortality		
unadjusted	3.90 [2.82–5.37]	<0.0001
adjusted	2.04 [1.47–2.83]	<0.0001
Cardiovascular Mortality		
unadjusted	6.49 [4.26–9.89]	<0.0001
adjusted	2.88 [1.88–4.43]	<0.0001

HR, hazard ratio; CI, confidence interval; incident AF was used as a time-dependent variable. Adjusted models included age, sex, history of hypertension, history of diabetes mellitus, heart failure, and LVEF.

4. Discussion

Interest is growing in analyzing outcomes in patients with chronic CAD [13–15]. Incident MI [16] or incident stroke [17] are probably the first events clinicians think of when assessing risk in these patients. However, other cardiovascular events may also affect management and may have significant prognostic implications. Our study documents a relatively high risk of real-life incident AF in chronic CAD patients, with a roughly linear increase of 1.6% per year. This result should be interpreted in the context of an unselected population of consecutive chronic CAD outpatients with a significant proportion of elderly individuals, and frequent history of hypertension, diabetes mellitus, and heart failure, all factors that are associated with incident AF in the present study as well as in the literature [7,18,19]. Incident AF is much less important in general population as reported by Vermond et al. in a large Dutch cohort with a cumulative incidence of 3% after a ten years mean follow-up and 3.3/1000 person-years [7]. In line with this, Wike et al. reported in a larger German cohort an incidence of 4.112/1000 person-years in the general population [20]. Importantly, to the best of our knowledge, no study assessed the incidence of AF in CAD outpatients. Of note, the interpretation of the rate of incident AF implies a need to consider screening strategies in this population. Our study protocol did not require specific screening for AF, so our data document incident AF diagnosed during routine real-life follow-up. Also, from a methodological point of view, we emphasize that our study may differ from earlier literature in that we present cumulative incidences, taking into account death as the competing event. We justify this choice by the high mortality rate of CAD patients at risk for AF. Indeed, inappropriate censoring of competing events may lead the Kaplan–Meier estimator to overestimate the cumulative incidence in the presence of competing risks, especially if the competing risk is frequent [11,12].

As stated above, the real-life design of our study yielded information on the diagnostic circumstances of incident AF. Such data are rarely available in the literature. An integral part of management for patients with chronic CAD is the planning of regular follow-up visits with the cardiologists. Although chronic CAD guidelines recommend an annual resting electrocardiogram (ECG), the level of evidence is acknowledged to be low [4,5]. Our data showed that incident AF was frequently diagnosed by a systematic ECG in the absence of AF-related symptoms. This high proportion of asymptomatic patients could be related to the wide use of betablockers prior to AF occurrence in our population. Moreover, it is plausible (although speculative) that patients with a history of CAD who experienced new symptoms had facilitated access to cardiology advice. This may have had important consequences by minimizing treatment delays. Concordant with these data is the relatively low number of incident AF discovered at time of hospitalization for an ischemic stroke (n = 5 for 5015 CAD patients followed-up during three years; 0.3/1000 patient-years).

International taskforces currently recommend against systematic screening for AF in the general population, citing the cost implications and uncertainty over the benefits of a systematic screening program compared to usual care [21]. However, screening in targeted high-risk groups remains to be questioned. Given the high incidence of AF compared to the general population and the proportion of asymptomatic AF in CAD outpatients reported in our study, extended screening strategies in such patients would be of interest.

One aim of our analysis was to describe the management strategy when incident AF is detected in chronic CAD patients. The present study focused on initial management at the time of AF diagnosis and, as such, clearly differs from previous analyses of registries reporting chronic medications in patients combining CAD and AF [3,22,23]. In addition, the 266 cases of incident AF occurred between 2013 and 2018, so our study describes the modern management of incident AF in patients with a history of CAD. First, we documented a very high use of anticoagulation, which is in accordance with the high thrombotic risk of the study population as documented by the CHA_2DS_2-VASc score. Indeed, according to current guidelines [24], anticoagulation would have to be considered in almost all CAD patients experiencing incident AF in the present study. Second, because almost all patients had a background of antiplatelet therapy before the AF event, the management of combinations of antithrombotic drugs was a matter of interest. When focusing the analysis on chronic patients, we found that cardiologists are still reluctant to stop all antiplatelet therapy in these patients. AF guidelines suggest going with anticoagulation alone if >1 year has passed with no acute events [24]. However, the level of evidence is limited, and expert consensus provides more modulated recommendations [25]. One recent randomized trial and many observational studies have shown that the addition of antiplatelet therapy is associated with a substantially increased risk of bleeding, with no clear benefit on ischemic events [3,22,23,26].

Finally, incident AF has been associated with increased mortality in general populations [7,8]. Our study extends these findings to a large population of outpatients with chronic CAD. In adjusted analyses, CAD patients who developed AF had a two-fold increased risk for all-cause mortality, largely similar to associations previously reported [7,8]. Incident AF should, therefore, be considered as an important warning sign for physicians working with CAD patients, even if anticoagulation is largely used. These data are concordant with previous findings suggesting that next to stroke prevention, further research is needed to improve the prognosis of patients with AF [7,27,28].

Study Limitations

Our study has some limitations. First, our data reflect the practice in a regional area, and we do not know whether these findings are generalizable for practices in other parts of the world. Second, because cardiologists determined inclusion, the data may not be generalizable to the overall population with CAD in the community. Finally, we present here initial management strategies for patients with incident AF and lack details on chronic management and antithrombotic modifications during follow-up. On the other hand, the absence of exclusion criteria, the very high follow-up rate, and the adjudication of clinical events can be considered strengths of the study.

5. Conclusions

Our study shows that real-life incident AF occurs at a stable annual rate of 1.6% in chronic CAD outpatients. Older age, heart failure, low LVEF, hypertension, and diabetes were associated with a higher risk of AF. In patients with chronic CAD, a substantial proportion of incident AF is diagnosed during a systematic cardiology outpatient visit in asymptomatic patients. In patients with chronic CAD and incident AF that were >1 year from their last MI and/or PCI, antiplatelets remain frequently combined with oral anticoagulation. Finally, we found that incident AF in patients with chronic CAD was associated with an increase in all-cause and cardiovascular mortality. Considering the high incidence of AF compared to the general population and the proportion of asymptomatic AF in CAD outpatients, extended screening strategies in such patients would be of interest.

Author Contributions: Conceptualization, S.N., G.L. and C.B.; Data curation, T.M. and O.T.; Formal analysis, S.N.; Funding acquisition, C.B.; Investigation, N.L. and C.B.; Methodology, S.N., G.L., T.M., N.L. and C.B.; Validation, N.L.; Writing—original draft, S.N. and C.B.; Writing—review & editing, G.L. and N.L. All authors have read and agreed to the published version of the manuscript.

Funding: This study was supported by the Fondation Coeur et Recherche, Paris, France.

Acknowledgments: Michel Deneve for monitoring the CARDIONOR study.

Conflicts of Interest: Lemesle reports personal fees from Amgen, Astra Zeneca, Bayer, Boehringer Ingelheim, Bristol-Myers Squibb, MSD, Novartis, Pfizer, Sanofi-Aventis, Servier, and The Medicine Co. Lamblin reports personal fees from Actelion, Akcea, Amicus therapeutics, Bayer, Novartis, MSD, Pfizer, and Sanofi-Aventis and travel grants from Amgen and Bristol-Myers Squibb. Ninni, Meurice, Tricot, and Bauters had nothing to disclose.

Abbreviations

ACT	anticoagulant therapy
APT	antiplatelet therapy
AF	atrial fibrillation
CAD	coronary artery disease
CI	confidence interval
DAPT	dual antiplatelet therapy
ECG	electrocardiogram
HF	heart failure
HR	hazard ratio
LVEF	left ventricular ejection fraction
MI	myocardial infarction
PCI	percutaneous coronary intervention
SAPT	single antiplatelet therapy

References

1. Goto, S.; Bhatt, D.L.; Rother, J. Prevalence, clinical profile, and cardiovascular outcomes of atrial fibrillation patients with atherothrombosis. *Am. Heart. J.* **2008**, *156*, 855–863. [CrossRef] [PubMed]
2. Aguilar, E.; Garcia-Diaz, A.M.; Sanchez Munoz-Torrero, J.F. Clinical outcome of stable outpatients with coronary, cerebrovascular or peripheral artery disease, and atrial fibrillation. *Thromb. Res.* **2012**, *130*, 390–395. [CrossRef] [PubMed]
3. Hamon, M.; Lemesle, G.; Tricot, O. Incidence, source, determinants, and prognostic impact of major bleeding in outpatients with stable coronary artery disease. *J. Am. Coll. Cardiol.* **2014**, *64*, 1430–1436. [CrossRef] [PubMed]
4. Fihn, S.D.; Gardin, J.M.; Abrams, J. 2012 ACCF/AHA/ACP/AATS/PCNA/SCAI/STS guideline for the diagnosis and management of patients with stable ischemic heart disease: A report of the American College of Cardiology Foundation/American Heart Association task force on practice guidelines, and the American College of Physicians, American Association for Thoracic Surgery, Preventive Cardiovascular Nurses Association, Society for Cardiovascular Angiography and Interventions, and Society of Thoracic Surgeons. *Circulation* **2012**, *126*, e354–e471. [CrossRef] [PubMed]
5. Montalescot, G.; Sechtem, U.; Achenbach, S. 2013 ESC guidelines on the management of stable coronary artery disease. *Eur. Heart J.* **2013**, *34*, 2949–3003. [CrossRef] [PubMed]
6. Schurtz, G.; Bauters, C.; Ducrocq, G. Effect of aspirin in addition to oral anticoagulants in stable coronary artery disease outpatients with an indication for anticoagulation. *Panminerva Med.* **2016**, *58*, 271–285. [PubMed]
7. Vermond, R.A.; Geelhoed, B.; Verweij, N. Incidence of Atrial Fibrillation and Relationship with Cardiovascular Events, Heart Failure, and Mortality: A Community-Based Study from The Netherlands. *J. Am. Coll. Cardiol.* **2015**, *66*, 1000–1007. [CrossRef]
8. Andersson, T.; Magnuson, A.; Bryngelsson, I.L. All-cause mortality in 272,186 patients hospitalized with incident atrial fibrillation 1995–2008: A Swedish nationwide long-term case-control study. *Eur. Heart J.* **2013**, *34*, 1061–1067. [CrossRef]
9. Lamblin, N.; Ninni, S.; Tricot, O. Secondary prevention and outcomes in outpatients with coronary artery disease, atrial fibrillation or heart failure: A focus on disease overlap. *Open Heart* **2020**, *7*, e001165. [CrossRef]
10. Bauters, C.; Tricot, O.; Meurice, T. Long-term risk and predictors of cardiovascular death in stable coronary artery disease: The CORONOR study. *Coron. Artery. Dis.* **2017**, *28*, 636–641. [CrossRef]
11. Wolbers, M.; Koller, M.T.; Stel, V.S. Competing risks analyses: Objectives and approaches. *Eur. Heart J.* **2014**, *35*, 2936–2941. [CrossRef] [PubMed]
12. Austin, P.C.; Lee, D.S.; Fine, J.P. Introduction to the Analysis of Survival Data in the Presence of Competing Risks. *Circulation* **2016**, *133*, 601–609. [CrossRef] [PubMed]
13. Daly, C.; Clemens, F.; Lopez Sendon, J.L. Gender differences in the management and clinical outcome of stable angina. *Circulation* **2006**, *113*, 490–498. [CrossRef] [PubMed]
14. Steg, P.G.; Greenlaw, N.; Tardif, J.C. Women and men with stable coronary artery disease have similar clinical outcomes: Insights from the international prospective CLARIFY registry. *Eur. Heart J.* **2012**, *33*, 2831–2840. [CrossRef]
15. Bauters, C.; Deneve, M.; Tricot, O. Prognosis of patients with stable coronary artery disease (from the CORONOR study). *Am. J. Cardiol.* **2014**, *113*, 1142–1145. [CrossRef]
16. Lemesle, G.; Tricot, O.; Meurice, T. Incident Myocardial Infarction and Very Late Stent Thrombosis in Outpatients with Stable Coronary Artery Disease. *J. Am. Coll. Cardiol.* **2017**, *69*, 2149–2156. [CrossRef]
17. Cordonnier, C.; Lemesle, G.; Casolla, B. Incidence and determinants of cerebrovascular events in outpatients with stable coronary artery disease. *Eur. Stroke J.* **2018**, *3*, 272–280. [CrossRef]
18. Alonso, A.; Krijthe, B.P.; Aspelund, T. Simple risk model predicts incidence of atrial fibrillation in a racially and geographically diverse population: The CHARGE-AF consortium. *J. Am. Heart Assoc.* **2013**, *2*, e000102. [CrossRef]
19. Smith, J.G.; Newton-Cheh, C.; Almgren, P. Assessment of conventional cardiovascular risk factors and multiple biomarkers for the prediction of incident heart failure and atrial fibrillation. *J. Am. Coll. Cardiol.* **2010**, *56*, 1712–1719. [CrossRef]

20. Wilke, T.; Groth, A.; Mueller, S. Incidence and Prevalence of Atrial Fibrillation: An Analysis Based on 8.3 Million Patients. *Europace* **2013**, *4*, 486–493. [CrossRef]
21. Jones, N.R.; Taylor, C.J.; Hobbs, F.D.R. Screening for atrial fibrillation: A call for evidence. *Eur. Heart J.* **2019**, *41*, 1075–1085. [CrossRef] [PubMed]
22. Lamberts, M.; Gislason, G.H.; Lip, G.Y. Antiplatelet therapy for stable coronary artery disease in atrial fibrillation patients taking an oral anticoagulant: A nationwide cohort study. *Circulation* **2014**, *129*, 1577–1585. [CrossRef] [PubMed]
23. Lemesle, G.; Ducrocq, G.; Elbez, Y. Vitamin K antagonists with or without long-term antiplatelet therapy in outpatients with stable coronary artery disease and atrial fibrillation: Association with ischemic and bleeding events. *Clin. Cardiol.* **2017**, *40*, 932–939. [CrossRef] [PubMed]
24. Kirchhof, P.; Benussi, S.; Kotecha, D. 2016 ESC Guidelines for the management of atrial fibrillation developed in collaboration with EACTS. *Eur. Heart J.* **2016**, *37*, 2893–2962. [CrossRef] [PubMed]
25. Angiolillo, D.J.; Goodman, S.G.; Bhatt, D.L. Antithrombotic Therapy in Patients with Atrial Fibrillation Undergoing Percutaneous Coronary Intervention: A North American Perspective-2016 Update. *Circ. Cardiovasc. Interv.* **2016**, *9*, e004395. [CrossRef] [PubMed]
26. Yasuda, S.; Kaikita, K.; Akao, M. Antithrombotic Therapy for Atrial Fibrillation with Stable Coronary Disease. *N. Engl. J. Med.* **2019**, *381*, 1103–1113. [CrossRef] [PubMed]
27. Piccini, J.P.; Hammill, B.G.; Sinner, M.F. Clinical course of atrial fibrillation in older adults: The importance of cardiovascular events beyond stroke. *Eur. Heart J.* **2014**, *35*, 250–256. [CrossRef]
28. Bassand, J.P.; Accetta, G.; Camm, A.J. Two-year outcomes of patients with newly diagnosed atrial fibrillation: Results from GARFIELD-AF. *Eur. Heart J.* **2016**, *37*, 2882–2889. [CrossRef]

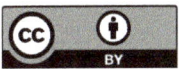

© 2020 by the authors. Licensee MDPI, Basel, Switzerland. This article is an open access article distributed under the terms and conditions of the Creative Commons Attribution (CC BY) license (http://creativecommons.org/licenses/by/4.0/).

Review
Mitochondrial Dysfunction in Atrial Fibrillation—Mechanisms and Pharmacological Interventions

Paweł Muszyński and Tomasz A. Bonda *

Department of General and Experimental Pathology, Medical University of Bialystok, Mickiewicza 2c, 15-222 Bialystok, Poland; Pawel.Muszynski@umb.edu.pl
* Correspondence: Tomasz.Bonda@umb.edu.pl; Tel.: +48-85-748-5593

Abstract: Despite the enormous progress in the treatment of atrial fibrillation, mainly with the use of invasive techniques, many questions remain unanswered regarding the pathomechanism of the arrhythmia and its prevention methods. The development of atrial fibrillation requires functional changes in the myocardium that result from disturbed ionic fluxes and altered electrophysiology of the cardiomyocyte. Electrical instability and electrical remodeling underlying the arrhythmia may result from a cellular energy deficit and oxidative stress, which are caused by mitochondrial dysfunction. The significance of mitochondrial dysfunction in the pathogenesis of atrial fibrillation remains not fully elucidated; however, it is emphasized by the reduction of atrial fibrillation burden after therapeutic interventions improving the mitochondrial welfare. This review summarizes the mechanisms of mitochondrial dysfunction related to atrial fibrillation and current pharmacological treatment options targeting mitochondria to prevent or improve the outcome of atrial fibrillation.

Keywords: atrial fibrillation; mitochondria; cardiac remodeling; pharmacotherapy

1. Introduction

Atrial fibrillation (AF) is the most frequent type of arrhythmia occurring, especially among patients with more advanced age. It is estimated that the prevalence of AF in the global population varies between 2% and 3.4% [1–3]. AF is 1.2 times more prevalent among males than females, less frequent at a younger age (0.12–0.16% > 49 y) and increases with age (3.7–4.2% 60–70 y and in 10–17% > 80 y.) [1]. The early onset of AF may be attributed to a genetic component or congenital heart defects [4–6]. In younger patients without structural heart defects, the pulmonary vein arrhythmogenesis frequently acts as the initiating trigger for AF, mostly paroxysmal, and recurrences can be successfully prevented by pulmonary vein ablation [7]. However, in elderly patients, the key initiating factors are atrial tissue degeneration and comorbidities affecting the atrial metabolism and atrial structure, more frequently leading to persistent or permanent AF [8,9].

AF significantly affects the quality of life, worsens morbidity and mortality and generates a significant socioeconomic burden [10]. Due to comorbidities caused by AF complications, a large proportion of people with AF are not able to function normally in society. Financial outlays for hospitalizations due to AF in 2005 cost USD 6.65 billion in the US [10]. The cost per patient per year was estimated from USD 2000 to USD 14200 in the US and from EUR 450 to EUR 3000 in Europe and was further increased by the introduction of non-vitamin K antagonist oral anticoagulants [11,12]. The aging of the population in developed countries will increase the number of people with AF. Therefore, advances in understanding the mechanisms leading to this arrhythmia for improving prevention and treatment are crucial to restrain the AF epidemic.

The pathophysiology of AF has been thoroughly investigated in the past decades, and the association between mitochondrial dysfunction and AF was proposed as early as the 1970s [13]. Mitochondria are organelles present in metabolically active cells, such as cardiomyocytes, in large numbers. They are responsible for synthesis of adenosine 5'-triphosphate (ATP), which provides energy for almost all intracellular processes, including mechanical work and active ion transport. Disturbance of mitochondrial energetics, oxidative stress and electrical remodeling was proposed to be associated with the occurrence of the arrhythmia [13,14]. Recent progress in scientific tools, including genomic, proteomic and metabolomic analyses, allow for further detailed investigation of the mechanisms linking consequences of mitochondrial dysfunction with development of AF [15–18].

This review summarizes the knowledge about the role of mitochondrial dysfunction in the pathogenesis of AF and gives an overview of the current treatment options to ameliorate the condition of mitochondria to prevent the arrhythmia or improve prognosis.

2. General Mechanisms of AF

The main mechanism of AF perpetuation is the re-entry phenomenon. It usually depends on the preexisting morphological substrate of enlarged atria, which are able to accommodate one or multiple depolarization waves or the spiral wave [19]. Premature atrial beats, originating most frequently from the myocardial sleeves within the pulmonary veins, trigger the re-entry and initiate AF [20]. However, in younger patients without significant morphological heart disease, rapid focal activity from the pulmonary veins may be more important as the underlying mechanism of AF. The arrhythmogenic foci may depend on diastolic calcium leak from the sarcoplasmic reticulum (SR) due to ryanodine receptor (RyR) hyperphosphorylation that promotes delayed afterdepolarizations and triggered activity to induce AF [21]. Re-entry and rapid focal activity both induce frequent atrial depolarizations and electrical remodeling that is characterized by slowed conduction and shortened atrial refractoriness, which promote re-entry and persistence of AF [20]. Electrical remodeling is induced by SR calcium overload and elevated cytoplasmic Ca^{2+} levels, reduced expression of the slow inward calcium channels, increased rectifier potassium current and altered expression of the connexins [22].

Many clinical risk factors promoting the development of AF were identified, such as older age, male sex, obesity, hypertension, coronary artery disease, heart failure (HF), chronic kidney disease, hyperthyroidism, diabetes mellitus (DM), chronic obstructive pulmonary disease (COPD) and valvular heart disease [23–25]. These disorders are responsible for the induction of unfavorable atrial structural remodeling and formation of the morphological substrate sustaining the arrhythmia. The pathomechanisms of structural remodeling include atrial pressure and volume overload leading to atrial dilation (valvular heart disease, HF), increased atrial epicardial fat tissue (obesity, metabolic syndrome), autonomic nervous system dysfunction (diabetes mellitus), systemic inflammation (coronary artery disease, HF, COPD), increased fibrosis, cellular ultrastructural defects and contractile proteins dysfunction [24,26].

3. Role of Mitochondria in the Physiology of the Heart

The mechanical work of the cardiac muscle relies on the contractile apparatus built up by the filaments of actin, myosin and dozens of regulatory proteins packed together into sarcomeres. Cardiac myocyte's contraction–relaxation cycle is coupled to the cytoplasmic calcium cycling, and both mechanical work and regulation of cytoplasmic calcium levels require uncompromised delivery of ATP [27]. The majority of ATP utilized by the cardiomyocyte is used for myosin ATPase of the contractile filaments, the sarcolemmal Na^+/K^+-ATPase and the Ca^{2+}-ATPase of the sarcoplasmic reticulum (SR) [28].

Cardiomyocytes rely on the aerobic metabolism, and the vast majority of ATP is synthesized in the mitochondria. The initial substrates for ATP synthesis include glucose and fatty acids. The mitochondrial respiration and beta-oxidation of fatty acids occur in the mitochondria and require constant delivery of oxygen [29,30]. The cytoplasmic phase, glycolysis, is anaerobic and it provides only a small amount of ATP. Its product, the pyruvate, is transported to the mitochondria and decarboxylated to form acetyl-coenzyme A (acetyl-CoA). Acetyl-CoA is also the end product of mitochondrial fatty-acid beta-oxidation. Next, acetyl-CoA acts as a donor of acetyl groups for the tricarboxylic acid cycle (TCA). Oxidation of the substrates provides energy and reduced nicotinamide adenine dinucleotide (NADH) and flavin adenine dinucleotide (FADH$_2$). These two compounds serve as electron donors for the mitochondrial electron transport chain (ETC). The flow of electrons along the ETC components, which have a gradually increasing redox potential, provides energy for the transfer of protons across the inner mitochondrial membrane. Protons collected in the intermembrane space generate the electrochemical gradient that is called the inner mitochondrial membrane (IMM) potential ($\Delta\Psi$m). ATP synthase located in the cristae of IMM uses the energy stored in this gradient to drive ATP synthesis in the process of oxidative phosphorylation [31].

In addition to involvement in ATP synthesis, mitochondria are an important regulator of intracellular calcium balance. The increased concentration of calcium ions in the cytoplasm increases its electrochemical gradient between the cytoplasm and the matrix, and promotes the influx of calcium via the mitochondrial calcium uniporter located in the inner mitochondrial membrane into the mitochondria. In this way, mitochondria can buffer the excess of cytosolic Ca^{2+} or release it via the sodium/calcium symporter (NCLX) when its concentration in the cytoplasm falls down [32].

4. Involvement of Mitochondrial Dysfunction in the Pathogenesis of AF

Recent investigations link mitochondrial dysfunction with the pathogenesis of AF [33]. Frequent depolarizations of atrial myocardium increase energetic demands of the cells. In paroxysmal or short-lasting persistent AF, mitochondria are able to increase the synthesis of ATP, but with time the production of ATP decreases, suggesting mitochondrial dysfunction [33]. Low ATP levels affect the intracellular ionic equilibrium, decrease the efficiency of all energy-requiring enzymatic reactions and impair contraction, relaxation and ionic homeostasis of the cell. Diminished levels of ATP lead to activation of cytoplasmic glycolytic enzymes and increased synthesis of lactate that may be considered a mechanism similar to the Warburg effect found in rapidly growing tumors [34,35]. Cellular metabolic stress results in the lowering of the ATP/AMP ratio, which activates the energy sensor adenosine monophosphate protein kinase (AMPK). Activation of this enzyme shifts metabolic pathways toward glycolysis and inhibits the anabolic processes. AMPK can also affect the ionic channels, for example, the ATP-sensitive potassium channel and slow inward calcium channel, and thus modify electrophysiological properties of the cardiac myocytes [14,36]. AMPK is activated in the atrial myocardium in paroxysmal but not long-lasting AF, and is considered the compensatory response to the metabolic stress induced by the arrhythmia [14].

Dysfunctional mitochondria are the source of a large amount of free radicals, especially the superoxide anion (O$_2^-$), which oxidizes many intracellular targets including RyR2 of the SR and the sarcolemmal inward sodium channel [37]. These changes directly alter cardiomyocyte's excitability and intercellular coupling and build-up the functional background to maintain the reentrant circuits. In addition, mitochondrial dysfunction leads to cytokine release, activation of fibroblasts, deposition of the connective tissue and enhancement of automaticity, promoting development of the arrhythmia [38]. Indeed, experimental and clinical data reveal the association between altered mitochondrial function and the risk of atrial fibrillation [39].

4.1. Mitochondrial Ultrastructural Abnormalities

Mitochondrial dysfunction is characterized by both functional and morphological changes. Modification of mitochondrial shape, volume and remodeling of the cristae ultrastructure is coupled to cellular bioenergetic balance and requires the involvement of several mitochondrial proteins [40]. A rapid depolarization rate during AF increases demands for the generation of high-energy compounds and implies additional stress to the cardiomyocytes.

Persistent atrial fibrillation induced in goat initially induced degradation of myofibrils and accumulation of glycogen that were followed by mitochondrial elongation and changes in the cristae orientation; however, no further ultrastructural mitochondrial changes were evident after 16 weeks of the arrhythmia in this animal model [41]. In the mouse with AF and HF, atrial cardiomyocytes contained defective mitochondria with matrix edema and interruption of the inner and outer membrane structures that were related to diminished ATP synthesis [42]. Ozcan et al. described increased volume and number of mitochondria in AF accompanying HF in mice.

In atrial samples collected from patients during cardiac surgery, the ultrastructural examination suggested an increased number of mitochondria frequently having changed shape during AF, but without obvious swelling and cristae derangement [43]. In the model of atrial tachycardia using human atrial samples subjected to rapid pacing, there was an increased number of swollen mitochondria with partial cristaeolysis and completely disrupted mitochondria, which were prevented by verapamil, which suggests calcium-related mechanisms of these ultrastructural changes [44]. Indeed, elevated sarcoplasmic Ca^{2+} levels, secondary to Ca^{2+} leak from the SR in RyR2 mutant mice, leads to mitochondrial dysmorphology [45]. The mitochondrial matrix volume can be additionally influenced by potassium fluxes through the Ca^{2+}-dependent (K-Ca) and ATP-dependent potassium channels (mitoK$_{ATP}$) that promote edema, whereas K^+/H^+ exchanger (KHE) allowing for potassium efflux prevents mitochondrial swelling [46].

4.2. Disturbed Mitochondrial Biogenesis

Mitochondrial biogenesis is a complex process of increasing the global mass of mitochondria within the cell. The process of mitochondrial biogenesis includes the fusion and fission events and concomitant control of mitochondria quality.

The primary mitochondrial biogenesis is induced by environmental stress, such as exercise, caloric restriction, low temperature, oxidative stress, cell division, renewal and differentiation, through the cyclic adenosine monophosphate (cAMP) and protein kinase A (PKA) pathways.

The biogenesis of mitochondria is strictly connected with the mitochondrial ultrastructural changes and requires involvement of many regulatory proteins, which are involved in the division (fission) and contribute to a build-up of the structural and functional basis. The majority of proteins are encoded by nuclear DNA, but some of them are based on autonomous mitochondrial DNA [47,48]. The master regulator of mitochondrial biogenesis is PGC-1α (peroxisome proliferator-activated receptor-γ coactivator 1-α, the product of the PPARGC1A gene). High energetic demand augments the expression of PGC-1α [49]. Activation of PGC-1α is achieved through its deacetylation by sirtuin 1 (SIRT1) or phosphorylation by AMPK and is inhibited by histone acetyltransferase GCN5 (general control of amino-acid synthesis 5) [47,49]. PGC-1α directly adjusts transcription, ribosome formation and assembly of the mitochondrial structural proteins, but also stimulates expression of the nuclear respiratory factors 1 and 2 (NRF-1 and NRF-2), through which it promotes the mitochondrial biogenesis indirectly [50]. PGC1-α together with NRFs promote transcription of mitochondrial genes, starting with the activation of mitochondrial transcription factors, such as mitochondrial transcription factor A (Tfam), Yin-Yang 1 (YY1), mitochondrial DNA-directed RNA polymerase (POLRMT), mitochondrial dimethyladenosine transferase 1 (Tfb1m) and transducer of regulated cAMP response element-binding protein (TORC) [51].

In a rabbit model of pacing-induced AF, mitochondrial DNA content and the expression of transcription factors involved in mitochondrial biogenesis were decreased [52]. In another study, examining rats with streptozotocin-induced diabetes mellitus, Shao et al. found impaired expression of the regulators of mitochondrial biogenesis in diabetic animals that was related to high inducibility of atrial fibrillation, and pharmacological improvement of the indices of mitochondrial biogenesis blunts propensity to AF [39]. Impaired expression of PGC-1α was also found among other disturbances before development of postoperative AF [53].

4.3. Mitochondria-Related Oxidative Stress

Reactive oxygen species (ROS) in normal cardiac myocytes originate from mitochondria [54]. The electron transfer chain is the source of small amounts of ROS even under physiological conditions, but any disturbance in the proton gradient across the inner mitochondrial membrane leads to diminished ATP and excessive ROS generation [42].

Atrial fibrillation is characterized by excessive ROS generation due to mitochondrial dysfunction but also due to activation of other mechanisms, such as NADPH oxidase [45,55–58]. In the atrial muscle of patients with AF, reduction of complex I and II activity with increased activity of complex V was found, which was paralleled by increased production of superoxide [59]. Excessive ROS production and diminished superoxide dismutase promoting oxidative stress in atrial samples were also found in patients in whom AF developed during postoperative follow-up [44,55]. Oxidative stress was linked to changes in gene transcription, damage to mitochondrial DNA, increased activity of NADPH oxidase and xanthine oxidase and local induction of inflammatory processes. Oxidation of ryanodine receptors causes their dysfunction and leakage of Ca^{2+} from the SR [60]. On the other hand, disturbed intracellular Ca^{2+} homeostasis, occurring due to genetic manipulations or under metabolic stress, is related to increased synthesis of ROS by mitochondria [45]. Oxidative stress induces proinflammatory pathways via activation of NF-κB, caspase-1 and NLRP-3 inflammasome [44,61,62]. Moreover, both oxidative stress and inflammation upregulate expression of transforming growth factor β1 (TGF-β1) that leads to proliferation of fibroblasts, their recruitment into myofibroblasts and fibrosis of the atrial myocardium, which is an important constituent of atrial structural remodeling promoting AF [30].

AF development and atrial remodeling can be successfully prevented by treatment with an antioxidant probucol, which in addition to attenuated oxidative stress, also inhibits NF-κB and proinflammatory and profibrotic cytokines release [63]. Potentiation of mitochondrial free radical scavenging mechanisms induced by overexpression of catalase in transgenic mice was sufficient to prevent mitochondrial dysmorphology, SR Ca^{2+} leak and inducibility of AF [45]. Attenuation of oxidative stress by the silencing of the NADPH oxidase 2 with a gene-based approach successfully prevented the electrical remodeling of atrial myocardium and maintenance of the arrhythmia in a canine model of AF [64], and gene therapy directed at the improvement of mitochondrial antioxidative capacity may also be effective in prevention of AF.

5. Pharmacological Interventions Improving Mitochondrial Function in AF

Among pharmacological agents that improve the function of mitochondria and the energetic balance of cardiomyocytes, there are several groups of drugs used in the contemporary practice, mostly in the treatment of diabetes mellitus, and newly developed medications targeting mitochondria more specifically. The clinical benefits achieved by improvement of the mitochondrial function are presented in Figure 1. This chapter describes the effects of these drugs on the mechanisms related to atrial fibrillation.

5.1. The Dipeptidyl Peptidase-4 (DDP-4) Inhibitors

The Dipeptidyl peptidase-4 (DDP-4) inhibitors are a new group of oral antidiabetic drugs acting on the incretin system. DDP-4 is an enzyme that inactivates gastric inhibitory polypeptide (GIP) and glucagon-like peptide-1 (GLP-1). Blocking DDP-4 increases the levels of the above hormones, inhibits glucagon and upregulates insulin release.

In cardiomyocytes, hypoxia increases the expression of DDP-4, which triggers the generation of free radicals and $\Delta\Psi m$ reduction [65]. Thus, the cardioprotective effects of DDP-4 are related to attenuation of oxidative stress and amelioration of mitochondrial function [65]. A DDP-4 inhibitor, alogliptin, was shown to reduce the duration of burst pacing-induced atrial fibrillation by 73% in the rabbit model of HF [66]. The exact cellular mechanisms were not evaluated, but alogliptin reduced the extent of atrial fibrosis, improved left atrial capillary density and promoted the activity of endothelial NOS [66]. In another animal study using the model of alloxan-induced diabetes mellitus, treatment with alogliptin resulted in improved ΔΨm and mitochondrial biogenesis via activation of the PGC-1α/NRF1/Tfam signaling pathway that was paralleled by preservation of the left atrial diameter, lowering of hs-CRP levels, upregulation of superoxide dismutase and improved atrial electrical function [67]. Linagliptin, another DDP-4 inhibitor, prevented atrial electrical remodeling, reduced oxidative stress and suppressed AF inducibility in a canine model of atrial fibrillation [68]. The protective effects of DDP4 inhibitors against AF seems to be related to lowering ROS, preserving mitochondrial biogenesis and reducing inflammation [69]. The therapeutic potential of DDP4 inhibitors was confirmed in a large observational study involving over 90,000 diabetic patients, in whom the addition of a DDP-4 inhibitor as a second-line anti-diabetic treatment reduced new onset AF by 35% [70].

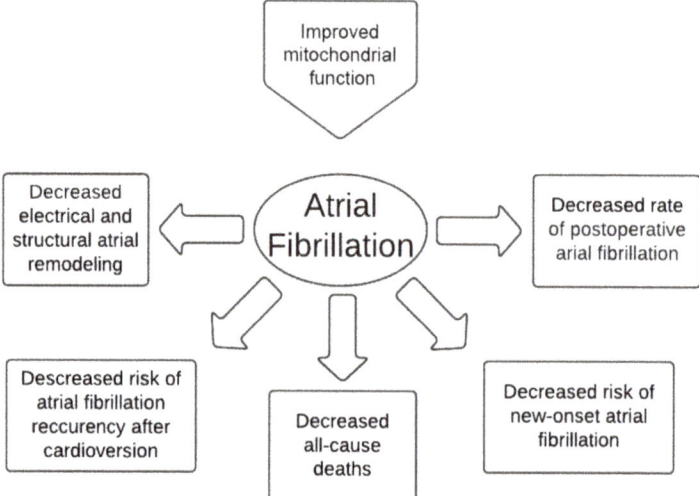

Figure 1. Clinical benefits expected from improvement of the mitochondrial function in atrial fibrillation.

5.2. Selective Inhibitors of the Sodium-Glucose Co-Transporter 2

Gliflozines are selective inhibitors of the sodium-glucose co-transporter 2 (SGLT2) initially introduced for the treatment of type 2 diabetes mellitus. However, recent studies revealed the cardioprotective potential of these medications. The EMPA-REG OUTCOME trial showed that among patients with DM and HF, SGLT2 inhibitors lead to a significant reduction of hospitalization rate by 35% and cardiovascular deaths by 38% [71]. The CVD-REAL study compared the influence of newly initiated antidiabetic therapy with SGLT2 inhibitors versus other glucose-lowering drugs in a huge cohort of patients with diabetes. The SGLT2 inhibitor was superior to other antidiabetic treatments, decreasing the risk of HF-related hospitalization rates by 39%, all-cause mortality by 51% and combined HF hospitalizations and all-cause death by 46% [72].

The beneficial cardiovascular outcomes initiated further research aimed at establishing the mechanisms of the cardioprotective action of SGLT2 inhibitors. Kidney-dependent volume contraction resulting from glycosuria and osmotic diuresis is the obvious candidate for cardioprotection, but there may also be vascular and direct cardiac actions of these medications that significantly contribute to the observed advantages.

SGLT2-i can reduce arterial resistance, which is related to flow-mediated dilation, suggesting improvement of endothelial function [73]. Research performed by Zhou et al. indeed showed the ameliorating effect of the SGLT2 inhibitor on endothelial cells. In mice with streptozotocin-induced diabetes, treatment with empagliflozin preserved cardiac microvascular barrier function and integrity, sustained eNOS phosphorylation and endothelium-dependent relaxation, as well as higher microvessel density and perfusion. Inhibition of mitochondrial fission, induced by activation of AMPK and attenuated ROS production, were proposed as the mechanism for the observed endothelial effects [74].

Direct effects of SGLT2-i on cardiomyocytes were described in both animal and human studies. SGLT2 inhibitors block an Na^+/H^+ exchanger (NHE-1) and normalize cytosolic Na^+ and Ca^{2+} concentrations [75] independently from the presence of DM. Elevated cytoplasmic sodium levels may negatively affect energy supply and demand matching and can even induce mitochondrial oxidative stress [76]. Low cytosolic sodium augments mitochondrial Na^+/Ca^{2+} exchange, increases mitochondrial calcium concentration and improves mitochondrial function [77]. Prompt binding and blocking of the NHE-1 by SGLT2 inhibitors were proposed, but pharmacological approaches also suggest an indirect effect on the exchanger via the stimulation of AMPK [78].

The results of improved mitochondrial function after empagliflozin treatment were shown in the rat model of STZ-induced diabetes [39]. Shao et al. observed in their study that SGLT2 inhibition restores the mitochondrial $\Delta\Psi m$ and mitochondrial respiratory rate with concomitant increased expression of PGC-1α, NRF-1 and Mfn-1, suggesting promotion of mitochondrial biogenesis. Ameliorated mitochondrial function was related to attenuation of the synthesis of ROS, lower systemic inflammation, inhibition of atrial fibrosis and cardiomyocyte hypertrophy [39]. Involvement of these mechanisms resulted in the reduction of tachypacing-induced AF susceptibility by about 50% in the group treated with empagliflozin [39]. In another experimental study with empagliflozin, Li et al. showed its suppressing activity on oxidative stress and myocardial fibrosis through inhibition of the TGF-β/Smad pathway and activation of Nrf2/ARE signaling [79].

Clinical data from patients with diabetes and present AF show benefits of treatment with SGLT2 inhibitors. The EMPA-REG OUTCOME trial subanalysis revealed that the use of the SGLT2 inhibitors in these patients brings 50% reduction of all-cause deaths, 48% reduction of cardiovascular deaths and significantly decreases the risk of new edema or nephropathy development [80]. A recent analysis of pooled nine cardiovascular and renal outcome clinical trials conducted in patients with and without diabetes revealed 21% relative risk reduction of AF in patients treated with SGLT2 inhibitors as compared to placebo [81].

SGLT2 inhibitors seem to be more effective in reducing the risk of AF than DDP-4 inhibitors in patients with diabetes. The observational study showed that treatment with SGLT2-i was associated with a 39% lower risk of new-onset AF as compared to treatment with DPP4 inhibitors [82].

To date, the majority of both experimental and clinical studies with gliflozins were conducted in diabetic subjects. The improvement of mitochondrial function and cellular energetics, protecting against the development of electrical and structural atrial remodeling, brought by SGLT2 inhibitors is clear in diabetics. The recent study showed that the cardioprotective effect of gliflozins is independent from glycated hemoglobin A1c concentration or from pre-existence of other comorbidities, such as AF, HF or atherosclerotic cardiovascular disease [83]. However, the exact mechanism in which SGLT2 inhibitors reduce the risk of AF in patients without diabetes was not established and requires further investigation [81].

5.3. Ubiquinone

Ubiquinone (coenzyme Q10, CoQ10) is an important mitochondrial cofactor involved in the electron transport from complex I to complex II and from complex II to complex III of the respiratory chain. In addition, CoQ10 is an effective antioxidant, membrane stabilizer, cofactor of mitochondrial uncoupling proteins, a stabilizer of calcium-dependent channels, metabolic regulator and an indirect regulator of signaling molecule formation and cell growth [84]. The levels of CoQ10 in the myocardium are relatively high, but can decrease with age, statin treatment or due to genetic defects. Diminished plasma CoQ10 levels are seen in advanced HF and are associated with the severity of symptoms [85]. Although the majority of studies have looked at the effect of CoQ10 treatment in HF, there are premises for considering CoQ10 in AF prevention [86].

Atrial samples collected from patients after a two-week CoQ10 treatment showed better respiratory function and lower levels of oxidative stress marker malonyldialdehyde [87]. In patients with HF, treatment with CoQ10 significantly reduced the incidence of AF during a 12-month follow-up, which was attributed to its antioxidative capacity [88]. In a small, double-blind, randomized controlled trial, short-term CoQ10 treatment reduced incidence of postoperative AF by about half [89]; however, these results were not confirmed by other studies, as summarized by the meta-analysis by de Frutos et al. [90].

Taking into account a good tolerability and favorable safety profile, CoQ10 can be considered an adjuvant therapy reducing the risk of AF in certain situations; however, further studies are required to elucidate its clinical effectiveness.

5.4. Metformin

Metformin, the first-line antidiabetic medication, can prevent AF by attenuation of atrial remodeling [91,92]. The analysis of data from 645,710 patients with type 2 DM during a 13-year follow-up collected in the Taiwan National Health Insurance Research Database showed that metformin decreased the incidence of AF by 19% [93]. The mechanisms of this clinical effect are not clear and a possible explanation is brought by experimental studies with pacing-induced AF. In one study, metformin activated AMPK, Src kinase and normalized connexin expression to attenuate the pacing-induced increase in the refractory period, AF inducibility and AF duration [94]. In another study it prevented atrial electrical and structural remodeling by activating the AMPK/PGC-1α/PPAR-α pathway and normalizing the metabolic pathway activities [92]. Due to its electronegativity, metformin becomes concentrated in mitochondria and, thus, orchestration of cellular energy metabolism may play a role in AF development. Preservation of mitochondrial function by metformin was related to improved oxygen consumption and enhanced function of complexes I, II and IV [95]. In addition, in rodents subjected to myocardial infarction, metformin improved cardiac function via preservation of mitochondrial respiration and mitochondrial biogenesis, which was paralleled by upregulation of PGC-1α [91].

Metformin remains the first choice of treatment in DM, and with no doubt, it reduces cardiovascular risks in diabetes patients. Animal experiments suggest that metformin has cardioprotective effects, including prevention of AF, even without DM. The question remains whether metformin has a significant cardioprotective effect also in people without diabetes.

5.5. Thiazolidinediones

Thiazolidinediones (TZDs) are the next group of medications used in treatment of DM influencing mitochondrial function, introduced as agonists PPAR-γ to reduce insulin resistance. In an experimental model of alloxan-induced DM in rabbits, TZDs attenuated atrial remodeling and AF inducibility and improved function of ion channels (I_{Ca} and I_{Na}) and activation of pERK, TGF-β1, TLR4, NF-κB and HSP70 [96]. In the Wistar AF model, pretreatment with pioglitazone decreased AF duration, and upregulation of antioxidant mechanisms and inhibition of mitochondrial apoptotic signaling pathways were proposed as the protective mechanisms [97]. A few registries and clinical trials suggest the effectiveness of TZD in preventing atrial fibrillation. The analysis of Danish nationwide registries of over 100,000 diabetic patients with no prior AF showed that TZD reduced the incidence of AF by 24% when adjusted for age, sex and comorbidities, compared to other second-line antidiabetic treatments [98]. Another suggestion for TZDs preventive potential against AF was provided by a meta-analysis of three randomized clinical trials and four observational studies, in which TZDs reduced the risk of AF incidence by 23% (for new-onset AF) and provided a 59% risk reduction of AF recurrence [99]. Nevertheless, in patients with coronary artery disease treated with either TZD or other second-line medications during a median follow-up of 4.2 years, TZDs did not affect the prevalence of AF [100].

Furthermore, TZDs improved the recurrence of AF after electrical cardioversion in a small randomized prospective study [101]. Thus, there is a need for prospective randomized trials to determine the usefulness and safety of TZDs in AF prevention.

5.6. Fibrates

Fibrates are agonists of PPARα, and they are used in treatment of hypertriglyceridemia via attenuation of hepatic apoC-III and promotion of lipoprotein lipase-mediated lipolysis [102]. They may also influence mitochondrial function through the PPARα/PGC-1α pathway [103]. In the experimental animal model of AF, fenofibrate was found to decrease metabolic remodeling by regulating the PPAR-α/sirtuin 1/PGC-1α pathway and reversed shortened atrial refractory period [104]. Bezafibrate induced beneficial effects on mitochondrial biogenesis, increasing expression of PPARGC1A, GFAP, S100B, DCX NRF1 and TFAM genes and an mtDNA copy number [105]. The lipid lowering medications, including fibrates, were connected with a significant decrease in AF prevalence in patients with reduced left ventricular ejection fraction, independently from lipid profile, possibly via anti-inflammatory and antioxidant effects [106]; however, the clinical benefits of this treatment for AF outcomes were not evaluated.

5.7. Trimetazidine

Trimetazidine (TMZ) is an anti-anginal drug that was approved for the treatment of ischemic heart disease, and its beneficial effects are related to improvement of cellular energetic balance. TMZ inhibits the long-chain 3-ketoacyl CoA thiolase, which is involved in fatty acid oxidation. It was originally proposed that inhibition of beta-oxidation shifts mitochondrial substrate utilization toward glucose and improves ATP synthesis; however, recent studies challenge this traditional paradigm, showing lack of changes in fatty acid or carbohydrate metabolism in the myocardium in either acute or chronic treatment with TMZ and suggest other mechanisms to be responsible for the protective activity of this drug [107,108].

In ischemic conditions, TMZ directly acts on the respiratory chain activity via activation of the complex I [109,110]. Improved function of the ETC increases consumed the ADP/O_2 ratio and reduced the generation of ROS [111]. In ischemic conditions, TMZ normalizes the expression of factors regulating mitochondrial biogenesis, such as PPARγ and PGC-1α, and also adjusts the expression of Mfn-1, Drp1 and Opa-1 to the normal levels, which suggests the impact on the mitochondrial fusion/fission dynamics [110]. TMZ was, however, not proven to induce any beneficial effects on the mitochondrial function without the ischemic context, but regardless of the precise metabolic mechanisms of action, its antiarrhythmic activity was postulated. In a series of studies, TMZ improved the electrocardiographic parameters reflecting susceptibility to atrial and ventricular arrhythmias, such as P-wave duration and P-wave dispersion [112], heart rate variability [113] and Tpeak–Tend duration and dispersion [114]. The preliminary report using the tachypacing model suggests that TMZ prevents tachycardia-induced atrial ultrastructural remodeling, decreases AF inducibility and shortens AF duration [112,115]. It is unknown if these protective effects of TMZ in conditions without an ischemic context are related to improvement in mitochondrial function. In a chronic atrial pacing model in dogs, TMZ did not affect the levels of creatine phosphate, ATP, ADP, AMP and total adenosine, and it also did not prevent ultrastructural changes, such as mitochondrial swelling and cristae derangements, myolysis and karyopynkosis, but reduced oxidative stress and promoted endothelial NO synthase expression [116,117].

The exact mechanisms of arrhythmic substrate modulation and clinical usefulness of TMZ in AF remain uncertain and require further studies.

5.8. Ranolazine

Ranolazine is an anti-anginal drug, which also has anti-arrhythmic properties due to selective inhibition of sodium currents [118]. As shown in the metanalyses, ranolazine decreases the probability of AF development in different clinical settings by about 50%, increases the cardioversion success rate of amiodarone and decreases time to restoration of the sinus rhythm [119,120]. The proposed mechanism of action of ranolazine is the prolongation of post-repolarization refractoriness and the slowing of the conduction velocity [121]. In addition to these electrophysiological effects, it was shown that ranolazine improves mitochondrial function, attenuates oxidative stress, suppresses apoptosis through augmentation of the Bcl-2/Bax ratio, reduction of the cleaved caspase-3 level and activation of the Akt/mTOR signaling pathway [122].

5.9. Experimental Treatments Targeting Mitochondria

Elamipretide (other names include Bendavia, MTP-131 or SS-31) is the first in the class of mitochondria-targeted drugs that entered clinical trials for treatment of HF. Elamipretide improves mitochondrial energetics and decreases generation of reactive oxygen species, possibly by stabilizing the mitochondrial membrane and cytochrome c [123]. Cardioprotective effects of the drug were shown in basic and human studies. In a dog model of chronic heart failure of ischemic etiology, elamipretide restored mitochondrial state-3 respiration, $\Delta\Psi m$, rate of ATP synthesis, normalized the ATP/ADP ratio, reduced levels of TNF-α and C-reactive protein and prevented decline of left ventricular systolic function [124]. Elamipretide treatment of samples of failing human ventricular myocardium significantly improved mitochondrial oxygen flux, complex I and complex IV of the ETC activities, and ETC-supercomplex-associated complex IV activity [123]. An initial randomized clinical trial using single elamipretide infusion in patients with heart failure with reduced ejection fraction demonstrated significant reduction of left ventricular end-diastolic volume following infusion [125]. Despite encouraging initial results, a recent phase 2 clinical trial on a small cohort of patients with heart failure showed a lack of improvement of left ventricular ejection fraction after repeated elamipretide administration for 28 days [126].

A few more medications specifically targeting mitochondria are currently being examined regarding their safety and efficacy. The potential of these still experimental therapies supporting mitochondrial function in the prevention of AF should be investigated after finishing outgoing safety and efficiency measurements. The list of these medications with a short description is provided in Table 1.

Table 1. Experimental medications targeting mitochondria. The efficacy of these medications in the treatment of AF was not tested. The clinical trial identifiers in the Clinicaltrial.org database are provided in the "References" column.

Medication	Mechanism of Action	Target Diseases	Current Research Stage	References
Elamipretide (MTP-131)	Improves mitochondrial ultrastructure and bioenergetics	Primary Mitochondrial Myopathy	Experimental studies; phase 3 randomized, double-blind, placebo-controlled trial—terminated; phase 2 randomized trials in heart failure—completed	Clinical trial, identifier: NCT03323749 NCT02788747 NCT02814097 NCT02914665
KL1333	The safety and efficiency measurements in progress, with potential effects on NAD+/NADH, FGF21 and GDF15 concentrations	Primary mitochondrial disease	Phase Ia/Ib trial (recruiting)	Clinical trial, identifier: NCT03888716
KH176	ROS level reduction and cell protection against redox stress	Mitochondrial disease	Phase IIb open-label, multi-center trial (planned ending date: June 2021)	Clinical trial [107,108] identifier: NCT02544217; NCT02909400; NCT04165239 NCT04604548

Table 1. Cont.

Medication	Mechanism of Action	Target Diseases	Current Research Stage	References
REN001	Selective PPAR delta agonist	Primary Mitochondrial Myopathy	Finished phase I due to COVID-19 pandemic but with sufficient data gathered to achieve the study objective	Clinical trial, identifier: NCT03862846
Idebenone	Antioxidant with ATP preserving properties: stimulates mitochondrial electron flux, increases respiratory function	Friedreich ataxia (FRDA) and Duchenne muscular dystrophy	Finished trial phase III in Duchenne muscular dystrophy and phase III study (IONIA)	[127,128]

KL1333 increases NAD$^+$ levels and activates SIRT1/AMPK/PGC-1α signaling, improves mitochondrial function and decreases oxidative stress in fibroblasts from mitochondrial encephalomyopathy, lactic acidosis and stroke-like episodes in patients [129].

Another medication, KH176, can effectively reduce increased cellular ROS levels and protect oxidative phosphorylation deficient primary cells against redox perturbations by interacting with the thioredoxin system/peroxiredoxin enzyme machinery [130].

Idebenone is a synthetic coenzyme Q10 analog and was tested to treat diverse diseases in which mitochondrial function is impaired [131]. It showed some cardioprotective potential in the animal model of ischemia/reperfusion, but other effects in heart diseases need to be examined [132]. The summary of the medications acting on the basic mechanisms linking mitochondrial dysfunction with atrial fibrillation is presented in Figure 2.

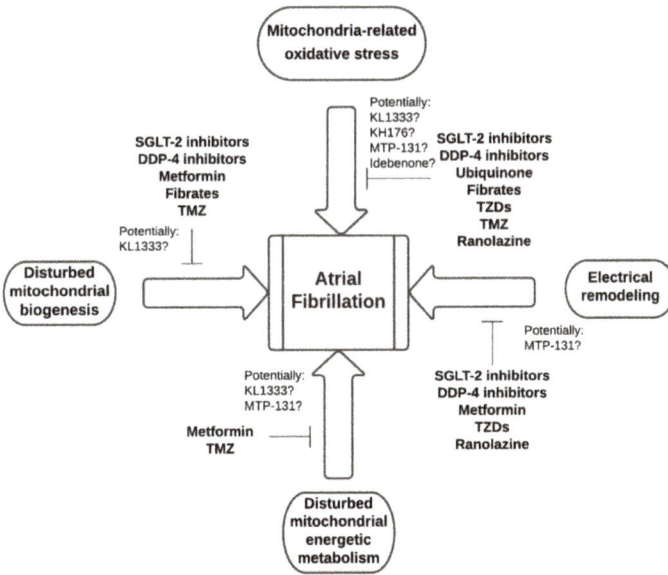

Figure 2. Pharmacological interventions targeting basic mechanisms of atrial fibrillation. Abbreviations: SGLT2—sodium-glucose co-transporter 2, DDP-4—dipeptidyl peptidase-4, TZDs—thiazolidinediones, TMZ—trimetazidine.

The impact of these medications targeting mitochondria in AF risk reduction or improvement of the AF outcomes are unknown. Most of the few trials conducted to date excluded patients with AF; thus, further basic and clinical investigations are required to establish the usefulness of these medications in patients with AF.

Gene therapy is another potential therapeutic approach; however, to date, it remains in an experimental phase. Genetic constructs, mostly inserted in adenoviral vectors, may be delivered to the myocardium by direct intramyocardial injection, by epicardial gene painting or via intracoronary infusion [133]. These gene-based approaches in animal models of AF were successful in the restoration of the sinus rhythm or improved control of the ventricular rate. Nevertheless, it is still too early for their introduction into clinical practice [133–135].

6. Conclusions

Preserved mitochondrial function is crucial for cardiomyocyte integrity and uncompromised cardiac performance. Atrial fibrillation may result from, induce or exaggerate energetic imbalance, disturbed metabolism and oxidative stress, and all of them are related to mitochondrial dysfunction, which can be targeted by currently available medications such as metformin, thiazolidinediones, fibrates, ranolazine or selective inhibitors of the sodium-glucose co-transporter 2. However, there is a gap in the knowledge about the significance of the effects in atrial fibrillation prevention and the impact of these treatments on the outcomes of the arrhythmia. Randomized double-blind placebo-controlled trials are needed for medications affecting the mitochondrial function in order to allow for more wide indications in clinical practice. The possible indications could include preservation of sinus rhythm in individuals with paroxysmal AF, or, after cardioversion, prevention or treatment of post-operative atrial fibrillation (POAF) with usage as a longitudinal additive in patients with persistent or permanent AF.

Author Contributions: Conceptualization, writing—original draft preparation, P.M. and T.A.B.; funding acquisition, P.M. All authors have read and agreed to the published version of the manuscript.

Funding: This research was funded by the research grant form Medical University of Bialystok, grant number SUB/1/DN/20/003/1124.

Institutional Review Board Statement: Not applicable.

Informed Consent Statement: Not applicable.

Data Availability Statement: Not applicable.

Conflicts of Interest: The authors declare no conflict of interest.

References

1. Zoni-Berisso, M.; Lercari, F.; Carazza, T.; Domenicucci, S. Epidemiology of atrial fibrillation: European perspective. *Clin. Epidemiol.* **2014**, *6*, 213–220. [CrossRef] [PubMed]
2. Kjerpeseth, L.J.; Igland, J.; Selmer, R.; Ellekjær, H.; Tveit, A.; Berge, T.; Kalstø, S.M.; Christophersen, I.E.; Myrstad, M.; Skovlund, E.; et al. Prevalence and incidence rates of atrial fibrillation in Norway 2004–2014. *Heart* **2021**, *107*, 201–207. [CrossRef] [PubMed]
3. Williams, B.A.; Chamberlain, A.M.; Blankenship, J.C.; Hylek, E.M.; Voyce, S. Trends in Atrial Fibrillation Incidence Rates Within an Integrated Health Care Delivery System, 2006 to 2018. *JAMA Netw. Open* **2020**, *3*, e2014874. [CrossRef] [PubMed]
4. Olesen, M.S.; Andreasen, L.; Jabbari, J.; Refsgaard, L.; Haunsø, S.; Olesen, S.-P.; Nielsen, J.B.; Schmitt, N.; Svendsen, J.H. Very early-onset lone atrial fibrillation patients have a high prevalence of rare variants in genes previously associated with atrial fibrillation. *Hear. Rhythm.* **2014**, *11*, 246–251. [CrossRef]
5. Staerk, L.; Sherer, J.A.; Ko, D.; Benjamin, E.J.; Helm, R.H. Atrial Fibrillation. *Circ. Res.* **2017**, *120*, 1501–1517. [CrossRef]
6. Mandalenakis, Z.; Rosengren, A.; Lappas, G.; Eriksson, P.; Gilljam, T.; Hansson, P.-O.; Skoglund, K.; Fedchenko, M.; Dellborg, M. Atrial Fibrillation Burden in Young Patients with Congenital Heart Disease. *Circulation* **2018**, *137*, 928–937. [CrossRef]
7. Saguner, A.M.; Maurer, T.; Wissner, E.; Santoro, F.; Lemes, C.; Mathew, S.; Sohns, C.; Heeger, C.H.; Reißmann, B.; Riedl, J.; et al. Catheter ablation of atrial fibrillation in very young adults: A 5-year follow-up study. *Europace* **2016**, *20*, 58–64. [CrossRef]
8. Lau, D.H.; Schotten, U.; Mahajan, R.; Antic, N.A.; Hatem, S.N.; Pathak, R.K.; Hendriks, J.; Kalman, J.M.; Sanders, P. Novel mechanisms in the pathogenesis of atrial fibrillation: Practical applications. *Eur. Hear. J.* **2015**, *37*, 1573–1581. [CrossRef]
9. Platonov, P.G.; Mitrofanova, L.B.; Orshanskaya, V.; Ho, S.Y. Structural Abnormalities in Atrial Walls Are Associated with Presence and Persistency of Atrial Fibrillation But Not With Age. *J. Am. Coll. Cardiol.* **2011**, *58*, 2225–2232. [CrossRef]
10. Wolowacz, S.E.; Samuel, M.; Brennan, V.K.; Jasso-Mosqueda, J.G.; Van Gelder, I.C. The cost of illness of atrial fibrillation: A systematic review of the recent literature. *Europace* **2011**, *13*, 1375–1385. [CrossRef]

11. Steffel, J.; Verhamme, P.; Potpara, T.S.; Albaladejo, P.; Antz, M.; Desteghe, L.; Haeusler, K.G.; Oldgren, J.; Reinecke, H.; Roldan-Schilling, V.; et al. The 2018 European Heart Rhythm Association Practical Guide on the use of non-vitamin K antagonist oral anticoagulants in patients with atrial fibrillation. *Eur. Heart J.* **2018**, *39*, 1330–1393. [CrossRef]
12. Kirchhof, P.; Benussi, S.; Kotecha, D.; Ahlsson, A.; Atar, D.; Casadei, B.; Castella, M.; Diener, H.C.; Heidbuchel, H.; Hendriks, J.; et al. 2016 ESC Guidelines for the management of atrial fibrillation developed in collaboration with EACTS. *Eur J. Cardiothorac. Surg.* **2016**, *50*, e1–e88. [CrossRef]
13. Thiedemann, K.U.; Ferrans, V.J. Left atrial ultrastructure in mitral valvular disease. *Am. J. Pathol.* **1977**, *89*, 575–604. [CrossRef]
14. Harada, M.; Tadevosyan, A.; Qi, X.; Xiao, J.; Liu, T.; Voigt, N.; Karck, M.; Kamler, M.; Kodama, I.; Murohara, T.; et al. Atrial Fibrillation Activates AMP-Dependent Protein Kinase and its Regulation of Cellular Calcium Handling: Potential Role in Metabolic Adaptation and Prevention of Progression. *J. Am. Coll. Cardiol.* **2015**, *66*, 47–58. [CrossRef]
15. Molvin, J.; Jujic, A.; Melander, O.; Pareek, M.; Råstam, L.; Lindblad, U.; Daka, B.; Leosdottir, M.; Nilsson, P.; Olsen, M.; et al. Exploration of pathophysiological pathways for incident atrial fibrillation using a multiplex proteomic chip. *Open Heart* **2020**, *7*, e001190. [CrossRef]
16. Kornej, J.; Büttner, P.; Hammer, E.; Engelmann, B.; Dinov, B.; Sommer, P.; Husser, D.; Hindricks, G.; Völker, U.; Bollmann, A. Circulating proteomic patterns in AF related left atrial remodeling indicate involvement of coagulation and complement cascade. *PLoS ONE* **2018**, *13*, e0198461. [CrossRef]
17. Ko, D.; Benson, M.D.; Ngo, D.; Yang, Q.; Larson, M.G.; Wang, T.J.; Trinquart, L.; McManus, D.D.; Lubitz, S.A.; Ellinor, P.T.; et al. Proteomics Profiling and Risk of New-Onset Atrial Fibrillation: Framingham Heart Study. *J. Am. Heart Assoc.* **2019**, *8*, e010976. [CrossRef]
18. Scholman, K.T.; Meijborg, V.M.F.; Galvez-Monton, C.; Lodder, E.M.; Boukens, B.J. From Genome-Wide Association Studies to Cardiac Electrophysiology: Through the Maze of Biological Complexity. *Front. Physiol.* **2020**, *11*, 557. [CrossRef]
19. Pandit, S.V.; Jalife, J. Rotors and the dynamics of cardiac fibrillation. *Circ. Res.* **2013**, *112*, 849–862. [CrossRef]
20. Khan, R. Identifying and understanding the role of pulmonary vein activity in atrial fibrillation. *Cardiovasc. Res.* **2004**, *64*, 387–394. [CrossRef]
21. Voigt, N.; Heijman, J.; Wang, Q.; Chiang, D.Y.; Li, N.; Karck, M.; Wehrens, X.H.T.; Nattel, S.; Dobrev, D. Cellular and molecular mechanisms of atrial arrhythmogenesis in patients with paroxysmal atrial fibrillation. *Circulation* **2014**, *129*, 145–156. [CrossRef]
22. Pellman, J.; Sheikh, F. Atrial fibrillation: Mechanisms, therapeutics, and future directions. *Compr. Physiol.* **2015**, *5*, 649–665. [CrossRef]
23. Schnabel, R.B.; Sullivan, L.M.; Levy, D.; Pencina, M.J.; Massaro, J.M.; D'Agostino, R.B., Sr.; Newton-Cheh, C.; Yamamoto, J.F.; Magnani, J.W.; Tadros, T.M.; et al. Development of a risk score for atrial fibrillation (Framingham Heart Study): A community-based cohort study. *Lancet* **2009**, *373*, 739–745. [CrossRef]
24. Wasmer, K.; Eckardt, L.; Breithardt, G. Predisposing factors for atrial fibrillation in the elderly. *J. Geriatr. Cardiol.* **2017**, *14*, 179–184. [CrossRef]
25. Tomaszuk-Kazberuk, A.; Koziński, M.; Kuźma, Ł.; Bujno, E.; Łopatowska, P.; Rogalska, E.; Dobrzycki, S.; Sobkowicz, B.; Lip, G.Y.H. Atrial fibrillation is more frequently associated with nonobstructive coronary lesions: The Bialystok Coronary Project. *Pol. Arch. Intern. Med.* **2020**, *130*, 1029–1036. [CrossRef]
26. Vlachos, K.; Letsas, K.P.; Korantzopoulos, P.; Liu, T.; Georgopoulos, S.; Bakalakos, A.; Karamichalakis, N.; Xydonas, S.; Efremidis, M.; Sideris, A. Prediction of atrial fibrillation development and progression: Current perspectives. *World J. Cardiol.* **2016**, *8*, 267–276. [CrossRef]
27. Pinnell, J.; Turner, S.; Howell, S. Cardiac muscle physiology. *Contin. Educ. Anaesth. Crit. Care Pain* **2007**, *7*, 85–88. [CrossRef]
28. Maack, C.; O'Rourke, B. Excitation-contraction coupling and mitochondrial energetics. *Basic Res. Cardiol.* **2007**, *102*, 369–392. [CrossRef]
29. Kohlhaas, M.; Nickel, A.G.; Maack, C. Mitochondrial energetics and calcium coupling in the heart. *J. Physiol.* **2017**, *595*, 3753–3763. [CrossRef]
30. Harada, M.; Melka, J.; Sobue, Y.; Nattel, S. Metabolic Considerations in Atrial Fibrillation-Mechanistic Insights and Therapeutic Opportunities. *Circ. J.* **2017**, *81*, 1749–1757. [CrossRef]
31. Hassanpour, S.H.; Dehghani, M.A.; Karami, S.Z. Study of respiratory chain dysfunction in heart disease. *J. Cardiovasc. Thorac. Res.* **2018**, *10*, 1–13. [CrossRef] [PubMed]
32. Liu, J.C. Is MCU dispensable for normal heart function? *J. Mol. Cell. Cardiol.* **2020**, *143*, 175–183. [CrossRef] [PubMed]
33. Wiersma, M.; van Marion, D.M.S.; Wust, R.C.I.; Houtkooper, R.H.; Zhang, D.; Groot, N.M.S.; Henning, R.H.; Brundel, B. Mitochondrial Dysfunction Underlies Cardiomyocyte Remodeling in Experimental and Clinical Atrial Fibrillation. *Cells* **2019**, *8*, 1202. [CrossRef] [PubMed]
34. Liu, Y.; Bai, F.; Liu, N.; Ouyang, F.; Liu, Q. The Warburg effect: A new insight into atrial fibrillation. *Clin. Chim. Acta* **2019**, *499*, 4–12. [CrossRef]
35. Hu, H.J.; Zhang, C.; Tang, Z.H.; Qu, S.L.; Jiang, Z.S. Regulating the Warburg effect on metabolic stress and myocardial fibrosis remodeling and atrial intracardiac waveform activity induced by atrial fibrillation. *Biochem. Biophys. Res. Commun.* **2019**, *516*, 653–660. [CrossRef]

36. Yoshida, H.; Bao, L.; Kefaloyianni, E.; Taskin, E.; Okorie, U.; Hong, M.; Dhar-Chowdhury, P.; Kaneko, M.; Coetzee, W.A. AMP-activated protein kinase connects cellular energy metabolism to KATP channel function. *J. Mol. Cell. Cardiol* **2012**, *52*, 410–418. [CrossRef]
37. Liu, M.; Liu, H.; Dudley, S.C., Jr. Reactive oxygen species originating from mitochondria regulate the cardiac sodium channel. *Circ. Res.* **2010**, *107*, 967–974. [CrossRef]
38. Karam, B.S.; Chavez-Moreno, A.; Koh, W.; Akar, J.G.; Akar, F.G. Oxidative stress and inflammation as central mediators of atrial fibrillation in obesity and diabetes. *Cardiovasc. Diabetol.* **2017**, *16*, 120. [CrossRef]
39. Shao, Q.; Meng, L.; Lee, S.; Tse, G.; Gong, M.; Zhang, Z.; Zhao, J.; Zhao, Y.; Li, G.; Liu, T. Empagliflozin, a sodium glucose co-transporter-2 inhibitor, alleviates atrial remodeling and improves mitochondrial function in high-fat diet/streptozotocin-induced diabetic rats. *Cardiovasc. Diabetol.* **2019**, *18*, 165. [CrossRef]
40. Cogliati, S.; Enriquez, J.A.; Scorrano, L. Mitochondrial Cristae: Where Beauty Meets Functionality. *Trends Biochem. Sci.* **2016**, *41*, 261–273. [CrossRef]
41. Ausma, J.; Litjens, N.; Lenders, M.H.; Duimel, H.; Mast, F.; Wouters, L.; Ramaekers, F.; Allessie, M.; Borgers, M. Time course of atrial fibrillation-induced cellular structural remodeling in atria of the goat. *J. Mol. Cell. Cardiol.* **2001**, *33*, 2083–2094. [CrossRef]
42. Ozcan, C.; Li, Z.; Kim, G.; Jeevanandam, V.; Uriel, N. Molecular Mechanism of the Association Between Atrial Fibrillation and Heart Failure Includes Energy Metabolic Dysregulation Due to Mitochondrial Dysfunction. *J. Card. Fail.* **2019**, *25*, 911–920. [CrossRef]
43. Sharma, S.; Sharma, G.; Hote, M.; Devagourou, V.; Kesari, V.; Arava, S.; Airan, B.; Ray, R. Light and electron microscopic features of surgically excised left atrial appendage in rheumatic heart disease patients with atrial fibrillation and sinus rhythm. *Cardiovasc. Pathol.* **2014**, *23*, 319–326. [CrossRef]
44. Bukowska, A.; Schild, L.; Keilhoff, G.; Hirte, D.; Neumann, M.; Gardemann, A.; Neumann, K.H.; Rohl, F.W.; Huth, C.; Goette, A.; et al. Mitochondrial dysfunction and redox signaling in atrial tachyarrhythmia. *Exp. Biol. Med. (Maywood)* **2008**, *233*, 558–574. [CrossRef]
45. Xie, W.; Santulli, G.; Reiken, S.R.; Yuan, Q.; Osborne, B.W.; Chen, B.X.; Marks, A.R. Mitochondrial oxidative stress promotes atrial fibrillation. *Sci. Rep.* **2015**, *5*, 11427. [CrossRef]
46. Yang, K.C.; Bonini, M.G.; Dudley, S.C., Jr. Mitochondria and arrhythmias. *Free Radic. Biol. Med.* **2014**, *71*, 351–361. [CrossRef]
47. Bouchez, C.; Devin, A. Mitochondrial Biogenesis and Mitochondrial Reactive Oxygen Species (ROS): A Complex Relationship Regulated by the cAMP/PKA Signaling Pathway. *Cells* **2019**, *8*, 287. [CrossRef]
48. Villena, J.A. New insights into PGC-1 coactivators: Redefining their role in the regulation of mitochondrial function and beyond. *FEBS J.* **2015**, *282*, 647–672. [CrossRef]
49. Jornayvaz, F.R.; Shulman, G.I. Regulation of mitochondrial biogenesis. *Essays Biochem.* **2010**, *47*, 69–84. [CrossRef]
50. Scarpulla, R.C. Nucleus-encoded regulators of mitochondrial function: Integration of respiratory chain expression, nutrient sensing and metabolic stress. *Biochim. Biophys. Acta* **2012**, *1819*, 1088–1097. [CrossRef]
51. Rimbaud, S.; Garnier, A.; Ventura-Clapier, R. Mitochondrial biogenesis in cardiac pathophysiology. *Pharmacol. Rep.* **2009**, *61*, 131–138. [CrossRef]
52. Dong, J.; Zhao, J.; Zhang, M.; Liu, G.; Wang, X.; Liu, Y.; Yang, N.; Liu, Y.; Zhao, G.; Sun, J.; et al. beta3-Adrenoceptor Impairs Mitochondrial Biogenesis and Energy Metabolism During Rapid Atrial Pacing-Induced Atrial Fibrillation. *J. Cardiovasc. Pharmacol. Ther.* **2016**, *21*, 114–126. [CrossRef]
53. Jeganathan, J.; Saraf, R.; Mahmood, F.; Pal, A.; Bhasin, M.K.; Huang, T.; Mittel, A.; Knio, Z.; Simons, R.; Khabbaz, K.; et al. Mitochondrial Dysfunction in Atrial Tissue of Patients Developing Postoperative Atrial Fibrillation. *Ann. Thorac. Surg.* **2017**, *104*, 1547–1555. [CrossRef]
54. Kowaltowski, A.J.; de Souza-Pinto, N.C.; Castilho, R.F.; Vercesi, A.E. Mitochondria and reactive oxygen species. *Free Radic. Biol. Med.* **2009**, *47*, 333–343. [CrossRef]
55. Montaigne, D.; Marechal, X.; Lefebvre, P.; Modine, T.; Fayad, G.; Dehondt, H.; Hurt, C.; Coisne, A.; Koussa, M.; Remy-Jouet, I.; et al. Mitochondrial dysfunction as an arrhythmogenic substrate: A translational proof-of-concept study in patients with metabolic syndrome in whom post-operative atrial fibrillation develops. *J. Am. Coll. Cardiol.* **2013**, *62*, 1466–1473. [CrossRef]
56. Korantzopoulos, P.; Kolettis, T.M.; Galaris, D.; Goudevenos, J.A. The role of oxidative stress in the pathogenesis and perpetuation of atrial fibrillation. *Int. J. Cardiol.* **2007**, *115*, 135–143. [CrossRef]
57. Mihm, M.J.; Yu, F.; Carnes, C.A.; Reiser, P.J.; McCarthy, P.M.; Van Wagoner, D.R.; Bauer, J.A. Impaired myofibrillar energetics and oxidative injury during human atrial fibrillation. *Circulation* **2001**, *104*, 174–180. [CrossRef]
58. Youn, J.Y.; Zhang, J.; Zhang, Y.; Chen, H.; Liu, D.; Ping, P.; Weiss, J.N.; Cai, H. Oxidative stress in atrial fibrillation: An emerging role of NADPH oxidase. *J. Mol. Cell. Cardiol.* **2013**, *62*, 72–79. [CrossRef]
59. Emelyanova, L.; Ashary, Z.; Cosic, M.; Negmadjanov, U.; Ross, G.; Rizvi, F.; Olet, S.; Kress, D.; Sra, J.; Tajik, A.J.; et al. Selective downregulation of mitochondrial electron transport chain activity and increased oxidative stress in human atrial fibrillation. *Am. J. Physiol. Heart Circ. Physiol.* **2016**, *311*, H54–H63. [CrossRef] [PubMed]
60. Shan, J.; Xie, W.; Betzenhauser, M.; Reiken, S.; Chen, B.X.; Wronska, A.; Marks, A.R. Calcium leak through ryanodine receptors leads to atrial fibrillation in 3 mouse models of catecholaminergic polymorphic ventricular tachycardia. *Circ. Res.* **2012**, *111*, 708–717. [CrossRef] [PubMed]

61. Rusciano, M.R.; Sommariva, E.; Douin-Echinard, V.; Ciccarelli, M.; Poggio, P.; Maione, A.S. CaMKII Activity in the Inflammatory Response of Cardiac Diseases. *Int. J. Mol. Sci.* **2019**, *20*, 4374. [CrossRef] [PubMed]
62. Suetomi, T.; Miyamoto, S.; Brown, J.H. Inflammation in nonischemic heart disease: Initiation by cardiomyocyte CaMKII and NLRP3 inflammasome signaling. *Am. J. Physiol. Heart Circ. Physiol.* **2019**, *317*, H877–H890. [CrossRef] [PubMed]
63. Fu, H.; Li, G.; Liu, C.; Li, J.; Wang, X.; Cheng, L.; Liu, T. Probucol prevents atrial remodeling by inhibiting oxidative stress and TNF-alpha/NF-kappaB/TGF-beta signal transduction pathway in alloxan-induced diabetic rabbits. *J. Cardiovasc. Electrophysiol.* **2015**, *26*, 211–222. [CrossRef] [PubMed]
64. Yoo, S.; Pfenniger, A.; Hoffman, J.; Zhang, W.; Ng, J.; Burrell, A.; Johnson, D.A.; Gussak, G.; Waugh, T.; Bull, S.; et al. Attenuation of Oxidative Injury With Targeted Expression of NADPH Oxidase 2 Short Hairpin RNA Prevents Onset and Maintenance of Electrical Remodeling in the Canine Atrium: A Novel Gene Therapy Approach to Atrial Fibrillation. *Circulation* **2020**, *142*, 1261–1278. [CrossRef]
65. Ma, Y.; Wang, J.; Wang, C.; Zhang, Q.; Xu, Y.; Liu, H.; Xiang, X.; Ma, J. DPP-4 inhibitor anagliptin protects against hypoxia-induced cytotoxicity in cardiac H9C2 cells. *Artif. Cells Nanomed. Biotechnol.* **2019**, *47*, 3823–3831. [CrossRef]
66. Yamamoto, T.; Shimano, M.; Inden, Y.; Takefuji, M.; Yanagisawa, S.; Yoshida, N.; Tsuji, Y.; Hirai, M.; Murohara, T. Alogliptin, a dipeptidyl peptidase-4 inhibitor, regulates the atrial arrhythmogenic substrate in rabbits. *Heart Rhythm* **2015**, *12*, 1362–1369. [CrossRef]
67. Zhang, X.; Zhang, Z.; Yang, Y.; Suo, Y.; Liu, R.; Qiu, J.; Zhao, Y.; Jiang, N.; Liu, C.; Tse, G.; et al. Alogliptin prevents diastolic dysfunction and preserves left ventricular mitochondrial function in diabetic rabbits. *Cardiovasc. Diabetol.* **2018**, *17*, 160. [CrossRef]
68. Igarashi, T.; Niwano, S.; Niwano, H.; Yoshizawa, T.; Nakamura, H.; Fukaya, H.; Fujiishi, T.; Ishizue, N.; Satoh, A.; Kishihara, J.; et al. Linagliptin prevents atrial electrical and structural remodeling in a canine model of atrial fibrillation. *Heart Vessels* **2018**, *33*, 1258–1265. [CrossRef]
69. Zhang, X.; Zhang, Z.; Zhao, Y.; Jiang, N.; Qiu, J.; Yang, Y.; Li, J.; Liang, X.; Wang, X.; Tse, G.; et al. Alogliptin, a Dipeptidyl Peptidase-4 Inhibitor, Alleviates Atrial Remodeling and Improves Mitochondrial Function and Biogenesis in Diabetic Rabbits. *J. Am. Heart Assoc.* **2017**, *6*. [CrossRef]
70. Chang, C.Y.; Yeh, Y.H.; Chan, Y.H.; Liu, J.R.; Chang, S.H.; Lee, H.F.; Wu, L.S.; Yen, K.C.; Kuo, C.T.; See, L.C. Dipeptidyl peptidase-4 inhibitor decreases the risk of atrial fibrillation in patients with type 2 diabetes: A nationwide cohort study in Taiwan. *Cardiovasc. Diabetol.* **2017**, *16*, 159. [CrossRef]
71. Fitchett, D.; Zinman, B.; Wanner, C.; Lachin, J.M.; Hantel, S.; Salsali, A.; Johansen, O.E.; Woerle, H.J.; Broedl, U.C.; Inzucchi, S.E.; et al. Heart failure outcomes with empagliflozin in patients with type 2 diabetes at high cardiovascular risk: Results of the EMPA-REG OUTCOME(R) trial. *Eur. Heart J.* **2016**, *37*, 1526–1534. [CrossRef]
72. Kosiborod, M.; Cavender, M.A.; Fu, A.Z.; Wilding, J.P.; Khunti, K.; Holl, R.W.; Norhammar, A.; Birkeland, K.I.; Jorgensen, M.E.; Thuresson, M.; et al. Lower Risk of Heart Failure and Death in Patients Initiated on Sodium-Glucose Cotransporter-2 Inhibitors Versus Other Glucose-Lowering Drugs: The CVD-REAL Study (Comparative Effectiveness of Cardiovascular Outcomes in New Users of Sodium-Glucose Cotransporter-2 Inhibitors). *Circulation* **2017**, *136*, 249–259. [CrossRef]
73. Batzias, K.; Antonopoulos, A.S.; Oikonomou, E.; Siasos, G.; Bletsa, E.; Stampouloglou, P.K.; Mistakidi, C.V.; Noutsou, M.; Katsiki, N.; Karopoulos, P.; et al. Effects of Newer Antidiabetic Drugs on Endothelial Function and Arterial Stiffness: A Systematic Review and Meta-Analysis. *J. Diabetes Res.* **2018**, *2018*, 1232583. [CrossRef]
74. Zhou, H.; Wang, S.; Zhu, P.; Hu, S.; Chen, Y.; Ren, J. Empagliflozin rescues diabetic myocardial microvascular injury via AMPK-mediated inhibition of mitochondrial fission. *Redox Biol.* **2018**, *15*, 335–346. [CrossRef]
75. Uthman, L.; Baartscheer, A.; Bleijlevens, B.; Schumacher, C.A.; Fiolet, J.W.T.; Koeman, A.; Jancev, M.; Hollmann, M.W.; Weber, N.C.; Coronel, R.; et al. Class effects of SGLT2 inhibitors in mouse cardiomyocytes and hearts: Inhibition of Na(+)/H(+) exchanger, lowering of cytosolic Na(+) and vasodilation. *Diabetologia* **2018**, *61*, 722–726. [CrossRef]
76. Bay, J.; Kohlhaas, M.; Maack, C. Intracellular Na(+) and cardiac metabolism. *J. Mol. Cell. Cardiol.* **2013**, *61*, 20–27. [CrossRef]
77. Kohlhaas, M.; Liu, T.; Knopp, A.; Zeller, T.; Ong, M.F.; Bohm, M.; O'Rourke, B.; Maack, C. Elevated cytosolic Na$^+$ increases mitochondrial formation of reactive oxygen species in failing cardiac myocytes. *Circulation* **2010**, *121*, 1606–1613. [CrossRef]
78. Ye, Y.; Jia, X.; Bajaj, M.; Birnbaum, Y. Dapagliflozin Attenuates Na(+)/H(+) Exchanger-1 in Cardiofibroblasts via AMPK Activation. *Cardiovasc. Drugs Ther.* **2018**, *32*, 553–558. [CrossRef]
79. Li, C.; Zhang, J.; Xue, M.; Li, X.; Han, F.; Liu, X.; Xu, L.; Lu, Y.; Cheng, Y.; Li, T.; et al. SGLT2 inhibition with empagliflozin attenuates myocardial oxidative stress and fibrosis in diabetic mice heart. *Cardiovasc. Diabetol.* **2019**, *18*, 15. [CrossRef]
80. Bohm, M.; Slawik, J.; Brueckmann, M.; Mattheus, M.; George, J.T.; Ofstad, A.P.; Inzucchi, S.E.; Fitchett, D.; Anker, S.D.; Marx, N.; et al. Efficacy of empagliflozin on heart failure and renal outcomes in patients with atrial fibrillation: Data from the EMPA-REG OUTCOME trial. *Eur. J. Heart Fail.* **2020**, *22*, 126–135. [CrossRef]
81. Okunrintemi, V.; Mishriky, B.M.; Powell, J.R.; Cummings, D.M. Sodium-glucose co-transporter-2 inhibitors and atrial fibrillation in the cardiovascular and renal outcome trials. *Diabetes Obes. Metab.* **2021**, *23*, 276–280. [CrossRef]
82. Ling, A.W.; Chan, C.C.; Chen, S.W.; Kao, Y.W.; Huang, C.Y.; Chan, Y.H.; Chu, P.H. The risk of new-onset atrial fibrillation in patients with type 2 diabetes mellitus treated with sodium glucose cotransporter 2 inhibitors versus dipeptidyl peptidase-4 inhibitors. *Cardiovasc. Diabetol.* **2020**, *19*, 188. [CrossRef] [PubMed]

83. Zelniker, T.A.; Bonaca, M.P.; Furtado, R.H.M.; Mosenzon, O.; Kuder, J.F.; Murphy, S.A.; Bhatt, D.L.; Leiter, L.A.; McGuire, D.K.; Wilding, J.P.H.; et al. Effect of Dapagliflozin on Atrial Fibrillation in Patients with Type 2 Diabetes Mellitus. *Circulation* **2020**, *141*, 1227–1234. [CrossRef] [PubMed]
84. Martelli, A.; Testai, L.; Colletti, A.; Cicero, A.F.G. Coenzyme Q10: Clinical Applications in Cardiovascular Diseases. *Antioxidants* **2020**, *9*, 341. [CrossRef] [PubMed]
85. Sharma, A.; Fonarow, G.C.; Butler, J.; Ezekowitz, J.A.; Felker, G.M. Coenzyme Q10 and Heart Failure: A State-of-the-Art Review. *Circ. Heart Fail.* **2016**, *9*, e002639. [CrossRef] [PubMed]
86. Mortensen, A.L.; Rosenfeldt, F.; Filipiak, K.J. Effect of coenzyme Q10 in Europeans with chronic heart failure: A sub-group analysis of the Q-SYMBIO randomized double-blind trial. *Cardiol. J.* **2019**, *26*, 147–156. [CrossRef] [PubMed]
87. Rosenfeldt, F.; Marasco, S.; Lyon, W.; Wowk, M.; Sheeran, F.; Bailey, M.; Esmore, D.; Davis, B.; Pick, A.; Rabinov, M.; et al. Coenzyme Q10 therapy before cardiac surgery improves mitochondrial function and in vitro contractility of myocardial tissue. *J. Thorac. Cardiovasc. Surg.* **2005**, *129*, 25–32. [CrossRef]
88. Zhao, Q.; Kebbati, A.H.; Zhang, Y.; Tang, Y.; Okello, E.; Huang, C. Effect of coenzyme Q10 on the incidence of atrial fibrillation in patients with heart failure. *J. Investig. Med.* **2015**, *63*, 735–739. [CrossRef]
89. Moludi, J.; Keshavarz, S.; Mohammad Javad, H.-a.; Rahimi Frooshani, A.; Sadeghpour, A.; Salarkia, S.; Gholizadeh, F. Coenzyme Q10 effect in prevention of atrial fibrillation after Coronary Artery Bypass Graft: Double-blind randomized clinical trial. *Tehran Univ. Med. J.* **2015**, *73*, 79–85.
90. De Frutos, F.; Gea, A.; Hernandez-Estefania, R.; Rabago, G. Prophylactic treatment with coenzyme Q10 in patients undergoing cardiac surgery: Could an antioxidant reduce complications? A systematic review and meta-analysis. *Interact. Cardiovasc. Thorac. Surg.* **2015**, *20*, 254–259. [CrossRef]
91. Sun, D.; Yang, F. Metformin improves cardiac function in mice with heart failure after myocardial infarction by regulating mitochondrial energy metabolism. *Biochem. Biophys. Res. Commun.* **2017**, *486*, 329–335. [CrossRef]
92. Liu, Y.; Bai, F.; Liu, N.; Zhang, B.; Qin, F.; Tu, T.; Li, B.; Li, J.; Ma, Y.; Ouyang, F.; et al. Metformin improves lipid metabolism and reverses the Warburg effect in a canine model of chronic atrial fibrillation. *BMC Cardiovasc. Disord.* **2020**, *20*, 50. [CrossRef]
93. Chang, S.H.; Wu, L.S.; Chiou, M.J.; Liu, J.R.; Yu, K.H.; Kuo, C.F.; Wen, M.S.; Chen, W.J.; Yeh, Y.H.; See, L.C. Association of metformin with lower atrial fibrillation risk among patients with type 2 diabetes mellitus: A population-based dynamic cohort and in vitro studies. *Cardiovasc. Diabetol.* **2014**, *13*, 123. [CrossRef]
94. Li, J.; Li, B.; Bai, F.; Ma, Y.; Liu, N.; Liu, Y.; Wang, Y.; Liu, Q. Metformin therapy confers cardioprotection against the remodeling of gap junction in tachycardia-induced atrial fibrillation dog model. *Life Sci.* **2020**, *254*, 117759. [CrossRef]
95. Barreto-Torres, G.; Parodi-Rullan, R.; Javadov, S. The role of PPARalpha in metformin-induced attenuation of mitochondrial dysfunction in acute cardiac ischemia/reperfusion in rats. *Int. J. Mol. Sci.* **2012**, *13*, 7694–7709. [CrossRef]
96. Liu, C.; Liu, R.; Fu, H.; Li, J.; Wang, X.; Cheng, L.; Korantzopoulos, P.; Tse, G.; Li, G.; Liu, T. Pioglitazone attenuates atrial remodeling and vulnerability to atrial fibrillation in alloxan-induced diabetic rabbits. *Cardiovasc. Ther.* **2017**, *35*. [CrossRef] [PubMed]
97. Xu, D.; Murakoshi, N.; Igarashi, M.; Hirayama, A.; Ito, Y.; Seo, Y.; Tada, H.; Aonuma, K. PPAR-gamma activator pioglitazone prevents age-related atrial fibrillation susceptibility by improving antioxidant capacity and reducing apoptosis in a rat model. *J. Cardiovasc. Electrophysiol.* **2012**, *23*, 209–217. [CrossRef]
98. Pallisgaard, J.L.; Lindhardt, T.B.; Staerk, L.; Olesen, J.B.; Torp-Pedersen, C.; Hansen, M.L.; Gislason, G.H. Thiazolidinediones are associated with a decreased risk of atrial fibrillation compared with other antidiabetic treatment: A nationwide cohort study. *Eur. Heart J. Cardiovasc. Pharmacother.* **2017**, *3*, 140–146. [CrossRef]
99. Zhang, Z.; Zhang, X.; Korantzopoulos, P.; Letsas, K.P.; Tse, G.; Gong, M.; Meng, L.; Li, G.; Liu, T. Thiazolidinedione use and atrial fibrillation in diabetic patients: A meta-analysis. *BMC Cardiovasc. Disord.* **2017**, *17*, 96. [CrossRef]
100. Pallisgaard, J.L.; Brooks, M.M.; Chaitman, B.R.; Boothroyd, D.B.; Perez, M.; Hlatky, M.A.; Bypass Angioplasty Revascularization Investigation 2 Diabetes Study, G. Thiazolidinediones and Risk of Atrial Fibrillation Among Patients with Diabetes and Coronary Disease. *Am. J. Med.* **2018**, *131*, 805–812. [CrossRef]
101. Gu, J.; Hu, W.; Song, Z.P.; Liu, X.; Zhang, D.D. PPARgamma agonist use and recurrence of atrial fibrillation after successful electrical cardioversion. *Hellenic. J. Cardiol.* **2017**, *58*, 387–390. [CrossRef] [PubMed]
102. Staels, B.; Dallongeville, J.; Auwerx, J.; Schoonjans, K.; Leitersdorf, E.; Fruchart, J.C. Mechanism of action of fibrates on lipid and lipoprotein metabolism. *Circulation* **1998**, *98*, 2088–2093. [CrossRef] [PubMed]
103. Kar, D.; Bandyopadhyay, A. Targeting Peroxisome Proliferator Activated Receptor alpha (PPAR alpha) for the Prevention of Mitochondrial Impairment and Hypertrophy in Cardiomyocytes. *Cell. Physiol. Biochem.* **2018**, *49*, 245–259. [CrossRef] [PubMed]
104. Liu, G.Z.; Hou, T.T.; Yuan, Y.; Hang, P.Z.; Zhao, J.J.; Sun, L.; Zhao, G.Q.; Zhao, J.; Dong, J.M.; Wang, X.B.; et al. Fenofibrate inhibits atrial metabolic remodelling in atrial fibrillation through PPAR-alpha/sirtuin 1/PGC-1alpha pathway. *Br. J. Pharmacol.* **2016**, *173*, 1095–1109. [CrossRef]
105. Augustyniak, J.; Lenart, J.; Gaj, P.; Kolanowska, M.; Jazdzewski, K.; Stepien, P.P.; Buzanska, L. Bezafibrate Upregulates Mitochondrial Biogenesis and Influence Neural Differentiation of Human-Induced Pluripotent Stem Cells. *Mol. Neurobiol.* **2019**, *56*, 4346–4363. [CrossRef]

106. Hanna, I.R.; Heeke, B.; Bush, H.; Brosius, L.; King-Hageman, D.; Dudley, S.C., Jr.; Beshai, J.F.; Langberg, J.J. Lipid-lowering drug use is associated with reduced prevalence of atrial fibrillation in patients with left ventricular systolic dysfunction. *Heart Rhythm* **2006**, *3*, 881–886. [CrossRef]
107. Cavar, M.; Ljubkovic, M.; Bulat, C.; Bakovic, D.; Fabijanic, D.; Kraljevic, J.; Karanovic, N.; Dujic, Z.; Lavie, C.J.; Wisloff, U.; et al. Trimetazidine does not alter metabolic substrate oxidation in cardiac mitochondria of target patient population. *Br. J. Pharmacol.* **2016**, *173*, 1529–1540. [CrossRef]
108. MacInnes, A.; Fairman, D.A.; Binding, P.; Rhodes, J.; Wyatt, M.J.; Phelan, A.; Haddock, P.S.; Karran, E.H. The antianginal agent trimetazidine does not exert its functional benefit via inhibition of mitochondrial long-chain 3-ketoacyl coenzyme A thiolase. *Circ. Res.* **2003**, *93*, e26–e32. [CrossRef]
109. Monteiro, P.; Duarte, A.I.; Goncalves, L.M.; Moreno, A.; Providencia, L.A. Protective effect of trimetazidine on myocardial mitochondrial function in an ex-vivo model of global myocardial ischemia. *Eur. J. Pharmacol.* **2004**, *503*, 123–128. [CrossRef]
110. Shi, W.; Shangguan, W.; Zhang, Y.; Li, C.; Li, G. Effects of trimetazidine on mitochondrial respiratory function, biosynthesis, and fission/fusion in rats with acute myocardial ischemia. *Anatol. J. Cardiol.* **2017**, *18*, 175–181. [CrossRef]
111. Dehina, L.; Vaillant, F.; Tabib, A.; Bui-Xuan, B.; Chevalier, P.; Dizerens, N.; Bui-Xuan, C.; Descotes, J.; Blanc-Guillemaud, V.; Lerond, L.; et al. Trimetazidine demonstrated cardioprotective effects through mitochondrial pathway in a model of acute coronary ischemia. *Naunyn Schmiedeberg's Arch. Pharmacol.* **2013**, *386*, 205–215. [CrossRef]
112. Gunes, Y.; Tuncer, M.; Guntekin, U.; Akdag, S.; Gumrukcuoglu, H.A. The effects of trimetazidine on p-wave duration and dispersion in heart failure patients. *Pacing Clin. Electrophysiol.* **2009**, *32*, 239–244. [CrossRef]
113. Zhang, J.; He, S.; Wang, X.; Wang, D. Effect of trimetazidine on heart rate variability in elderly patients with acute coronary syndrome. *Pak. J. Med. Sci.* **2016**, *32*, 75–78. [CrossRef]
114. Cera, M.; Salerno, A.; Fragasso, G.; Montanaro, C.; Gardini, C.; Marinosci, G.; Arioli, F.; Spoladore, R.; Facchini, A.; Godino, C.; et al. Beneficial electrophysiological effects of trimetazidine in patients with postischemic chronic heart failure. *J. Cardiovasc. Pharmacol. Ther.* **2010**, *15*, 24–30. [CrossRef]
115. Li, Z.; Chaolan, L.; Chengcheng, W.; Xi, H.; Yingying, W.; Jiaqiu, L.; Wei, H. GW28-e0789 Trimetazidine decreases inducibility and duration of atrial fibrillation in a dog model of congestive heart failure. *J. Am. Coll. Cardiol.* **2017**, *70*, C29. [CrossRef]
116. Han, W.; Yang, S.S.; Wei, N.; Huo, H.; Li, W.M.; Zhou, H.Y.; Zhou, G.; Cao, Y.; Dong, G.; Fu, S.B. Effects of chronic trimetazidine treatment on atrial energy metabolism in a canine model of chronic atrial fibrillation. *Zhonghua Xin Xue Guan Bing Za Zhi* **2008**, *36*, 556–559.
117. Han, W.; Li, W.M.; Zhou, H.Y.; Huo, H.; Wei, N.; Dong, G.; Cao, Y.; Zhou, G.; Yang, S.S. Effects of trimetazidine on atrial structural remodeling and platelet activation in dogs with atrial fibrillation. *Chin. Med. J.* **2009**, *122*, 2180–2183. [PubMed]
118. Francis, J.; Antzelevitch, C. Ranolazine as Antiarrhythmic Agent. *BMH Med. J.* **2019**, *56*, 58–64.
119. Guerra, F.; Romandini, A.; Barbarossa, A.; Belardinelli, L.; Capucci, A. Ranolazine for rhythm control in atrial fibrillation: A systematic review and meta-analysis. *Int. J. Cardiol.* **2017**, *227*, 284–291. [CrossRef]
120. Gong, M.; Zhang, Z.; Fragakis, N.; Korantzopoulos, P.; Letsas, K.P.; Li, G.; Yan, G.X.; Liu, T. Role of ranolazine in the prevention and treatment of atrial fibrillation: A meta-analysis of randomized clinical trials. *Heart Rhythm* **2017**, *14*, 3–11. [CrossRef]
121. Frommeyer, G.; Schmidt, M.; Clauß, C.; Kaese, S.; Stypmann, J.; Pott, C.; Eckardt, L.; Milberg, P. Further insights into the underlying electrophysiological mechanisms for reduction of atrial fibrillation by ranolazine in an experimental model of chronic heart failure. *Eur. J. Heart Fail.* **2012**, *14*, 1322–1331. [CrossRef] [PubMed]
122. Zou, D.; Geng, N.; Chen, Y.; Ren, L.; Liu, X.; Wan, J.; Guo, S.; Wang, S. Ranolazine improves oxidative stress and mitochondrial function in the atrium of acetylcholine-CaCl2 induced atrial fibrillation rats. *Life Sci.* **2016**, *156*, 7–14. [CrossRef] [PubMed]
123. Chatfield, K.C.; Sparagna, G.C.; Chau, S.; Phillips, E.K.; Ambardekar, A.V.; Aftab, M.; Mitchell, M.B.; Sucharov, C.C.; Miyamoto, S.D.; Stauffer, B.L. Elamipretide Improves Mitochondrial Function in the Failing Human Heart. *JACC Basic Transl. Sci.* **2019**, *4*, 147–157. [CrossRef]
124. Sabbah, H.N.; Gupta, R.C.; Kohli, S.; Wang, M.; Hachem, S.; Zhang, K. Chronic Therapy with Elamipretide (MTP-131), a Novel Mitochondria-Targeting Peptide, Improves Left Ventricular and Mitochondrial Function in Dogs With Advanced Heart Failure. *Circ. Heart Fail.* **2016**, *9*, e002206. [CrossRef]
125. Daubert, M.A.; Yow, E.; Dunn, G.; Marchev, S.; Barnhart, H.; Douglas, P.S.; O'Connor, C.; Goldstein, S.; Udelson, J.E.; Sabbah, H.N. Novel Mitochondria-Targeting Peptide in Heart Failure Treatment: A Randomized, Placebo-Controlled Trial of Elamipretide. *Circ. Heart Fail.* **2017**, *10*. [CrossRef]
126. Butler, J.; Khan, M.S.; Anker, S.D.; Fonarow, G.C.; Kim, R.J.; Nodari, S.; O'Connor, C.M.; Pieske, B.; Pieske-Kraigher, E.; Sabbah, H.N.; et al. Effects of Elamipretide on Left Ventricular Function in Patients With Heart Failure With Reduced Ejection Fraction: The PROGRESS-HF Phase 2 Trial. *J. Card. Fail.* **2020**, *26*, 429–437. [CrossRef]
127. Buyse, G.M.; Voit, T.; Schara, U.; Straathof, C.S.M.; D'Angelo, M.G.; Bernert, G.; Cuisset, J.-M.; Finkel, R.S.; Goemans, N.; McDonald, C.M.; et al. Efficacy of idebenone on respiratory function in patients with Duchenne muscular dystrophy not using glucocorticoids (DELOS): A double-blind randomised placebo-controlled phase 3 trial. *Lancet* **2015**, *385*, 1748–1757. [CrossRef]
128. Lagedrost, S.J.; Sutton, M.S.; Cohen, M.S.; Satou, G.M.; Kaufman, B.D.; Perlman, S.L.; Rummey, C.; Meier, T.; Lynch, D.R. Idebenone in Friedreich ataxia cardiomyopathy-results from a 6-month phase III study (IONIA). *Am. Heart J.* **2011**, *161*, 639–645. [CrossRef]

129. Seo, K.S.; Kim, J.H.; Min, K.N.; Moon, J.A.; Roh, T.C.; Lee, M.J.; Lee, K.W.; Min, J.E.; Lee, Y.M. KL1333, a Novel NAD(+) Modulator, Improves Energy Metabolism and Mitochondrial Dysfunction in MELAS Fibroblasts. *Front. Neurol.* **2018**, *9*, 552. [CrossRef]
130. Beyrath, J.; Pellegrini, M.; Renkema, H.; Houben, L.; Pecheritsyna, S.; van Zandvoort, P.; van den Broek, P.; Bekel, A.; Eftekhari, P.; Smeitink, J.A.M. KH176 Safeguards Mitochondrial Diseased Cells from Redox Stress-Induced Cell Death by Interacting with the Thioredoxin System/Peroxiredoxin Enzyme Machinery. *Sci. Rep.* **2018**, *8*, 6577. [CrossRef]
131. El-Hattab, A.W.; Zarante, A.M.; Almannai, M.; Scaglia, F. Therapies for mitochondrial diseases and current clinical trials. *Mol. Genet. Metab.* **2017**, *122*, 1–9. [CrossRef]
132. Perry, J.B.; Davis, G.N.; Allen, M.E.; Makrecka-Kuka, M.; Dambrova, M.; Grange, R.W.; Shaikh, S.R.; Brown, D.A. Cardioprotective effects of idebenone do not involve ROS scavenging: Evidence for mitochondrial complex I bypass in ischemia/reperfusion injury. *J. Mol. Cell. Cardiol.* **2019**, *135*, 160–171. [CrossRef]
133. Liu, Z.; Donahue, J.K. The Use of Gene Therapy for Ablation of Atrial Fibrillation. *Arrhythm. Electrophysiol. Rev.* **2014**, *3*, 139–144. [CrossRef]
134. Bikou, O.; Thomas, D.; Trappe, K.; Lugenbiel, P.; Kelemen, K.; Koch, M.; Soucek, R.; Voss, F.; Becker, R.; Katus, H.A.; et al. Connexin 43 gene therapy prevents persistent atrial fibrillation in a porcine model. *Cardiovasc. Res.* **2011**, *92*, 218–225. [CrossRef]
135. Trappe, K.; Thomas, D.; Bikou, O.; Kelemen, K.; Lugenbiel, P.; Voss, F.; Becker, R.; Katus, H.A.; Bauer, A. Suppression of persistent atrial fibrillation by genetic knockdown of caspase 3: A pre-clinical pilot study. *Eur. Heart J.* **2011**, *34*, 147–157. [CrossRef]

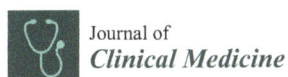 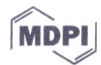

Review

RNAs and Gene Expression Predicting Postoperative Atrial Fibrillation in Cardiac Surgery Patients Undergoing Coronary Artery Bypass Grafting

Muhammad Shuja Khan [1], Kennosuke Yamashita [1,2], Vikas Sharma [3], Ravi Ranjan [1,2,4] and Derek James Dosdall [1,2,3,4,*]

1. Nora Eccles Harrison Cardiovascular Research and Training Institute, The University of Utah, Salt Lake City, UT 84112, USA; m.khan@utah.edu (M.S.K.); kennosuke.atmm3@gmail.com (K.Y.); ravi.ranjan@hsc.utah.edu (R.R.)
2. Division of Cardiovascular Medicine, The University of Utah-Health, Salt Lake City, UT 84132, USA
3. Division of Cardiothoracic Surgery, The University of Utah-Health, Salt Lake City, UT 84132, USA; vikas.sharma@hsc.utah.edu
4. Department of Biomedical Engineering, The University of Utah, Salt Lake City, UT 84112, USA
* Correspondence: derek.dosdall@utah.edu; Tel.: +1-801-587-2036

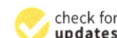

Received: 23 March 2020; Accepted: 14 April 2020; Published: 16 April 2020

Abstract: Postoperative atrial fibrillation (POAF) is linked with increased morbidity, mortality rate and financial liability. About 20–50% of patients experience POAF after coronary artery bypass graft (CABG) surgery. Numerous review articles and meta-analyses have investigated links between patient clinical risk factors, demographic conditions, and pre-, peri- and post-operative biomarkers to forecast POAF incidence in CABG patients. This narrative review, for the first time, summarize the role of micro-RNAs, circular-RNAs and other gene expressions that have shown experimental evidence to accurately predict the POAF incidence in cardiac surgery patients after CABG. We envisage that identifying specific genomic markers for predicting POAF might be a significant step for the prevention and effective management of this type of post-operative complication and may provide critical perspective into arrhythmogenic substrate responsible for POAF.

Keywords: postoperative atrial fibrillation; biomarkers; coronary artery bypass grafting; miRNA; circRNA; mtDNA; SNPs; atrial fibrillation

1. Introduction

Postoperative atrial fibrillation (POAF) occurs in 20–50% of coronary artery bypass graft (CABG) patients during postoperative stay [1]. It has been reported that the incidence of POAF is approximately 50% after combined CABG/valvular procedures, 30% after pure CABG surgery, and 40% following valve replacements or repair [2–4]. Although POAF is generally considered to be a transitory condition, it can be life-threatening and is associated with increased complications, morbidity, mortality rate and financial burden [4]. In cardiac patients that experienced an arrhythmia, 70% of them developed POAF before the end of the fourth postoperative day and 94% before the end of the sixth postoperative day [5]. Treatment of POAF is estimated to add an additional $1 billion in health care costs in the US alone [6]. Therefore, identifying patients at an early stage may help to define a population that is more likely to benefit from anti-arrhythmic drug therapy or additional surgical intervention during the open chest procedure and may lead to a substantial reduction in POAF in the highest risk patients [7–9]. Reducing the rate of POAF is linked with a decline in the extent of hospital stay and possible cost savings [4].

There have been several algorithms and theories used to forecast the complications of post-CABG surgery, however, current methods are established based-on patients' demographics and clinical co-morbidities, and preoperative performance status [3,10]. Recent literature has revealed many biomarkers that might be useful as a forecaster to predict post-CABG surgery atrial fibrillation [11,12]. The relationship of biomarkers that show tangible confirmation supporting clinical outcome has significantly advanced the field of medicine, helping clinicians in many medicine sub-specialties to forecast clinical course.

The potential for micro-RNAs (miRNAs) to evaluate cardiovascular disease as a non-invasive molecular biomarker is of increasing interest due to their abundant presence in in serum, plasma and urine [13–15]. Recently published literature showed that miRNAs that regulate gene expression are involved in the arrhythmogenic substrate of AF [16–18]. Further, experimental evidences reported the specific role of miRNAs in defining development or onset of arrhythmia and other cardiovascular disorders [18–27]. Several techniques have been established to compute miRNAs such as droplet digital polymerase chain reaction (PCR), quantitative stem-loop RT-PCR, chip-based digital PCR, quantitative real-time PCR (qRT-PCR) as well as RNAseq and microarrays [28–30].

Along with miRNAs, circular-RNAs (circRNAs) are greatly stable due to a resistance to their exonucleases and debranching enzymes [31,32]. Therefore, circRNAs hold distinctive benefits and may also be beneficial to identify a group of CABG patients who are at risk of POAF [11].

Besides miRNAs and circRNAs, the genomic biomarkers have also shed light on the molecular mechanisms that lead to structural and conductive atrial remodeling, creating an arrhythmogenic substrate for AF development [33]. Thus, the patient-specific genomic sequence may assist in finding the degree to which differentially expressed genes in the atrial tissue samples are linked with an increased risk for POAF in patients undergoing CABG.

To date, the relationship between the function of miRNAs, circRNAs, and gene expressions with POAF risk development in CABG patients has not been thoroughly reviewed in published literature. In this narrative review, we report the available experimental evidence of several miRNAs such as miRNA-483-5p [34], miRNA-29a [35], miRNA-23a [36], miRNA-26a [36], miRNA-199a [16], miRNA-1 [37], and miRNA-133a [37], one circRNA: circRNA-025016 [38], and selected gene expressions such as mitochondrial DNA (mtDNA) [39,40], and other single nucleotide polymorphisms (SNPs) such as vesicular overexpressed in cancer–prosurvival protein 1 gene (VOPP1) [41], rs3740563 [42], rs10504554 [43], rs2249825 [44], rs4572292 [45], rs11198893 [45], rs10033464 [46,47], rs2200733 [46–48] and rs13143308 [48] used previously as potential elements predicting POAF risk following CABG surgery.

2. Materials and Methods

2.1. Design of Study

We intended to assess relevant studies by examining the quality of the previously reported role of miRNA, circRNA and SNPs collected from either tissue, blood or plasma preoperatively and perioperatively among patients undergoing CABG surgery with and (or) without cardiopulmonary bypass (CPB). Articles were extracted using both PubMed and MEDLINE databases. The search strategy involved the MEsH keywords such as "atrial fibrillation", "Coronary Artery Bypass", "miRNAs", "circRNAs", "mtDNA", "SNP(s)", and the text keywords such as "postoperative atrial fibrillation" and "Coronary Artery Bypass Graft".

2.2. Data Extraction

An abstract's general information for each paper was assessed and studied to ensure both inclusion and exclusion criteria. Studies not published as full-text articles such as published abstracts, single case reports, opinion articles, editorial letters and articles not written in English were excluded. No article was excluded based on pre-existing antiarrhythmic drug therapy. Patient's w/wo AF history were included. Both prospective and retrospective studies were also included. Search was restricted to studies in adults (aged: 18 + years) w/wo POAF incidence after surgery but none of the studies were excluded based on sex, race/ethnicity, BMI, obesity, diabetes mellitus and myocardial infarction condition. This narrative review is focused on only CABG patients. However, to increase the number of studies and patient population, along with CABG, patients underwent CABG (with or without valve surgery procedures) were also considered and included in this narrative review. Studies reported data for patients underwent only valve surgery such as mitral valve replacement/repair (MVR/r) and aortic valve replacement/repair (AVR/r) were not included. Finally, studies reported the postoperative data for miRNA, circRNA, and gene expressions were included as long as their results exhibited preoperative data for the same parameters. Since this narrative review was focused on cardiac patients' samples (blood, serum and tissue) collected preoperatively and (or) intraoperatively, the previously reported in vivo studies investigating miRNA, circRNA, mtDNA and SNPs in small and large animal models were also excluded. Summaries of the clinical articles' selection, data extraction and evaluation are shown in Figure 1.

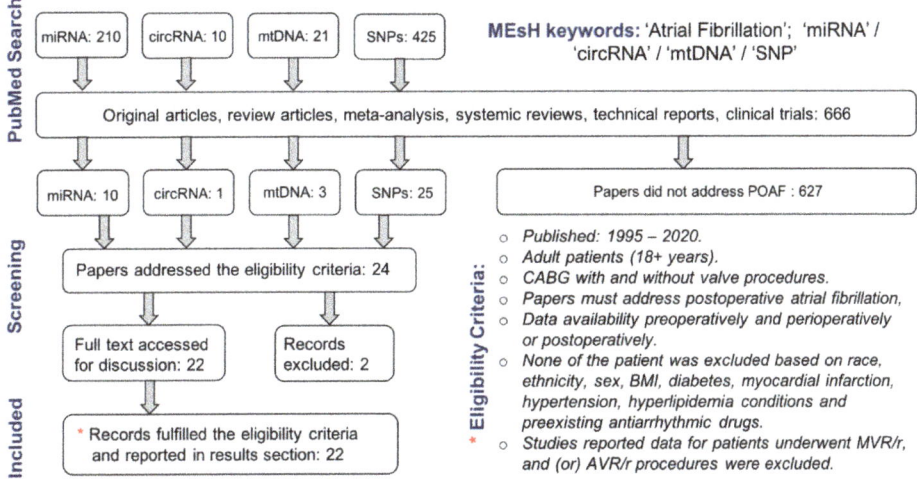

Figure 1. Flow diagram of selected studies searched and reported in this narrative review.

3. Results and Discussion

3.1. Micro-RNAs Predicting POAF

There are numerous studies reported that AF is associated with altered miRNA levels in atrial tissue and plasma [20,49–51]. miRNAs targeting pathways associated with the regulation of cardiomyocyte metabolism (miRNA-208a and miRNA-223) may alter the metabolic energy reserve required to maintain AF [23,52,53], whereas other miRNAs are thought to play a dominant role in changes related with structural (miRNA-133, miRNA-590, miRNA-29b, miRNA-208, miRNA-638, and miRNA-150) and electrical remodeling (miRNA-328, miRNA−1 and miRNA−26) [54]. Further miRNA−328 [55] and miRNA−29 [56] have also been demonstrated to be potential contributors in AF. Though numerous clinical studies have been reported, the detailed underlying mechanism of onset and persistence of POAF has not been completely elucidated. Mariscalco et al. explained numerous factors which could contribute to POAF risk development following CABG surgery such as atrial dilation, loss of connexins, autonomic imbalance, trauma, ischemia, mechanical myopericarditis, sutures, inflammation, and dysfunction caused by post- extra-corporeal circulation [57]. Similarly, Jalife & Kaur and Santulli et al. focused on a promising contribution of miRNA in similar circumstances [27,58,59]. On the contrary, Krogstad et al. studied plasma collected from 92 CABG patients, reported over 105 miRNAs [60].

In their work, 27 patients (29.4%) developed POAF, and interestingly, they did not find any single miRNA linked with the POAF onset. In the following sub-sections, we report selected miRNAs that have shown potential in predicting the POAF following CABG surgery.

3.1.1. miRNA−483−5p

miRNA−483−5p is a 22-nucleotide (AAGACGGGAGGAAA GAAGGGAG) intronic mature microRNA which is transcribed with its host gene, IGF2, located on chromosome 11p15.5 [61]. As reported that it has been isolated in several human samples such as brain tissue, myocardium, blood serum and hepatic [61,62]. At present, miRNA−483−5p remains relatively poorly examined. Harling et al. conducted a prospective study comprised of 34 patients undergoing non-emergent, on-pump CABG surgery at Imperial College Healthcare NHS Trust (London, UK), and evaluated the role of circulating miRNA−483−5p [34]. All these patients had no prior history of AF. They collected plasma samples at 24 h preoperatively and at day 2 and 4 postoperatively. Among 34 patients, 13 patients (38.2%) developed the POAF condition. These POAF patients tended to be older (64.4 ± 11.3 years), with a higher percentage being male (69.2%). After standard procedures and miRNAs isolation, they found sixteen miRNAs in POAF patients' atrial myocardium when compared with those maintaining SR. Specifically, miRNA−483−5p showed a 1.804-fold increase and was overexpressed in the preoperative serum samples. In comparison to preoperative samples, there was a substantial increase in the expression of miRNA−483−5p at 48 h time point in POAF-group, $p = 0.046$; however, in no-POAF group, there was no significant change in serum expression in samples collected preoperatively and 2-day postoperatively. Interestingly, both groups exhibited a major increase in miRNA−483−5p expression between 2- and 4- day postoperative time points (POAF group: $p = 0.0051$; no-POAF-group: $p = 0.0055$). In their study, the mean time to onset of AF was 2.5 days. In their findings, they further emphasized that the exact mechanistic role of miRNA−483−5p requires further examination with evaluation of its host gene transcription and protein expression. Thus, a large patient cohort is required to further examine the individual role of miRNA−483−5p as a potential biomarker for POAF risk prediction among CABG patients with no prior AF history.

3.1.2. miRNA−29a

miRNA−29 family targets a cadre of mRNAs that encode proteins involved in fibrosis, including multiple collagens, fibrillin, and elastin [63]. Thus, down-regulation of miRNA−29 would be predicted to derepress the expression of these mRNAs and enhance the fibrotic response. To explore the potential of miRNA−29a and its association in predicting POAF among CABG patients, recently Rizvi et al., conducted a study with 90 patients with no prior history of AF at Advocate Aurora Research Institute (Milwaukee, WI, USA) [35]. They collected fasted blood samples preoperatively in the morning of the cardiac surgery day. Thirty-four (37.8%) patients with average age of 72.04 ± 10.7 years developed POAF. In their findings, they did not report any significant difference in patients' baseline comorbidities. They further did not observe any significant differences in other risk factors such as diabetes, previous heart attack, high blood pressure, sleep apnea and stroke in patients who developed POAF compared with those who remained in sinus after cardiac surgery. Preoperative amino-terminal-procollagen-III-peptide (PIIINP) and carboxy-terminal-procollagen-I-peptide levels were low in group of patients that remained in sinus after cardiac surgery in comparison to those who developed POAAF with a decline in miRNA−29a. Therefore, this is the first prospective study exhibiting the role of miRNA−29a in association with POAF. Thus, combining age as the only significant clinical predictor with PIIINP and miRNA−29a provided a model that identified POAF patients with higher predictive accuracy. However, this study is limited to only 90 patients and thus, it does not allow to propose miRNA−29a that may be of high clinical relevance in predicting POAF risk development independently. Thus, a larger study is needed to confirm the diagnostic capacity of miRNA−29a in CABG patients with no prior history of AF.

3.1.3. miRNA–23a and miRNA–26a

miRNA–23a is a muscle specific miRNA and is richly expressed in myocardial cells [64]. It was revealed as a novel potential biomarker for diagnosing acute aortic dissection [65]. Similarly, Jansen et al. described the kinetics of another miRNA (miRNA–26a) to be involved in various cardiovascular pathologies [66]. The expression of miRNA–26a was noted to be significantly reduced in atrial samples collected from patients and large animals (dogs) with AF as compared to without AF (control group) [67]. Thus, to further explore the key role of miRNA–26a and miRNA–23a) in predicting POAF risk development, Feldman et al. reported a study to identify patients who developed POAF after undergoing CABG surgery and compared circulating blood levels of miRNA–23a and miRNA–26a between two groups (POAF, $n = 24$ vs. no-POAF, $n = 24$) at preoperative and postoperative time points [36]. They harvested peripheral venous blood preoperatively and 48 h after CABG surgery. The results revealed that the expression levels for miRNA–23a ($p = 0.02$) and –26a ($p = 0.01$) in the POAF group were reduced during the postoperative period in comparison to preoperative results with receiver operating curve of 0.63 (confidence interval [CI]: 0.51–0.74) and 0.66 (95% CI: 0.55–0.77), respectively. However, we envisage that a large prospective study assessing preoperative miRNA–23a and –26a in classifying patients' POAF risk is therefore essential before they can be recognized as potent biomarkers of predicting a high risk of POAF.

3.1.4. miRNA–199a

The cardiomyocyte-specific microRNA, miRNA–199a, is primary involved in the regulation of (Sirtuin1) SIRT1 expression in cardiac tissue [68]. SIRT1 is a cardioprotective protein involved in the regulation of angiogenesis, prevention of endothelial dysfunction, and counteraction of deleterious effects of ischemia reperfusion injury [68–70]. The level of miRNA–199a is lowered with cardiac ischemia, and thus allows an increase in SIRT1 in cardiomyocytes [71]. An enhanced SIRT1 expression is associated with the occurrence of AF [72–74]. Yamac et al. reported that an expression of miRNA–199a in 49 patients undergoing CABG procedure. Samples were collected from right atrial appendage tissue and miRNA–199a was lowered in 29 patients that developed POAF after surgery in comparison to 20 patients that remained in sinus ($p = 0.022$) [16]. Since, miRNA–199a was drastically downregulated in tissue probes of patients suffering from POAF, SIRT1 protein was significantly upregulated in tissue probes of patients with POAF ($p < 0.001$). This was the only study that reported the miRNA–199a of patients undergoing CABG surgery. Further work is warranted to develop a multicenter study comprised of large cohort of patients for reproducibility, and its clinical applicability at large.

3.1.5. miRNA–1 and miRNA–133a

Both miRNA–1 and miRNA–133 are the most abundant miRNAs in the heart as they are expressed from bicistronic transcripts containing miRNA clusters [75]. Specifically, patients with persistent AF, miRNA–1 is downregulated in comparison with patients that remain in sinus [76]. Tsoporsis et al. conducted a small prospective patient study ($n = 42$) and collected right atrial appendage samples and venous blood pre- and post-CABG to evaluate the effectiveness of miRNA–1 and –133 [37]. In comparison to patients ($n = 24$, 77.7%) who remained in sinus after cardiac surgery, the group of patients who developed POAF expressed no differences in pre and post CABG levels for both miRNA–1 and miRNA–1. Similarly, in their findings, they did not observe any statistically significant differences in plasma samples collected pre- and post CABG in either of the group (POAF vs. no-POAF). All of the consented patients had no preoperative AF history.

3.2. circRNA Predicting POAF

circRNAs have distinctive advantages in comparison to miRNAs in identifying POAF risk among cardiac surgery patients with no preoperative history of AF [11]. Zhang et al. demonstrated a retrospective study with 13,617 plasma circRNAs expression profiles in group of patients that developed POAF and those who remained in sinus after cardiac procedures [38]. Interestingly, their selected circRNAs that were associated with POAF risk development were further validated in two separate and independent cohorts of patients who underwent isolated off-pump CABG. In their work, specifically, an independent cohort of 284 patients (CABG surgery with no prior history of AF) was included to investigate the functioning of the specific circRNA i.e., circRNA_025016). After filtering 31 circRNAs, only nine of them revealed a fold change of more than four in patients who developed POAF as compared to those who remained in sinus. All analyses were conducted via standard qPCR. With further analysis of patient plasma samples, circRNA_025016 revealed the strongest linked with POAF risk and was also found to be elevated in all CABG patients in comparison with healthy controls. Nevertheless, these findings should be further assessed in larger prospective multicenter studies to clarify its role in predicting POAF risk development.

3.3. Gene Expressions Predicting POAF

To investigate electrical and structural atrial remodeling, genetic association could be helpful in defining the molecular mechanisms in creating a substrate for AF [33]. The gene expression pattern in atrial tissue might be useful in determining the extent to which the differentially expressed gene(s) in the human atrium are linked with a high POAF risk in CABG surgery patients.

3.3.1. Mitochondrial DNA (mtDNA)

In peripheral blood, mtDNA is found to be linked with a patient's oxidative stress [77] and is traced in close vicinity of the main cellular source of reactive oxygen species [78]. It has also been reported that oxidative stress plays a critical role in post-surgery AF development in cardiac surgery patients [11,79–81]. Zhang et al. measured mtDNA retrospectively using the standard qRT-PCR in peripheral blood collected preoperatively from 485 CABG patients without prior history of AF [39]. The mtDNA copy number was drastically higher in patients with POAF ($n = 101$, 21%) than in those who remained in sinus following CABG procedure ($p < 0.001$). They further investigated that age was not a critical parameter for POAF development in their study. This may imply that mtDNA copy number can be an independent preoperative biomarker for POAF risk. The presented results in their study highly indicate that patients with increase mtDNA copy number may be prone to POAF after cardiac surgery. In another study reported by Sandler et. al., [40], mtDNA was investigated at three different time points (preoperatively, after CPB within 90 min of decannulation, and postoperatively at day 1 and day 2) from 16 patients enrolled prospectively. In comparison to preoperative results, mtDNA in their blood samples was significantly elevated following CPB (six-fold increase post-CPB, $p = 0.008$ and five-fold increase 1–2 days postoperatively, $p = 0.02$). Patients with POAF showed an increase in mtDNA post-CPB than those with no-POAF. Further, patients who developed POAF exhibited at least a two-fold increase of mtDNA postoperatively, whereas this happened in less than 50% of patients without POAF ($p = 0.037$). Their results indicated that the tissue damage and the relevant inflammation initiated by surgery on CPB play a critical function in POAF development, and thus, this confirms that there may be a mechanistic existence at molecular level between mtDNA and POAF. Consequently, future studies are required to assess oxidative stress that impacts mtDNA copy number in the development of POAF risk among CABG patients with no prior history of AF.

3.3.2. Single Nucleotide Polymorphisms (SNPs)

Genetic variation in the G protein-coupled receptor kinase 5 genes (GRK5) potentially acts as a physiological regulator of β-adrenergic receptor activity [82–85] and is associated with POAF development in CABG (on-pump) patients that are treated with β-blockers (BBs) perioperatively [42]. BBs are used to prevent post-surgery AF developments and as the treatment as well; however, about 20% patients still develop AF following CABG despite having BBs [86]. Kertai et al. noted the same and reported that genetic variation in GRK5 is strongly linked with POAF despite perioperative BB therapy in patients undergoing CABG surgery [42]. In their study with 245 on-pump CABG patients, they isolated genomic DNA from whole blood using standard procedures at Duke Genomic Analysis Facility and tested 492 SNPs. Of the 492 SNPs examined, three SNPs (rs11198893, rs3740563 and rs10787959), belong to the intragenic region of GRK5, showed an increased risk for POAF in 42 patients (17.1%) despite preoperative BBs therapy. Further, among three SNPs, rs3740563 revealed the most significant marker statistically associated with an increased risk for POAF development. Later the same group extended the study with RAA tissue samples. They analyzed the raw data from gene expression profiling in 45 patients with no prior AF history and underwent on-pump CABG surgery [41]. Among 45 patients, 13 (28.9%) developed POAF in spite of preoperative BB therapy. Finally, to further investigate that how sets of genes might be systematically changed their behavior in patients with POAF in comparison with no-POAF, they demonstrated gene set enrichment scrutiny. The most significant search was vesicular overexpressed in cancer - prosurvival protein 1 gene (VOPP1) which showed 1.83-fold change ($p < 0.01$) and was found to be up-regulated in patients that developed POAF. The second most significant probe was LOC389286 gene which revealed 0.49-fold change ($p < 0.01$) and was found to be down-regulated in patients that developed POAF. These results depict that patients undergoing CABG surgery, RAA gene expression profiling can be helpful scientifically to study VOPP1 as it has a critical role in the development of POAF despite using BBs therapy preoperatively. Therefore, the mechanisms that connect atrial VOPP1 expression with the development of POAF in cardiac surgery patients remains unclear.

Kertai et al. conducted a gene-wide association study in two cohorts of patients (diversity, $n = 877$ and validation, $n = 304$) to investigate the link of a genetic polymorphism in lymphocyte antigen 96 (LY96) with POAF incidence in CABG patients [43]. Based on SNPs selection criteria, they recognized only the minor allele of rs10504554, in the intronic region of the LY96, which exhibited a lower risk for POAF in both data sets (discovery data set: OR 0.48, 95% CI 0.34–0.68, $p < 0.01$, and replication dataset: OR 0.55, 95% CI 0.31–0.99, $p = 0.046$). These evidences in two different groups: discovery and validation, conclude that a SNP (rs10504554) is associated with decreased risk of POAF in patients undergoing CABG surgery. A prospective cohort study with 128 patients was conducted by Qu et al. to study the relationship between rs2249825 (C/G) polymorphism in high-mobility group box protein 1 (HMGB1) and POAF in patients who underwent CABG under CPB [44]. POAF incidence occurred in 37 (28.9%) patients. Blood samples were collected before, and after (at 4, and 24 h) CPB. Enzyme immunoassay was used to quantify HMGB1 level. In their findings, they reported that plasma HMGB1 level was increased 4 h after CPB ($p < 0.0001$) and was still increased at 24 h ($p < 0.0001$) in comparison to HMGB1 levels quantified in pre-CPB blood samples. Several epidemiologic cohorts have shown an association between SNPs in the chromosome 4q25 region and the development of AF [87–90]. The SNPs in the same region have also been associated with an increased risk of AF recurrence after catheter ablation [89]. Earlier retrospective studies reported that polymorphisms in chromosome 4q25 are associated with the development of POAF [46,48].

In the study of 1166 white participants from the TexGen genetic registry conducted by Virani et al., [46] the overall POAF incidence after CABG was 36.45% and variants in 4q25 were associated with an increased risk of POAF. In their findings, both rs2200733 and rs10033464 were associated with POAF (OR 1.41, 95% CI 1.04 to 1.91, and OR 1.47, 95% CI 1.05 to 2.06, respectively). Similarly, in two independently collected cardiac surgery cohorts (discovery, $n = 959$ and validation, $n = 494$) conducted by Body et al., non-coding SNPs within the chromosome 4q25 region were independently associated with POAF following CABG surgery [48]. They prospectively collected genomic data from patients undergoing primary CABG surgery with CPB at three major United States cardiovascular centers. They identified rs2200733 and rs13143308 as two SNPs by deCODE8 in the discovery cohort in POAF group ($n = 289$, 30.1%) and were also validated in the validation cohort ($n = 151$, 30.6%). Both rs2200733 and rs13143308 were significantly associated with POAF (rs2200733, OR = 1.97, 95% CI = 1.24–3.15 and rs13143308, OR = 1.76, 95% CI = 1.2–2.52). On the contrary, based on another prospective study conducted by Sodhi et al. [47] with 160 patients undergoing both on/off-pump CABG surgery, SNP markers (rs2200733 and rs10033464) were not predictors of POAF incidence following cardiac surgery. In their findings, POAF occurred in 16% (23) of the patients. Interestingly, in their quantitative results, 30% of total patients revealed a positive genetic test and these patients did not develop POAF. This reduced the positive predictive value to 8% and a negative predictive value increased to 86%. Therefore, this implies that genetic testing cannot be utilized on an individual level to predict the development of POAF risk. Thus, the reported results in different prospective and retrospective studies require detailed validation through multicenter studies in a large cohort.

4. Limitations

In the reported literature, we observed significant inconsistencies between tissue studies and plasma samples that could be the result of the biological variation among the patients enrolled in the respective studies. Most of the presented results were extracted based on small cohort population. We also noted that most of the studies have shown only discovery group and the results were not validated in the independent validation group. Only two studies showed results for both the discovery and the validation groups [48], [43]. Most of the studies have patient population w/wo preexisting AF. Further, it has been observed that miRNA expression can be tissue specific and the expression levels for these tissue samples are highly dependent on their origin which can be right atria (RA) or left atria (LA).

Collecting a tissue sample from RAA has some limitations that could limit the contribution to predicting POAF risk development following CABG surgery. First, the RAA tissue used for gene expression profiling was sampled at the time of venous cannulation before sCPB, but a second RAA tissue sample was not collected aright fter terminating CPB. Thus, possible acute alterations in the pre-existing gene expression patterns that may result from myocardial ischemia/reperfusion injury and has not been studied in some of the reports.

Atrial fibrillation frequently originates from the pulmonary veins in LA, while only a small portion originates from the superior vena cava or the inferior vena cava, or in the RA [91]. Therefore, those studies that collected tissue samples from RAA and exhibited gene expression profiles may not completely reveal the gene expression patterns that could truly contribute to POAF development [92]. There were also studies that reported the results based on tissue sample collected from LA in CABG patients. Nevertheless, this would increase the risk of complications, and these studies may be helpful for research only, but they are not easy to implement clinically.

There are several drugs that could potentially add bias in the results such as the most commonly used one is heparin. It has also been observed that sometimes, the patient blood samples may have been stored in holding tubes containing heparin. It is commonly seen that heparin obstructs the enzymes in the PCR and thus may affect its results. As shown in Table 1, results for sensitivity, specificity and AUC have not been reported, and this limits the repeatability of the given data.

Table 1. mi/circRNAs and other gene expressions recently reported to be used as predictors of POAF development among CABG patients.

RNAs and Gene Expression	Protein/Gene/Loci	CABG	Source	All Patients	Study Type	With POAF	p Value	AUC	Sensitivity	Specificity	Technique	Ref.
miRNA−483−5p		On-pump	Blood	34	Prospective	12 (35.3%)	0.046	0.78	77.78	77.27	qPCR	[34]
miRNA−26a		On-pump	Serum	48	Prospective	24 (50.0%)	0.010	0.66	-	-	qPCR	[36]
miRNA−23a		On-pump	Serum	48	Prospective	24 (50.0%)	0.020	0.63	-	-	qPCR	[36]
miRNA−199a	SIRT1	On-pump	RAA	63	Prospective	20 (31.7%)	0.022	-	-	-	qPCR	[16]
miRNA−1 and miRNA−133a		On/Off-pump	RAA	42	Prospective	14 (33.3%)	<0.05	-	-	-	qPCR	[37]
circRNA−025016		Off-pump	Plasma	284	Prospective	68 (23.9%)	<0.01	-	73.52	77.83	qPCR	[38]
mtDNA		Off-pump	Blood	485	Prospective	101 (20.8%)	<0.01	0.81	70.3	80.2	qPCR	[39]
mtDNA		On-pump	Plasma	16	Prospective	6 (37.5%)	<0.01	-	-	-	qPCR	[40]
SNP (VOPP1)		Off-pump	RAA	45	Prospective	13 (28.9%)	<0.01	-	-	-	eQTL	[41]
SNP (rs3740563)		On-pump	Blood	245	Prospective	42 (17.1%)	0.011	-	-	-	OMNI1-Quad BeadChip	[42]
SNP (rs2249825)	HMGB1	On-pump	Blood	128	Prospective	37 (29.9%)	<0.001	-	-	-	qPCR	[44]
SNP (rs4572292 and rs11198693)	GRK5	On/Off-pump	Blood	1348	Reterospective	405 (30.0%)	<0.01	-	-	-	qPCR	[45]
SNP (rs2200733 and rs10033464)#	4q25	On/Off-pump	Buccal swabs	143	Prospective	23 (16.1%)	NS	-	16	71	deCODE	[17]
SNP (rs2200733 and rs10033464)	4q25	On/Off-pump	Blood	1166	Reterospective	425 (36.4%)	0.048	-	-	-	qPCR	[46]
SNP (rs2200733 and rs13143308)	4q25	On-pump	Blood	959 * 494 **	Prospective	289 (30.1%) * 151 (30.6%) **	<0.01	0.72	-	-	deCODE	[48]
SNP (rs10504554)	LY96	On-pump	Blood	877 * 304 **	Prospective	84 (27.6%)	<0.01	-	-	-	OMNI1-Quad BeadChip	[43]

mtDNA: mitochondrial DNA; VOPP1: vesicular overexpressed in cancer, prosurvival protein 1; SNP: single-nucleotide polymorphism; qPCR: quantitative polymerase chain reaction; eQTL: expression quantitative trait loci; RAA: right atrial appendage. # In this work, genetic testing exhibited a low sensitivity and positive predictive value in assessing the risk of developing postoperative AF in an individual patient. * and ** represent discovery and validation groups, respectively. NS represents not significant.

5. Future Perspective

This narrative review demonstrated experimental evidence of miRNAs, circRNA and selected gene expressions of mtDNA and SNPs as valuable predictors of POAF risk development in cardiac surgery patients following CABG. Although our knowledge of the roles of mi/circ-RNAs and selected gene expressions has significantly improved, additional research is highly recommended with larger patient cohorts to validate these selected mi/circRNAs and gene expressions as potential biomarkers for diagnosing POAF risk development. Finding appropriate miRNAs in serum/blood samples preoperatively may provide more details on molecular mechanisms that lead to electrical and structural atrial remodeling, revealing which cardiac surgery patients are at greatest risk for POAF development.

Preoperative miRNAs, circRNA and SNPs may also uncover patients that would benefit from increased post-surgical monitoring, pre-emptive antiarrhythmic therapy, and further personalized treatment strategies, such as prophylactic surgical interventions (surgical Maze, surgical pulmonary vein isolation, etc.) to minimizing the risk of developing long-term AF. Future studies may emphasis on improved understanding the multifactorial mechanisms of POAF risk development. This narrative review suggests an important need to focus on the mechanisms of changes in signaling pathways in patients who are at POAF risk. Further, we suggest the following outlines to develop translational clinical research to assess and authenticate the validity of the reported miRNAs, circRNA, mtDNA and SNPs:

- A large cohort study is warranted to investigate multivariate aforementioned parameters (miRNA, circRNA and gene expressions).
- Prospective study should be established with cardiac surgery patients with no preoperative AF history.
- Multicenter studies should enroll cardiac surgery patients regardless of their race, ethnicity, sex, BMI, diabetes, COPD, hypertension, hyperlipidemia, PVD, PAD, myocardial infarction, PCI, TIA and CAD.
- For each patient, pre-, intra- and post-operative antiarrhythmic drug record must be reported.
- Each patient blood sample must be collected preoperatively at two time points (24 h and 6 h) before surgery. RAA tissue sample can also collected intraoperatively.
- Same technique (qPCR, eQTL or OMNI1-Quad BeadChip) must be implemented to test assay.
- Electrophysiology findings such as conduction velocity and refractive period should be co-related with the levels for miRNA, circRNA and SNPs.
- Patients must be categorized as 'no-POAF' for those who do not develop post-surgery atrial fibrillation and 'POAF' for those who develop post-surgery AF within 1–4 days cardiac surgery.
- Results must be reported for both discovery and validated groups.

Author Contributions: Conceptualization, D.J.D.; methodology, M.S.K. and K.Y.; writing—original draft preparation, M.S.K.; writing—review and editing, M.S.K., K.Y. and D.J.D.; clinical relevance, R.R. and V.S. supervision, D.J.D. All authors have read and agreed to the published version of the manuscript.

Funding: Research reported in this publication was supported by National Heart, Lung, and Blood Institute of the National Institutes of Health, NIH under award: R01HL128752 (D.J.D.), a research grant from the Nora Eccles Treadwell Foundation (D.J.D.) and American Heart Association, AHA under award: 9POST34450115 (M.S.K.). The content is solely the responsibility of the authors and does not necessarily represent the official views of the NIH and AHA.

Conflicts of Interest: The authors declare no conflict of interest.

References

1. Gillinov, A.M.; Bagiella, E.; Moskowitz, A.J.; Raiten, J.M.; Groh, M.A.; Bowdish, M.E.; Ailawadi, G.; Kirkwood, K.A.; Perrault, L.P.; Parides, M.K.; et al. Rate Control versus Rhythm Control for Atrial Fibrillation after Cardiac Surgery. *N. Engl. J. Med.* **2016**, *374*, 1911–1921. [CrossRef]
2. Bidar, E.; Bramer, S.; Maesen, B.; Maessen, J.G.; Schotten, U. Post-operative atrial fibrillation-Pathophysiology, treatment and prevention. *J. Atr. Fibrillation* **2013**, *5*, 781. [PubMed]
3. Bessissow, A.; Khan, J.; Devereaux, P.J.; Alvarez-Garcia, J.; Alonso-Coello, P. Postoperative atrial fibrillation in non-cardiac and cardiac surgery: An overview. *J. Thromb. Haemost.* **2015**, *13*, S304–S312. [CrossRef] [PubMed]
4. Yin, L.; Ling, X.; Zhang, Y.; Shen, H.; Min, J.; Xi, W.; Wang, J.; Wang, Z. CHADS2 and CHA2DS2-VASc Scoring Systems for Predicting Atrial Fibrillation following Cardiac Valve Surgery. *PLoS ONE* **2015**, *10*, e0123858. [CrossRef] [PubMed]
5. Aranki, S.F.; Shaw, D.P.; Adams, D.H.; Rizzo, R.J.; Couper, G.S.; VanderVliet, M.; Collins, J.J.; Cohn, L.H.; Burstin, H.R. Predictors of Atrial Fibrillation After Coronary Artery Surgery: Current Trends and Impact on Hospital Resources. *Circulation* **1996**, *94*, 390–397. [CrossRef] [PubMed]
6. Steinberg, J.S. Postoperative atrial fibrillation: A billion-dollar problem. *J. Am. Coll. Cardiol.* **2004**, *43*, 1001–1003. [CrossRef]
7. Badhwar, V.; Rankin, J.S.; Damiano, R.J.; Gillinov, A.M.; Bakaeen, F.G.; Edgerton, J.R.; Philpott, J.M.; McCarthy, P.M.; Bolling, S.F.; Roberts, H.G.; et al. The Society of Thoracic Surgeons 2017 Clinical Practice Guidelines for the Surgical Treatment of Atrial Fibrillation. *Ann. Thorac. Surg.* **2017**, *103*, 329–341. [CrossRef]
8. Mavroudis, C.; Deal, B.J. Prophylactic arrhythmia surgery in association with congenital heart disease. *Transl. Pediatrics* **2016**, *5*, 148–159. [CrossRef]
9. Stulak, J.M.; Suri, R.M.; Dearani, J.A.; Sundt, T.M.; Schaff, H.V. When Should Prophylactic Maze Procedure Be Considered in Patients Undergoing Mitral Valve Surgery? *Ann. Thorac. Surg.* **2010**, *89*, 1395–1401. [CrossRef]
10. Yamashita, K.; Selzman, C.; Ranjan, R.; Hu, N.; Dosdall, D. Clinical Risk Factors for Post-operative Atrial Fibrillation among Patients after Cardiac Surgery. *Thorac. Cardiovasc. Surg.* **2019**, *67*, 107–116.
11. Reckman, Y.J.; Creemers, E.E. Circulating circles predict postoperative atrial fibrillation. *J. Am. Heart Assoc.* **2018**, *7*, 1–4. [CrossRef] [PubMed]
12. Khan, M.S.; Yamashita, K.; Sharma, V.; Ranjan, R.; Selzman, C.H.; Dosdall, D.J. Perioperative Biomarkers Predicting Postoperative Atrial Fibrillation Risk After Coronary Artery Bypass Grafting: A Narrative Review. *J. Cardiothorac. Vasc. Anesth.* **2019**. [CrossRef] [PubMed]
13. Kondkar, A.A.; Abu-Amero, K.K. Utility of circulating MicroRNAs as clinical biomarkers for cardiovascular diseases. *BioMed Res. Int.* **2015**, *2015*, 821823. [CrossRef] [PubMed]
14. Sayed, A.S.M.; Xia, K.; Salma, U.; Yang, T.; Peng, J. Diagnosis, prognosis and therapeutic role of circulating miRNAs in cardiovascular diseases. *Heart Lung Circ.* **2014**, *23*, 503–510. [CrossRef]
15. Ono, K.; Kuwabara, Y.; Han, J. MicroRNAs and cardiovascular diseases. *FEBS J.* **2011**, *278*, 1619–1633. [CrossRef]
16. Yamac, A.H.; Kucukbuzcu, S.; Ozansoy, M.; Gok, O.; Oz, K.; Erturk, M.; Yilmaz, E.; Ersoy, B.; Zeybek, R.; Goktekin, O.; et al. Altered expression of micro-RNA 199a and increased levels of cardiac SIRT1 protein are associated with the occurrence of atrial fibrillation after coronary artery bypass graft surgery. *Cardiovasc. Pathol.* **2016**, *25*, 232–236. [CrossRef]
17. Slagsvold, K.H.; Rognmo, O.; Hoydal, M.; Wisloff, U.; Wahba, A. Remote ischemic preconditioning preserves mitochondrial function and influences myocardial MicroRNA expression in atrial myocardium during coronary bypass surgery. *Circ. Res.* **2014**, *114*, 851–859. [CrossRef]
18. McManus, D.D.; Lin, H.; Tanriverdi, K.; Quercio, M.; Yin, X.; Larson, M.G.; Ellinor, P.T.; Levy, D.; Freedman, J.E.; Benjamin, E.J. Relations between circulating microRNAs and atrial fibrillation: Data from the Framingham Offspring Study. *Heart Rhythm* **2014**, *11*, 663–669. [CrossRef]
19. Gurha, P. MicroRNAs in cardiovascular disease. *Curr. Opin. Cardiol.* **2016**, *31*, 249–254. [CrossRef]
20. Zhou, S.-S.; Jin, J.-P.; Wang, J.-Q.; Zhang, Z.-G.; Freedman, J.H.; Zheng, Y.; Cai, L. miRNAS in cardiovascular diseases: Potential biomarkers, therapeutic targets and challenges. *Acta Pharmacol. Sin.* **2018**, *39*, 1073–1084. [CrossRef]

21. Claudia, B.; Fiedler, J.; Thum, T. Cardiovascular Importance of the MicroRNA−23/27/24 Family. *Microcirculation* **2012**, *19*, 208–214.
22. Van Rooij, E.; Sutherland, L.B.; Liu, N.; Williams, A.H.; McAnally, J.; Gerard, R.D.; Richardson, J.A.; Olson, E.N. A signature pattern of stress-responsive microRNAs that can evoke cardiac hypertrophy and heart failure. *Proc. Natl. Acad. Sci. USA* **2006**, *103*, 18255–18260. [CrossRef] [PubMed]
23. Grueter, C.E.; Van Rooij, E.; Johnson, B.A.; Deleon, S.M.; Sutherland, L.B.; Qi, X.; Gautron, L.; Elmquist, J.K.; Bassel-Duby, R.; Olson, E.N. A cardiac MicroRNA governs systemic energy homeostasis by regulation of MED13. *Cell* **2012**, *149*, 671–683. [CrossRef]
24. Yang, B.; Lin, H.; Xiao, J.; Lu, Y.; Luo, X.; Li, B.; Zhang, Y.; Xu, C.; Bai, Y.; Wang, H.; et al. The muscle-specific microRNA miR−1 regulates cardiac arrhythmogenic potential by targeting GJA1 and KCNJ2. *Nat. Med.* **2007**, *13*, 486–491. [CrossRef] [PubMed]
25. Wang, Z.; Lu, Y.; Yang, B. MicroRNAs and atrial fibrillation: New fundamentals. *Cardiovasc. Res.* **2011**, *89*, 710–721. [CrossRef] [PubMed]
26. Van den Berg, N.W.E.; Kawasaki, M.; Berger, W.R.; Neefs, J.; Meulendijks, E.; Tijsen, A.J.; de Groot, J.R. MicroRNAs in Atrial Fibrillation: From Expression Signatures to Functional Implications. *Cardiovasc. Drugs Ther.* **2017**, *2017*, 345–365. [CrossRef] [PubMed]
27. Gomes Da Silva, A.M.; Silbiger, V.N. MiRNAs as biomarkers of atrial fibrillation. *Biomarkers* **2014**, *19*, 631–636. [CrossRef] [PubMed]
28. Vester, B.; Wengel, J. MicroRNA assay methods: A review of current technologies. *Biochemistry* **2004**, *43*, 13233–13241. [CrossRef]
29. Moody, L.; He, H.; Pan, Y.-X.; Chen, H. Methods and novel technology for microRNA quantification in colorectal cancer screening. *Clin. Epigenetics* **2017**, *9*, 119. [CrossRef]
30. Garcia-Elias, A.; Alloza, L.; Puigdecanet, E.; Nonell, L.; Tajes, M.; Curado, J.; Enjuanes, C.; Díaz, O.; Bruguera, J.; Martí-Almor, J.; et al. Defining quantification methods and optimizing protocols for microarray hybridization of circulating microRNAs. *Sci. Rep.* **2017**, *7*, 7725. [CrossRef]
31. Chen, Y.; Li, C.; Tan, C.; Liu, X. Circular RNAs: A new frontier in the study of human diseases. *J. Med. Genet.* **2016**, *53*, 359–365. [CrossRef] [PubMed]
32. Guo, Y.; Luo, F.; Liu, Q.; Xu, D. Regulatory non-coding RNAs in acute myocardial infarction. *J. Cell. Mol. Med.* **2017**, *21*, 1013–1023. [CrossRef] [PubMed]
33. Carnes, C.A.; Janssen, P.M.L.; Ruehr, M.L.; Nakayama, H.; Nakayama, T.; Haase, H.; Bauer, J.A.; Chung, M.K.; Fearon, I.M.; Gillinov, A.M.; et al. Atrial Glutathione Content, Calcium Current, and Contractility. *J. Biol. Chem.* **2007**, *282*, 28063–28073. [CrossRef] [PubMed]
34. Harling, L.; Lambert, J.; Ashrafian, H.; Darzi, A.; Gooderham, N.J.; Athanasiou, T. Elevated serum microRNA 483−5p levels may predict patients at risk of post-operative atrial fibrillation. *Eur. J. Cardiothorac Surg.* **2017**, *51*, 73–78. [CrossRef] [PubMed]
35. Rizvi, F.; Mirza, M.; Olet, S.; Albrecht, M.; Edwards, S.; Emelyanova, L.; Kress, D.; Ross, G.R.; Holmuhamedov, E.; Tajik, A.J.; et al. Noninvasive biomarker-based risk stratification for development of new onset atrial fibrillation after coronary artery bypass surgery. *Int. J. Cardiol.* **2020**. [CrossRef]
36. Feldman, A.; Moreira, D.A.R.; Gun, C.; Wang, H.-T.L.; Hirata, M.H.; de Freitas Germano, J.; Leite, G.G.S.; Farsky, P. Analysis of Circulating miR−1, miR−23a, and miR−26a in Atrial Fibrillation Patients Undergoing Coronary Bypass Artery Grafting Surgery. *Ann. Hum. Genet.* **2017**, *81*, 99–105. [CrossRef]
37. Tsoporis, J.N.; Fazio, A.; Rizos, I.K.; Izhar, S.; Proteau, G.; Salpeas, V.; Rigopoulos, A.; Sakadakis, E.; Toumpoulis, I.K.; Parker, T.G. Increased right atrial appendage apoptosis is associated with differential regulation of candidate MicroRNAs 1 and 133A in patients who developed atrial fibrillation after cardiac surgery. *J. Mol. Cell. Cardiol.* **2018**, *121*, 25–32. [CrossRef]
38. Zhang, J.; Xu, Y.; Xu, S.; Liu, Y.; Yu, L.; Li, Z.; Xue, X.; Wang, H. Plasma Circular RNAs, Hsa_circRNA_025016, Predict Postoperative Atrial Fibrillation After Isolated Off-Pump Coronary Artery Bypass Grafting. *J. Am. Heart Assoc.* **2018**, *7*, e006642. [CrossRef]
39. Zhang, J.; Xu, S.; Xu, Y.; Liu, Y.; Li, Z.; Zhang, Y.; Jin, Y.; Xue, X.; Wang, H. Relation of Mitochondrial DNA Copy Number in Peripheral Blood to Postoperative Atrial Fibrillation After Isolated Off-Pump Coronary Artery Bypass Grafting. *Am. J. Cardiol.* **2017**, *119*, 473–477. [CrossRef]

40. Sandler, N.; Kaczmarek, E.; Itagaki, K.; Zheng, Y.; Otterbein, L.; Khabbaz, K.; Liu, D.; Senthilnathan, V.; Gruen, R.L.; Hauser, C.J. Mitochondrial DAMPs Are Released During Cardiopulmonary Bypass Surgery and Are Associated With Postoperative Atrial Fibrillation. *Heart Lung Circ.* **2018**, *27*, 122–129. [CrossRef]
41. Kertai, M.D.; Qi, W.; Li, Y.-J.; Lombard, F.W.; Liu, Y.; Smith, M.P.; Stafford-Smith, M.; Newman, M.F.; Milano, C.A.; Mathew, J.P.; et al. Gene signatures of postoperative atrial fibrillation in atrial tissue after coronary artery bypass grafting surgery in patients receiving β-blockers. *J. Mol. Cell. Cardiol.* **2016**, *92*, 109–115. [CrossRef] [PubMed]
42. Kertai, M.D.; Li, Y.-W.; Li, Y.-J.; Shah, S.H.; Kraus, W.E.; Fontes, M.L.; Stafford-Smith, M.; Newman, M.F.; Podgoreanu, M.V.; Mathew, J.P. G Protein-Coupled Receptor Kinase 5 Gene Polymorphisms Are Associated With Postoperative Atrial Fibrillation After Coronary Artery Bypass Grafting in Patients Receiving -Blockers. *Circ. Cardiovasc. Genet.* **2014**, *7*, 625–633. [CrossRef] [PubMed]
43. Kertai, M.D.; Li, Y.J.; Ji, Y.; Qi, W.; Lombard, F.W.; Shah, S.H.; Kraus, W.E.; Stafford-Smith, M.; Newman, M.F.; Milano, C.A.; et al. Genome-wide association study of new-onset atrial fibrillation after coronary artery bypass grafting surgery. *Am. Heart J.* **2015**, *170*, 580.e28–590.e28. [CrossRef] [PubMed]
44. Qu, C.; Wang, X.W.; Huang, C.; Qiu, F.; Xiang, X.Y.; Lu, Z.Q. High mobility group box 1 gene polymorphism is associated with the risk of postoperative atrial fibrillation after coronary artery bypass surgery. *J. Cardiothorac. Surg.* **2015**, *10*, 88. [CrossRef]
45. Liu, L.; Zhang, L.; Liu, M.; Zhang, Y.; Han, X.; Zhang, Z. GRK5 polymorphisms and Postoperative Atrial Fibrillation following Coronary Artery Bypass Graft Surgery. *Sci. Rep.* **2015**, *5*, 12768. [CrossRef]
46. Virani, S.S.; Brautbar, A.; Lee, V.V.; Elayda, M.; Sami, S.; Nambi, V.; Frazier, L.; Wilson, J.M.; Willerson, J.T.; Boerwinkle, E.; et al. Usefulness of single nucleotide polymorphism in chromosome 4q25 to predict in-hospital and long-term development of atrial fibrillation and survival in patients undergoing coronary artery bypass grafting. *Am. J. Cardiol.* **2011**, *107*, 1504–1509. [CrossRef]
47. Gurpreet, S.; Shea, J.; Najam, F.; Solomon, A.J. Can a Genetic Test Predict the Development of Postoperative Atrial Fibrillation. *Int. J. Clin. Cardiol.* **2015**, *2*, 32.
48. Body, S.C.; Collard, C.D.; Shernan, S.K.; Fox, A.A.; Liu, K.Y.; Ritchie, M.D.; Perry, T.E.; Muehlschlegel, J.D.; Aranki, S.; Donahue, B.S.; et al. Variation in the 4q25 chromosomal locus predicts atrial fibrillation after coronary artery bypass graft surgery. *Circ. Cardiovasc. Genet.* **2009**, *2*, 499–506. [CrossRef]
49. Luo, X.; Yang, B.; Nattel, S. MicroRNAs and atrial fibrillation: Mechanisms and translational potential. *Nat. Rev. Cardiol.* **2015**, *12*, 80–90. [CrossRef]
50. Arora, P.; Wu, C.; Khan, A.M.; Bloch, D.B.; Davis-Dusenbery, B.N.; Ghorbani, A.; Spagnolli, E.; Martinez, A.; Ryan, A.; Tainsh, L.T.; et al. Atrial natriuretic peptide is negatively regulated by microRNA–425. *J. Clin. Investig.* **2013**, *123*, 3378–3382. [CrossRef]
51. Heneghan, H.M.; Miller, N.; Kerin, M.J. MiRNAs as biomarkers and therapeutic targets in cancer. *Curr. Opin. Pharmacol.* **2010**, *10*, 543–550. [CrossRef] [PubMed]
52. Lu, H.; Buchan, R.J.; Cook, S.A. MicroRNA–223 regulates Glut4 expression and cardiomyocyte glucose metabolism. *Cardiovasc. Res.* **2010**, *86*, 410–420. [CrossRef] [PubMed]
53. Mayr, M.; Yusuf, S.; Weir, G.; Chung, Y.-L.; Mayr, U.; Yin, X.; Ladroue, C.; Madhu, B.; Roberts, N.; De Souza, A.; et al. Combined Metabolomic and Proteomic Analysis of Human Atrial Fibrillation. *J. Am. Coll. Cardiol.* **2008**, *51*, 585–594. [CrossRef]
54. Sharma, D.; Li, G.; Xu, G.; Liu, Y.; Xu, Y. Atrial remodeling in atrial fibrillation and some related microRNAs. *Cardiology* **2011**, *120*, 111–121. [CrossRef] [PubMed]
55. Lu, Y.; Zhang, Y.; Wang, N.; Pan, Z.; Gao, X.; Zhang, F.; Zhang, Y.; Shan, H.; Luo, X.; Bai, Y.; et al. MicroRNA–328 contributes to adverse electrical remodeling in atrial fibrillation. *Circulation* **2010**, *122*, 2378–2387. [CrossRef] [PubMed]
56. Dawson, K.; Wakili, R.; Örd́ög, B.; Clauss, S.; Chen, Y.; Iwasaki, Y.; Voigt, N.; Qi, X.Y.; Sinner, M.F.; Dobrev, D.; et al. MicroRNA29: A mechanistic contributor and potential biomarker in atrial fibrillation. *Circulation* **2013**, *127*, 1466–1475. [CrossRef]
57. Mariscalco, G.; Musumeci, F.; Banach, M. Factors influencing post-coronary artery bypass grafting atrial fibrillation episodes. *Kardiol. Pol.* **2013**, *71*, 1115–1120. [CrossRef]
58. Santulli, G.; Iaccarino, G.; De Luca, N.; Trimarco, B.; Condorelli, G. Atrial fibrillation and microRNAs. *Front. Physiol.* **2014**, *5*, 15. [CrossRef]

59. Jalife, J.; Kaur, K. Atrial remodeling, fibrosis, and atrial fibrillation. *Trends Cardiovasc. Med.* **2015**, *25*, 475–484. [CrossRef]
60. Krogstad, L.E.B.; Slagsvold, K.H.; Wahba, A. Remote ischemic preconditioning and incidence of postoperative atrial fibrillation. *Scand. Cardiovasc. J.* **2015**, *49*, 117–122. [CrossRef]
61. Lutter, D.; Marr, C.; Krumsiek, J.; Lang, E.W.; Theis, F.J. Intronic microRNAs support their host genes by mediating synergistic and antagonistic regulatory effects. *BMC Genom.* **2010**, *11*, 224. [CrossRef] [PubMed]
62. Qiao, Y.; Ma, N.; Wang, X.; Hui, Y.; Li, F.; Xiang, Y.; Zhou, J.; Zou, C.; Jin, J.; Lv, G.; et al. MiR–483–5p controls angiogenesis in vitro and targets serum response factor. *FEBS Lett.* **2011**, *585*, 3095–3100. [CrossRef] [PubMed]
63. Van Rooij, E.; Sutherland, L.B.; Thatcher, J.E.; DiMaio, J.M.; Naseem, R.H.; Marshall, W.S.; Hill, J.A.; Olson, E.N. Dysregulation of microRNAs after myocardial infarction reveals a role of miR–29 in cardiac fibrosis. *Proc. Natl. Acad. Sci. USA* **2008**, *105*, 13027–13032. [CrossRef]
64. Di, Y.; Zhang, D.; Hu, T.; Li, D. miR–23 regulate the pathogenesis of patients with coronary artery disease. *Int. J. Clin. Exp. Med.* **2015**, *8*, 11759–11769. [PubMed]
65. Dong, J.; Bao, J.; Feng, R.; Zhao, Z.; Lu, Q.; Wang, G.; Li, H.; Su, D.; Zhou, J.; Jing, Q.; et al. Circulating microRNAs: A novel potential biomarker for diagnosing acute aortic dissection. *Sci. Rep.* **2017**, *7*, 12784. [CrossRef] [PubMed]
66. Jansen, F.; Schäfer, L.; Wang, H.; Schmitz, T.; Flender, A.; Schueler, R.; Hammerstingl, C.; Nickenig, G.; Sinning, J.-M.; Werner, N. Kinetics of Circulating MicroRNAs in Response to Cardiac Stress in Patients With Coronary Artery Disease. *J. Am. Heart Assoc.* **2017**, *6*, e005270. [CrossRef] [PubMed]
67. Luo, X.; Pan, Z.; Shan, H.; Xiao, J.; Sun, X.; Wang, N.; Lin, H.; Xiao, L.; Maguy, A.; Qi, X.-Y.; et al. MicroRNA–26 governs profibrillatory inward-rectifier potassium current changes in atrial fibrillation. *J. Clin. Investig.* **2013**, *123*, 1939–1951. [CrossRef]
68. Kukreja, R.C.; Yin, C.; Salloum, F.N. MicroRNAs: New players in cardiac injury and protection. *Mol. Pharmacol.* **2011**, *80*, 558–564. [CrossRef]
69. Kilic, U.; Gok, O.; Bacaksiz, A.; Izmirli, M.; Elibol-Can, B.; Uysal, O. SIRT1 gene polymorphisms affect the protein expression in cardiovascular diseases. *PLoS ONE* **2014**, *9*, e90428. [CrossRef]
70. Choi, S.E.; Kemper, J.K. Regulation of SIRT1 by microRNAs. *Mol. Cells* **2013**, *36*, 385–392. [CrossRef]
71. Yamac, A.H.; Huyut, M.A.; Yilmaz, E.; Celikkale, I.; Bacaksiz, A.; Demir, Y.; Demir, A.R.; Erturk, M.; Bakhshaliyev, N.; Ozdemir, R.; et al. MicroRNA 199a is downregulated in patients after coronary artery bypass graft surgery and is associated with increased levels of sirtuin 1 (SIRT 1) protein and major adverse cardiovascular events at 3-year follow-up. *Med. Sci. Monit.* **2018**, *24*, 6245–6254. [CrossRef]
72. Rane, S.; He, M.; Sayed, D.; Vashistha, H.; Malhotra, A.; Sadoshima, J.; Vatner, D.E.; Vatner, S.F.; Abdellatif, M. Downregulation of MiR–199a derepresses hypoxia-inducible factor–1α and sirtuin 1 and recapitulates hypoxia preconditioning in cardiac myocytes. *Circ. Res.* **2009**, *104*, 879–886. [CrossRef] [PubMed]
73. Sun, X.L.; Bu, P.L.; Liu, J.N.; Wang, X.; Wu, X.N.; Zhao, L.X. Expression of SIRT1 in right auricle tissues and the relationship with oxidative stress in patients with atrial fibrillation. *Xi Bao Yu Fen Zi Mian Yi Xue Za Zhi Chin. J. Cell. Mol. Immunol.* **2012**, *28*, 972–974.
74. Vegter, E.L.; Ovchinnikova, E.S.; van Veldhuisen, D.J.; Jaarsma, T.; Berezikov, E.; van der Meer, P.; Voors, A.A. Low circulating microRNA levels in heart failure patients are associated with atherosclerotic disease and cardiovascular-related rehospitalizations. *Clin. Res. Cardiol.* **2017**, *106*, 598–609. [CrossRef] [PubMed]
75. Clauss, S.; Sinner, M.F.; Kääb, S.; Wakili, R. The role of MicroRNAs in antiarrhythmic therapy for atrial fibrillation. *Arrhythmia Electrophysiol. Rev.* **2015**, *4*, 146–155. [CrossRef]
76. Girmatsion, Z.; Biliczki, P.; Bonauer, A.; Wimmer-Greinecker, G.; Scherer, M.; Moritz, A.; Bukowska, A.; Goette, A.; Nattel, S.; Hohnloser, S.H.; et al. Changes in microRNA–1 expression and IK1 up-regulation in human atrial fibrillation. *Heart Rhythm* **2009**, *6*, 1802–1809. [CrossRef] [PubMed]
77. Ide, T.; Tsutsui, H.; Hayashidani, S.; Kang, D.; Suematsu, N.; Nakamura, K.; Utsumi, H.; Hamasaki, N.; Takeshita, A. Mitochondrial DNA damage and dysfunction associated with oxidative stress in failing hearts after myocardial infarction. *Circ. Res.* **2001**, *88*, 529–535. [CrossRef]
78. Shokolenko, I.; Venediktova, N.; Bochkareva, A.; Wilson, G.L.; Alexeyev, M.F. Oxidative stress induces degradation of mitochondrial DNA. *Nucleic Acids Res.* **2009**, *37*, 2539–2548. [CrossRef]

79. Phan, K.; Khuong, J.N.; Xu, J.; Kanagaratnam, A.; Yan, T.D. Obesity and postoperative atrial fibrillation in patients undergoing cardiac surgery: Systematic review and meta-analysis. *Int. J. Cardiol.* **2016**, *217*, 49–57. [CrossRef]
80. Turagam, M.K.; Mirza, M.; Werner, P.H.; Sra, J.; Kress, D.C.; Tajik, A.J.; Jahangir, A. Circulating biomarkers predictive of postoperative atrial fibrillation. *Cardiol. Rev.* **2016**, *24*, 76–87. [CrossRef]
81. Perrier, S.; Meyer, N.; Hoang Minh, T.; Announe, T.; Bentz, J.; Billaud, P.; Mommerot, A.; Mazzucotelli, J.-P.; Kindo, M. Predictors of Atrial Fibrillation After Coronary Artery Bypass Grafting: A Bayesian Analysis. *Ann. Thorac. Surg.* **2017**, *103*, 92–97. [CrossRef] [PubMed]
82. Philipp, M.; Berger, I.M.; Just, S.; Caron, M.G. Overlapping and opposing functions of G protein-coupled receptor kinase 2 (GRK2) and Grk5 during heart development. *J. Biol. Chem.* **2014**, *289*, 26119–26130. [CrossRef] [PubMed]
83. Liggett, S.B.; Cresci, S.; Kelly, R.J.; Syed, F.M.; Matkovich, S.J.; Hahn, H.S.; Diwan, A.; Martini, J.S.; Sparks, L.; Parekh, R.R.; et al. A GRK5 polymorphism that inhibits β-adrenergic receptor signaling is protective in heart failure. *Nat. Med.* **2008**, *14*, 510–517. [CrossRef] [PubMed]
84. Zhang, Y.; Matkovich, S.J.; Duan, X.; Gold, J.I.; Koch, W.J.; Dorn, G.W. Nuclear effects of G-protein receptor kinase 5 on histone deacetylase 5-regulated gene transcription in heart failure. *Circ. Heart Fail.* **2011**, *4*, 659–668. [CrossRef]
85. Gold, J.I.; Martini, J.S.; Hullmann, J.; Gao, E.; Chuprun, J.K.; Lee, L.; Tilley, D.G.; Rabinowitz, J.E.; Bossuyt, J.; Bers, D.M.; et al. Nuclear Translocation of Cardiac G Protein-Coupled Receptor Kinase 5 Downstream of Select Gq-Activating Hypertrophic Ligands Is a Calmodulin-Dependent Process. *PLoS ONE* **2013**, *8*, e57324. [CrossRef]
86. Crystal, E.; Garfinkle, M.S.; Connolly, S.; Ginger, T.; Sleik, K.; Yusuf, S. Interventions for preventing post-operative atrial fibrillation in patients undergoing heart surgery. In *Cochrane Database of Systematic Reviews*; Crystal, E., Ed.; John Wiley & Sons, Ltd.: Chichester, UK, 2004; p. CD003611.
87. Kääb, S.; Darbar, D.; Van Noord, C.; Dupuis, J.; Pfeufer, A.; Newton-Cheh, C.; Schnabel, R.; Makino, S.; Sinner, M.F.; Kannankeril, P.J.; et al. Large scale replication and meta-analysis of variants on chromosome 4q25 associated with atrial fibrillation. *Eur. Heart J.* **2009**, *30*, 813–819. [CrossRef]
88. Anselmi, C.V.; Novelli, V.; Roncarati, R.; Malovini, A.; Bellazzi, R.; Bronzini, R.; Marchese, G.; Condorelli, G.; Montenero, A.S.; Puca, A.A. Association of rs2200733 at 4q25 with atrial flutter/fibrillation diseases in an Italian population. *Heart* **2008**, *94*, 1394–1396. [CrossRef]
89. Chen, F.; Yang, Y.; Zhang, R.; Zhang, S.; Dong, Y.; Yin, X.; Chang, D.; Yang, Z.; Wang, K.; Gao, L.; et al. Polymorphism rs2200733 at chromosome 4q25 is associated with atrial fibrillation recurrence after radiofrequency catheter ablation in the Chinese Han population. *Am. J. Transl. Res.* **2016**, *8*, 688–697.
90. Lubitz, S.A.; Sinner, M.F.; Lunetta, K.L.; Makino, S.; Pfeufer, A.; Rahman, R.; Veltman, C.E.; Barnard, J.; Bis, J.C.; Danik, S.P.; et al. Independent susceptibility markers for atrial fibrillation on chromosome 4q25. *Circulation* **2010**, *122*, 976–984. [CrossRef]
91. Oral, H. Post-Operative Atrial Fibrillation and Oxidative Stress. *J. Am. Coll. Cardiol.* **2008**, *51*, 75–76. [CrossRef]
92. Hsu, J.; Hanna, P.; Van Wagoner, D.R.; Barnard, J.; Serre, D.; Chung, M.K.; Smith, J.D. Whole Genome Expression Differences in Human Left and Right Atria Ascertained by RNA Sequencing. *Circ. Cardiovasc. Genet.* **2012**, *5*, 327–335. [CrossRef] [PubMed]

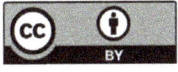

© 2020 by the authors. Licensee MDPI, Basel, Switzerland. This article is an open access article distributed under the terms and conditions of the Creative Commons Attribution (CC BY) license (http://creativecommons.org/licenses/by/4.0/).

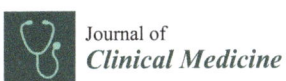 Journal of *Clinical Medicine*

Article

Left Atrial Remodeling and Brain Natriuretic Peptide Levels Variation after Left Atrial Appendage Occlusion

Thibaut Pommier [1,2,*], Thibault Leclercq [1], Charles Guenancia [1,2], Carole Richard [1,2], Guillaume Porot [1], Gabriel Laurent [1] and Luc Lorgis [1,2]

1. Department of Cardiology, University Hospital, 21000 Dijon, France; thibault.leclercq@chu-dijon.fr (T.L.); charles.guenancia@chu-dijon.fr (C.G.); carole.richard@chu-dijon.fr (C.R.); guillaume.porot@chu-dijon.fr (G.P.); gabriel.laurent@chu-dijon.fr (G.L.); luc.lorgis@chu-dijon.fr (L.L.)
2. Laboratory of Cerebro-Vascular Pathophysiology and Epidemiology (PEC2), University of Burgundy, 21000 Dijon, France
* Correspondence: thibaut.pommier@chu-dijon.fr; Tel.: +33-06-26-45-61-90

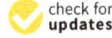

Citation: Pommier, T.; Leclercq, T.; Guenancia, C.; Richard, C.; Porot, G.; Laurent, G.; Lorgis, L. Left Atrial Remodeling and Brain Natriuretic Peptide Levels Variation after Left Atrial Appendage Occlusion. *J. Clin. Med.* 2021, 10, 3443. https://doi.org/10.3390/jcm10153443

Academic Editor: Patrizio Mazzone

Received: 11 July 2021
Accepted: 31 July 2021
Published: 3 August 2021

Publisher's Note: MDPI stays neutral with regard to jurisdictional claims in published maps and institutional affiliations.

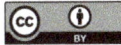

Copyright: © 2021 by the authors. Licensee MDPI, Basel, Switzerland. This article is an open access article distributed under the terms and conditions of the Creative Commons Attribution (CC BY) license (https://creativecommons.org/licenses/by/4.0/).

Abstract: Background: Few data are available about brain natriuretic peptide (BNP) variation and left atrial remodeling after the left atrial appendage occlusion (LAAO) technique. Methods: Prospective study included all consecutive patients successfully implanted with an LAAO device. Contrast-enhanced cardiac computed tomography (CT) was performed before and 6 weeks after the procedure with reverse left atrial remodeling defined by an increase in LA volume >10%, together with blood sampling obtained before, 48 h after device implantation and at the first visit after discharge (30–45 days) for BNP measurement. Results: Among the 43 patients implanted with a complete dataset, mean end-diastolic LA volume was 139 ± 64 mL and 141 ± 62 mL at baseline and during follow-up (45 ± 15 days), respectively, showing no statistical difference ($p = 0.45$). No thrombus was seen on the atrial side of the device. Peridevice leaks (defined as presence of dye in the LAA beyond the device) were observed in 17 patients (40%) but were trivial or mild. Reverse atrial remodeling (RAR) at 6 weeks was observed in six patients (14%). Despite no difference in BNP levels on admission, median BNP levels at 48 h were slightly increased in RAR patients when compared with controls. During FU, BNP levels were strictly identical in both groups. These results were not modified even when each RAR case was matched with two controls on age, LVEF, creatinine levels and ACE inhibitors treatment to avoid potential confounders. Conclusion: Our study showed that despite the fact that the LAAO technique can induce left atrial remodeling measured by a CT scan, it does not seem to impact BNP levels on the follow-up. The results need to be transposed to clinical outcomes of this expanding population in future studies.

Keywords: left atrial appendage occlusion; bleeding risk; BNP; atrial remodeling; atrial fibrillation; atrial cardiopathy

1. Introduction

Atrial fibrillation (AF) is the most common heart rhythm disorder and the second most common cause of stroke [1]. Atrial fibrillation prevalence increases with age, and the current demographic evolution with an elderly population makes it a major cause of morbidity [2]. Thrombus that emerges inside the left atrial appendage (LAA) is the most common cause of ischemic stroke in non-valvular atrial fibrillation patients [3]. Anticoagulation effectively reduces the risk of ischemic stroke and all-cause death in patients with AF and is still currently the reference treatment of thromboembolic risk prevention in patients with atrial fibrillation but sometimes represents an inappropriate option for some patients [4]. Firstly, anticoagulation also increases the risk of hemorrhage complications in patients at high risk of bleeding, and several studies confirm that the AF population is under-treated with nearly 40% of patients at risk for stroke who do not receive any form of oral anticoagulation [5].

Moreover, approximately 10% of the patients have a contraindication to anticoagulation, and 2% have an absolute contraindication.

In patients with non-valvular AF, percutaneous left atrial appendage occlusion (LAAO) has emerged as an alternative approach to reduce the risk of stroke, especially in patients with high bleeding risk or a contraindication of oral anticoagulation [6]. LAA is a frequent source of systemic embolism due to blood stasis in the LAA in the fibrillating atrium leading to thrombus formation, and it is the reason why an occlusion or removal of the LAA may decrease the risk of systemic embolization. Nearly 92% of LA thrombi are localized in the LAA [7]. There are several methods of LAA closure, including percutaneous [8] and surgical approaches [9]. Concerning the interventional approach, left atrial appendage occlusion is performed with the implantation of a device excluding the LAA [10,11]. Nowadays, according to ESC Guidelines, LAAO may be considered for stroke prevention in patients with AF and contraindications for long-term anticoagulant treatment (those with a previous life-threatening bleeding without a reversible cause) [12].

LAAO is therefore effective to reduce the risk of stroke in well-selected AF patients. However, few data are available about the potential hemodynamic consequences of left atrial appendage occlusion. The role of the LAA in cardiac hemodynamics has been previously investigated in both animal and human studies [7]. LAA is a complex structure with variable shape and size and with effective contractions during sinus rhythm, but contractions disappear during AF, leading to the formation of thrombi. Left atrial appendage has several important mechanical and endocrine functions. It is a reservoir chamber due to its distensible ability, allowing a response to an increase in the volume or the overload of the left atrium [13]; an exclusion of the LAA may encourage an increase in the volume of the left atrium. Then, the LAA has a neurohormonal activity and is known as the source of the atrial natriuretic peptide (ANP) with secretion in response to an increased atrial volume or pressure, allowing a vasodilator and diuretic activity and a decrease of blood pressure. Studies found that patients with LAAO have significantly lower ANP secretion and concomitant increase of cardiac congestion.

Therefore, LAA functions will be changed after LAAO. Consequently, these modifications can affect cardiac function and structure, but there are few data about the impact of percutaneous LAAC on left atrial functional and structural remodeling.

In our center, the first patients who had undergone an LAA occlusion experienced a rise in the brain natriuretic peptide (BNP) associated with cardiac congestion. Nevertheless, even if the relationship between the ANP and the LAA is established, there are limited data about BNP variation and left atrium remodeling after the left atrial appendage occlusion technique. The objectives of our study were to assess the relationship between BNP variation and left atrium remodeling after the left appendage occlusion (LAAO) technique.

2. Materials and Methods

2.1. Study Flow Chart

All consecutive patients successfully implanted with an LAAO device using either the Amplatzer Cardiac Plug (ACP) device (St. Jude Medical, Minneapolis, MN, USA) or the Watchman device (Boston Scientific, Natick, MA, USA) were included in a prospective single-center study at Dijon University Hospital for a period of four years. A complete screening with all clinical and paraclinical signs of the implanted patients was noted before the procedure, just like the data concerning the percutaneous intervention. A contrast-enhanced cardiac computed tomography (CT) was performed before and 6 weeks after the procedure with reverse left atrial remodeling defined by an increase in LA volume >10%. A blood sampling was obtained before, 48 h after device implantation and at the first visit after discharge (30–45 days) for BNP measurement. Major adverse cardiac events (MACEs) were collected after device implantation and during the follow-up.

After 6 weeks, patients were classified according to the presence or absence of left atrial remodeling, based on the second CT evaluation.

The study sample consisted of 43 patients, with at least one-year follow-up. The flow chart is shown in Figure 1.

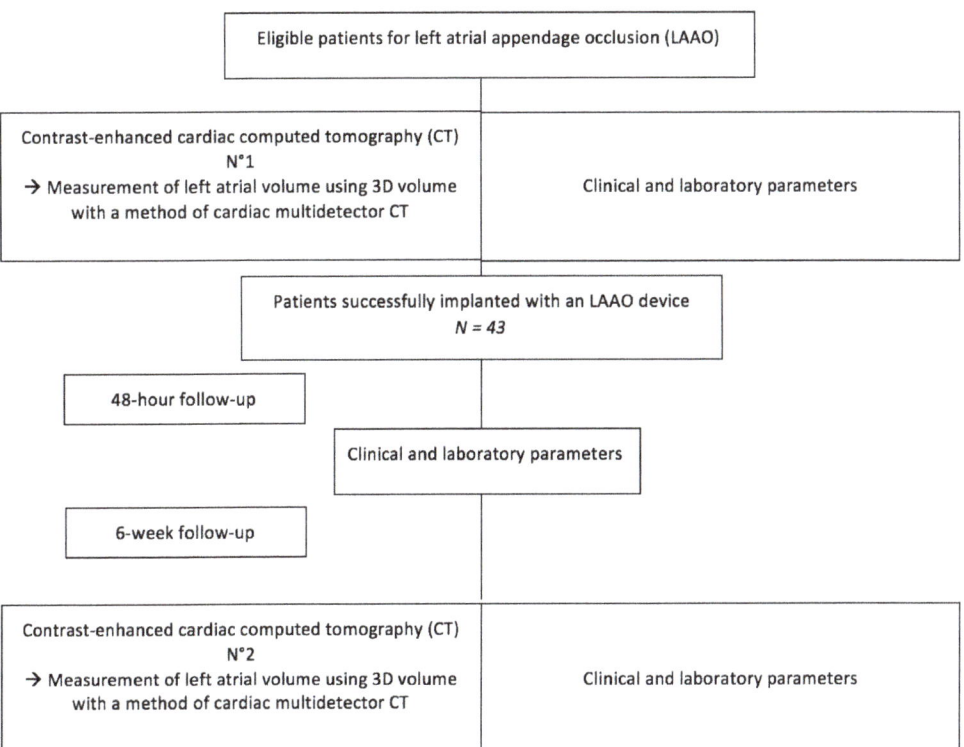

Figure 1. Flow chart of the study.

2.2. Cardiac CT Analysis

All cardiac CT images were analyzed by experienced practitioners using syngo.via software. An automated 3D region-growing segmentation algorithm was used to calculate the volumes of the left atrium [14] (Figure 2). Left atrial volumes were estimated by two experienced practitioners because of the novelty of the technique, and there was a difference of less than 5% between the two measurements proving the reproducibility of the technique. CT was performed pre-procedurally and 6 weeks post-procedurally to evaluate left atrial volumes but also device position, device thrombus or the presence of residual peridevice leaks.

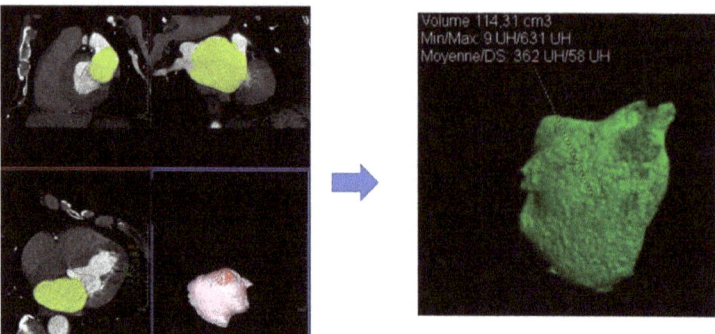

Figure 2. Left Atrial volume assessment using ECG-gated cardiac multidetector CT.

2.3. Statistical Analysis

Statistical analyses were performed using SPSS version 12.0.1 (Statistical Package for the Social Sciences, IBM Inc., Armonk, NY, USA). Dichotomous variables were expressed as *n* (%) and continuous variables as mean and standard deviation. A Kolmogorov–Smirnov test was performed to analyze the normality of continuous variables. Mann–Whitney test (skewed data) or Student's *t*-test (unskewed data) was used to compare continuous data, and the Chi 2 test or Fisher's test was used for dichotomous data. Significance threshold was set at 5%.

3. Results

3.1. Patients Baseline Characteristics

Baseline characteristics on admission to the hospital are summarized in Table 1.

The study included 43 patients, with a median age of 75, with a male predominance (65%). In the implanted patients, the median CHA_2DS_2-VASc score was nearly 4 while the median HAS-BLED score was also nearly 4. Most patients had permanent atrial fibrillation (70%), and most patients had a prior stroke (70%) in the medical history. Eighty-four percent of the patients reported a prior bleeding, most of whom had normal left ventricular function.

In the cohort, four indications for LAAO were revealed: previous bleeding under OAC (84%), cerebral amyloid angiopathy (12%), high risk of bleeding (2%) or stroke despite OAC (2%).

3.2. CT Results and Left Atrial Remodeling

The baseline CT examination was performed less than a month before the procedure, and the second CT was performed 48 ± 36 days after the device implantation. Results are shown in Table 2. At 6 weeks, 6 patients (14%) exhibited left atrial remodeling on CT, while the remaining 37 patients (86%) did not have a significant increase in left atrial volume. There were no statistically significant differences between the two groups according to left atrial remodeling in age, sex, demographic data or symptoms. The HAS-BLED score and the CHA_2DS_2-VASc score were the same in the two groups, the same as atrial fibrillation class, prior stroke or prior bleeding.

In the global population, mean LA volume was respectively 139 ± 64 mL at baseline and 140 ± 63 mL during follow-up, showing no statistical difference. Interestingly, reverse left atrial remodeling was found in six patients, with a median volume increase of 26 mL. No thrombus was found on the atrial side of the device. Peridevice leaks (defined as presence of dye in the LAA beyond the device) were observed in four patients, with no statistical difference between both groups (adverse remodeling or not).

Table 1. Patients' characteristics (according to the presence or absence of reverse atrial remodeling).

	RAR Group N = 6	No RAR Group N = 37	p
Age, years	80 ± 5.7	75 ± 8.2	0.120
Sex (male)	5 (84)	23 (62)	0.304
Hypertension	5 (84)	36 (98)	0.262
Diabetes	3 (50)	8 (22)	0.164
CHA_2DS_2-VASc score	4.3 ± 1.21	4.2 ± 1.4	0.873
HAS BLED score	4 ± 0.9	4.3 ± 1.26	0.498
Paroxysmal AF	1 (16)	12 (33)	0.401
Permanent AF	5 (84)	25 (67)	0.401
Prior stroke	5 (84)	25 (67)	0.401
Congestive heart failure	1 (16)	6 (16)	0.681
History of CAD	1 (16)	10 (27)	0.512
History of CABG	0 (0)	4 (11)	0.535
Prior bleeding	5 (84)	31 (84)	0.681
Prior TAVR	0 (0)	1 (3)	0.857
LVEF, %	60 ± 4	56 ± 9	0.110
Creatinine clearance, mL/min	66 ± 14	66 ± 26	0.919
Pre-procedural NT-proBNP, pg/mL	486 ± 392	2987 ± 6766	0.054
Post-procedural NT-proBNP, pg/mL	1274 ± 1316	2156 ± 3248	0.402
FU NT-proBNP, pg/mL	1255 ± 1603	2574 ± 3309	0.308
Post-procedural troponin, pg/mL	0.26 ± 0.17	0.34 ± 0.39	0.370
Indication for LAAO			
Previous bleeding under OAC	5 (84)	31 (84)	0.681
Cerebral amyloid angiopathy	1 (16)	4 (11)	
High risk of bleeding	0 (0)	1 (3)	
Stroke despite OAC	0 (0)	1 (3)	

Data are presented as n (%) and mean ± SD. AF, Atrial Fibrillation; CAD, Coronary Artery Disease; CABG, Coronary Artery Bypass Graft; ICE, Intracardiac Echocardiography; LVEF, left ventricular ejection fraction; TAVR, Transaortic Valve Replacement; TOE: Transesophageal Echocardiography; OAC, Oral Anticoagulant.

3.3. Procedural and Post-Procedural Characteristics

Interventional LAA closure was successful in all the patients, and no procedure-related major complications were observed. At one year, six patients had died. Other complications included major bleeding (four patients) and congestive heart failure (eight patients). There was no significant difference between the two groups regarding procedural and post-procedural characteristics and results (Table 2).

3.4. Atrial Remodeling and Natriuretic Peptides

Blood samples including natriuretic peptides (B-type natriuretic peptide (BNP)) were collected according to a standardized method before the procedure, 48 h after the procedure and at distance. Firstly, the concentration of the BNP is not different between the two groups according to the presence or not of adverse remodeling of the left atrium, whatever the time of blood sampling. The results are summarized in Table 3. However, we noted that the patients with RAR had a trend of BNP increasing just after the device implantation, then stabilizing, while in those without RAR, a decrease in the BNP level after LAAO was observed (Figure 3). This correlation between RAR and increase of the BNP level after LAAO could be explained by the loss of reservoir function of the left atrium after LAAO, before an adaptation.

Table 2. Procedural and post-procedural characteristics (according to the presence or absence of reverse atrial remodeling).

	RAR Group N = 6	No RAR Group N = 37	p
Procedure			
Device success	6 (100)	37 (100)	1.00
Technical success	6 (100)	36 (97)	0.875
Procedural success	6 (100)	35 (95)	0.758
Total time in the lab, min	81 ± 25	94 ± 33	0.346
Fluoroscopy time, min	30 ± 18	23 ± 13	0.407
Contrast used (mL)	57 ± 19	59 ± 34	0.868
Mean number of devices used	1.2 ± 0.5	1.2 ± 0.4	0.522
Size of the device used	21 ± 4	23 ± 4	0.507
In-Hospital MACE			
Vascular complication	0 (0)	0 (0)	1.00
Cardiac tamponnade	0 (0)	1 (3)	0.860
Device migration	0 (0)	1 (3)	0.860
Device thrombus	1 (16)	3 (8)	0.465
Stroke/TIA	0 (0)	0 (0)	1.00
Post-procedure CT			
Time delay CT_1-LAAO	27 ± 41	40 ± 44	0.502
Time delay LAAO-CT_2	50 ± 16	48 ± 38	0.839
Left atrial volume CT_1	127 ± 46	141 ± 66	0.551
Left atrial volume CT_2	151 ± 51	138 ± 64	0.597
Device thrombus	0	0	1.00
No peridevice leak	6 (100)	33 (89)	0.349
Small peridevice leak	0 (0)	3 (8)	0.630
Large peridevice leak	0 (0)	1 (3)	0.860
MACE at 1Y-FU			
FU in days	801 ± 474	736 ± 383	0.761
Stroke/TIA	0 (0)	0 (0)	1.00
Cardiac death	0 (0)	2 (6)	0.381
Non cardiac death	0 (0)	4 (11)	0.063
Major bleeding	1 (16)	3 (8)	0.465
Device migration	0	1 (3)	0.860
Heart failure	0 (0)	3 (8)	0.622

Data are presented as n (%) or Mean ± SD.

Table 3. Pre-procedural and post-procedural characteristics on CT.

	Pre-Procedure CT	Post-Procedure CT
Time delay CT-LAAO (day)	39 ± 43	48 ± 36
Left atrial volume CT (mL)	139 ± 64	140 ± 63
Reverse remodeling (LA)	-	6 (14%)

Data are presented as n (%) or Mean ± SD.

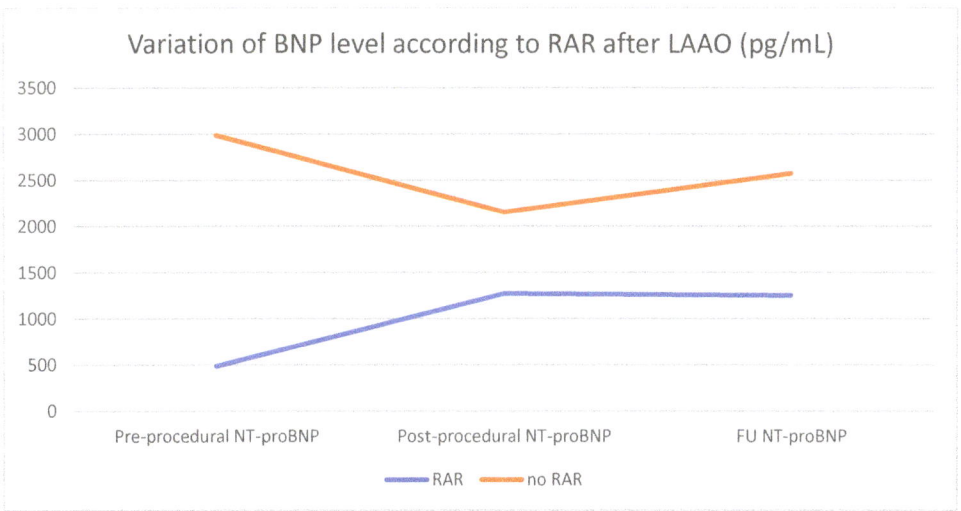

Figure 3. Variation of BNP level according to RAR after LAAO (pg/mL).

4. Discussion

In this study, we aimed to evaluate the impact of LAAO on cardiac hemodynamics based on imaging parameters using LA volume on cardiac CT over time.

We therefore noted that a proportion of patients had left atrial remodeling after an LAAO, even if this was clearly just a trend without statistical difference. However, the presence of cardiac remodeling associated with symptoms suggests that LAA removal can potentially induce heart failure. Obviously, this is the loss of the reservoir function of the LAA after closure which can explain post-procedural LA remodeling.

Percutaneous LAAO is sometimes the only option for ischemic stroke prevention, especially in patients with contraindication for long-term OAC or high risk of bleeding. Although the safety and efficacy of this treatment have been demonstrated in randomized controlled trials and real-world experience [15], data about the impacts of LAAO on cardiac remodeling are not well established with a small number of studies, and the present study brings additional data on this topic.

4.1. Left Atrial Remodeling after LAAO

In 2017, Jalal et al. [16] were the first to non-invasively evaluate the left atrial hemodynamic impact of percutaneous LAA closure and showed no early significant LA remodeling but a trend toward an increase in LV filling pressure. In their population of 63 patients, mean LA volume was 145 ± 55 mL and 144 ± 50 mL at baseline and during follow-up, respectively, without statistical difference. However, regarding echocardiographic assessment of diastolic function, a significant difference was observed in the E/E' ratio which increased after LAA closure.

In the same line, Tan Phan et al. [17] showed in 2018 that there was a significant increase in LA size and LV filling pressure (also significant increase in the E/e' ratio) among NVAF patients after LAAO. The authors concluded that the impact of LAA closure on cardiac functional and structural remodeling observed on echocardiography may have potential clinical implications.

Finally, Luani et al. [18] observed once again in cardiac echography that left atrial volume increased significantly after interventional LAA closure, but left atrial enlargement was not correlated with clinical progression of heart failure in this study.

Our study is in agreement with previous studies highlighting an increase in LA size in cardiac CT in some patients, as well as variations in natriuretic peptide levels, even if no significant difference or correlation was observed. This new study confirms the real potential for left atrial remodeling after LAAO, in agreement with previous studies. These hypotheses will have to be confirmed with future randomized controlled trials with regular follow-up by CT scan and also by echocardiography.

4.2. Natriuretic Peptide Variation after LAAC

The LAA allows production of the atrial natriuretic peptide (ANP) [19], which plays an important role in natriuresis and regulation of heart-filling pressures. With the emergence of LAA occlusion, we can expect variations in the levels of natriuretic peptides and thus changes in cardiac physiology. Unfortunately, although the LAA is a source of the ANP, the impact of LAAO on natriuretic peptide levels remains largely unknown. In his study, Lakkireddy [20] compared the levels of natriuretic peptides before LAAO then during the follow-up with several measurements for three months. In comparison with pre-endocardial LAA device levels, the concentration of the ANP was significantly higher immediately after the procedure. Twenty-four hours after the procedure and at 3 months, the levels of the ANP were not significantly different when compared with the pre-endocardial LAA device baseline. BNP levels displayed similar changes.

In our study, ANP was not available, and we therefore opted for the BNP assay in blood sampling to search for a link between left atrial remodeling and heart failure. Having data on the ANP would have been better.

Moreover, the role of natriuretic peptides is not only about cardiac congestion. ANP and BNP act on the heart, blood vessels and also on the kidneys. The natriuretic peptides have an important role in regulating the circulation. LAAO can therefore also cause changes in the levels of natriuretic peptides not linked to heart failure but potentially linked to vascular and renal changes, in particular, linked to changes in volemia after procedures such as LAAO, where the patients may benefit from vascular replenishment for hypotension or alternatively diuretics for congestion, with a variable intensity of production of natriuretic peptides according to the situation.

4.3. Limitations of the Study

The study was retrospective with a limited number of patients. It would have been interesting to have in addition an echocardiography follow-up and another measurement of the left atrial size and also an evaluation of the filling pressures. Furthermore, changes in medication that may affect cardiac remodeling were not evaluated. A limitation of this study is the lack of dosage of the ANP, a specific marker of the left atrial, produced by the atria, which was not available at the start of the study on the blood sampling of the patients.

The present study provided, however, new insights regarding the interaction between natriuretic peptides, atrial remodeling and left appendage occlusion and had the advantage to benefit a short-time follow-up, with many cardiac CTs in association with a clinical and biological follow-up.

5. Conclusions

Our study showed a trend in favor of remodeling of the left atrial measured by CT scan after an LAAO, just like some modifications in the BNP level around the device implantation without statistical difference with a low number of patients. The potential impact of LAAO concerning cardiac remodeling is, however, real. The results need to be transposed to clinical outcomes of this expanding population in future studies.

Author Contributions: Conceptualization, T.P. and L.L.; Methodology, T.P., L.L. and C.G.; Formal analysis, L.L. and T.P.; Investigation, T.P., T.L., L.L., C.R. and G.P.; Supervision, C.G., G.L. and L.L.; Writing—original draft, T.P. and L.L.; Writing—review and editing, T.P., L.L. and C.G. All authors have read and agreed to the published version of the manuscript.

Funding: This research received no external funding.

Informed Consent Statement: Informed consent was obtained from all subjects involved in the study.

Data Availability Statement: The data that support the findings of this study are available on request from the corresponding author. The data are not publicly available due to privacy or ethical restrictions.

Acknowledgments: We wish to thank Florence Bichat and Anais Hamon for their research and editorial assistance.

Conflicts of Interest: The authors declare no conflict of interest.

Abbreviations

AF	atrial fibrillation
BNP	brain natriuretic peptide
LAA	left atrial appendage
LAAO	left atrial appendage occlusion
OAC	oral anticoagulant

References

1. Chugh, S.S.; Havmoeller, R.; Narayanan, K.; Singh, D.; Rienstra, M.; Benjamin, E.J.; Gillum, R.F.; Kim, Y.H.; McAnulty, J.H., Jr.; Zheng, Z.J.; et al. Worldwide epidemiology of atrial fibrillation: A Global Burden of Disease 2010 Study. *Circulation* **2014**, *129*, 837–847. [CrossRef] [PubMed]
2. Go, A.S.; Hylek, E.M.; Phillips, K.A.; Chang, Y.; Henault, L.E.; Selby, J.V.; Singer, D.E. Prevalence of diagnosed atrial fibrillation in adults: National implications for rhythm management and stroke prevention: The AnTicoagulation and Risk Factors in Atrial Fi-brillation (ATRIA) Study. *JAMA* **2001**, *285*, 2370–2375. [CrossRef] [PubMed]
3. Regazzoli, D.; Ancona, F.; Trevisi, N.; Guarracini, F.; Radinovic, A.; Oppizzi, M.; Agricola, E.; Marzi, A.; Sora, N.C.; Della Bella, P.; et al. Left Atrial Appendage: Physiology, Pathology, and Role as a Therapeutic Target. *BioMed Res. Int.* **2015**, *2015*, 1–13. [CrossRef] [PubMed]
4. Bungard, T.J.; Ghali, W.A.; Teo, K.K.; McAlister, F.A.; Tsuyuki, R.T. Why do patients with atrial fibrillation not receive warfarin? *Arch. Intern. Med.* **2000**, *160*, 41–46. [CrossRef] [PubMed]
5. Saving the Brain: Proper Anticoagulation Therapy for Patients with Atrial Fibrillation. Medical Update. 2016. Available online: https://medicalupdate.pennstatehealth.org/cardiology/saving-the-brain-proper-anticoagulation-therapy-for-patients-with-atrial-fibrillation/ (accessed on 1 May 2020).
6. Meier, B.; Blaauw, Y.; Khattab, A.A.; Lewalter, T.; Sievert, H.; Tondo, C.; Glikson, M. EHRA/EAPCI expert consensus statement on catheter-based left atrial appendage occlusion. *Europace* **2014**, *16*, 1397–1416. [CrossRef] [PubMed]
7. Naksuk, N.; Padmanabhan, D.; Yogeswaran, V.; Asirvatham, S.J. Left Atrial Appendage: Embryology, Anatomy, Physiology, Arrhythmia and Therapeutic Intervention. *JACC Clin. Electrophysiol.* **2016**, *2*, 403–412. [CrossRef] [PubMed]
8. Block, P.C.; Burstein, S.; Casale, P.N.; Kramer, P.H.; Teirstein, P.; Williams, D.O.; Reisman, M. Percutaneous left atrial appendage transcatheter occlusion to prevent stroke in high-risk patients with atrial fibrillation: Early clinical experience. *Circulation* **2002**, *105*, 1887–1889.
9. Blackshear, J.L.; Odell, J.A. Appendage obliteration to reduce stroke in cardiac surgical patients with atrial fibrillation. *Ann. Thorac. Surg.* **1996**, *61*, 755–759. [CrossRef]
10. Reddy, V.Y.; Sievert, H.; Halperin, J.; Doshi, S.K.; Buchbinder, M.; Neuzil, P.; Huber, K.; Whisenant, B.; Kar, S.; Swarup, V.; et al. Percutaneous left atrial appendage closure vs. warfarin for atrial fibrillation: A randomized clinical trial. *JAMA* **2014**, *312*, 1988–1998. [CrossRef] [PubMed]
11. Holmes, D.R.; Kar, S.; Price, M.J.; Whisenant, B.; Sievert, H.; Doshi, S.K.; Huber, K.; Reddy, V.Y. Prospective randomized evaluation of the Watchman Left Atrial Appendage Closure device in patients with atrial fibrillation versus long-term warfarin therapy: The PREVAIL trial. *J. Am. Coll. Cardiol.* **2014**, *64*, 1–12. [CrossRef] [PubMed]
12. Kirchhof, P.; Benussi, S.; Kotecha, D.; Ahlsson, A.; Atar, D.; Casadei, B.; Castella, M.; Diener, H.C.; Heidbuchel, H.; Hendriks, J.; et al. 2016 ESC Guidelines for the management of atrial fibrillation developed in collaboration with EACTS. *Eur. Heart J.* **2016**, *37*, 2893–2962. [CrossRef] [PubMed]
13. Davis, C.A.; Rembert, J.C.; Greenfield, J.C. Compliance of left atrium with and without left atrium appendage. *Am. J. Physiol. Circ. Physiol.* **1990**, *259*, H1006–H1008. [CrossRef] [PubMed]
14. Mühlenbruch, G.; Das, M.; Hohl, C.; Wildberger, J.E.; Rinck, D.; Flohr, T.G.; Koos, R.; Knackstedt, C.; Günther, R.W.; Mahnken, A.H. Global left ventricular function in cardiac CT. Evaluation of an automated 3D region-growing segmentation algorithm. *Eur. Radiol.* **2005**, *16*, 1117–1123. [CrossRef] [PubMed]
15. Reddy, V.Y.; Doshi, S.K.; Kar, S.; Gibson, D.N.; Price, M.J.; Huber, K.; Horton, R.P.; Buchbinder, M.; Neuzil, P.; Gordon, N.T.; et al. 5-Year Outcomes after Left Atrial Appendage Closure: From the PREVAIL and PROTECT AF Trials. *J. Am. Coll. Cardiol.* **2017**, *70*, 2964–2975. [CrossRef] [PubMed]
16. Jalal, Z.; Iriart, X.; Dinet, M.; Corneloup, O.; Pillois, X.; Cochet, H.; Thambo, J. Evaluation of left atrial remodelling following percuta-neous left atrial appendage closure. *J. Geriatr. Cardiol.* **2017**, *14*, 496–500. [PubMed]

17. Phan, Q.T.; Shin, S.Y.; Cho, I.-S.; Lee, W.-S.; Won, H.; Sharmin, S.; Lee, D.-Y.; Kim, T.-H.; Kim, C.-J.; Kim, S.-W. Impact of left atrial appendage closure on cardiac functional and structural remodeling: A difference-in-difference analysis of propensity score matched samples. *Cardiol. J.* **2019**, *26*, 519–528. [CrossRef] [PubMed]
18. Luani, B.; Groscheck, T.; Genz, C.; Tanev, I.; Rauwolf, T.; Herold, J.; Medunjanin, S.; Schmeisser, A.; Braun-Dullaeus, R.C. Left atrial enlargement and clinical considerations in pa-tients with or without a residual interatrial shunt after closure of the left atrial appendage with the WATCH-MANTM-device. *BMC Cardiovasc. Disord.* **2017**, *17*, 294. [CrossRef] [PubMed]
19. Chapeau, C.; Gutkowska, J.; Schiller, P.W.; Milne, R.W.; Thibault, G.; Garcia, R.; Genest, J.; Cantin, M. Localization of immunoreactive synthetic atrial natriuretic factor (ANF) in the heart of various animal species. *J. Histochem. Cytochem.* **1985**, *33*, 541–550. [CrossRef] [PubMed]
20. Lakkireddy, D.; Turagam, M.; Afzal, M.R.; Rajasingh, J.; Atkins, D.; Dawn, B.; Di Biase, L.; Bartus, K.; Kar, S.; Natale, A.; et al. Left Atrial Appendage Closure and Systemic Homeostasis: The LAA HOMEOSTASIS Study. *J. Am. Coll. Cardiol.* **2018**, *71*, 135–144. [CrossRef] [PubMed]

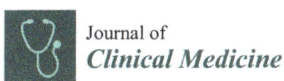 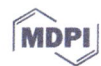

Article

Major Bleeding Predictors in Patients with Left Atrial Appendage Closure: The Iberian Registry II

José Ramón López-Mínguez [1,*], Juan Manuel Nogales-Asensio [1], Eduardo Infante De Oliveira [2], Lino Santos [3], Rafael Ruiz-Salmerón [4], Dabit Arzamendi-Aizpurua [5], Marco Costa [6], Hipólito Gutiérrez-García [7], Jose Antonio Fernández-Díaz [8], Xavier Freixa [9], Ignacio Cruz-González [10], Raúl Moreno [11], Andrés Íñiguez-Romo [12] and Fernando Alfonso-Manterola [13]

1. Cardiology Department, Interventional Cardiology Section, Hospital Universitario de Badajoz, 06080 Badajoz, Spain; juanmanogales@yahoo.es
2. Cardiology Department, Interventional Cardiology Section, Hospital de Santa María, 1649-028 Lisbon, Portugal; e.infante.de.oliveira@gmail.com
3. Cardiology Department, Interventional Cardiology Section, Centro Hospitalario de Vila Nova de Gaia, 4430-999 Vila Nova de Gaia Oporto, Portugal; ljsantos30@gmail.com
4. Cardiology Department, Interventional Cardiology Section, Hospital Virgen de la Macarena, 41009 Seville, Spain; rjruizsalmeron@yahoo.es
5. Cardiology Department, Interventional Cardiology Section, Hospital Santa Creu i San Pau, 08041 Barcelona, Spain; dabitarza@gmail.com
6. Cardiology Department, Interventional Cardiology Section, Centro Hospitalar e Universitário de Coimbra, 3004-561 Coimbra, Portugal; marcocostacard@sapo.pt
7. Cardiology Department, Interventional Cardiology Section, Hospital Clínico de Valladolid, 47003 Valladolid, Spain; hggmaire@gmail.com
8. Cardiology Department, Interventional Cardiology Section, Hospital Puerta de Hierro, Majadahona, 28222 Madrid, Spain; joseantoniofer@gmail.com
9. Cardiology Department, Interventional Cardiology Section, Hospital Clínic de Barcelona, 08036 Barcelona, Spain; xavierfreixa@hotmail.com
10. Cardiology Department, Interventional Cardiology Section, Hospital Universitario de Salamanca, 37007 Salamanca, Spain; cruzgonzalez.ignacio@gmail.com
11. Cardiology Department, Interventional Cardiology Section, Hospital La Paz, 28046 Madrid, Spain; raulmorenog@hotmail.com
12. Cardiology Department, Interventional Cardiology Section, Hospital Álvaro Cunqueiro, 36213 Vigo, Pontevedra, Spain; Andres.Iniguez.Romo@sergas.es
13. Cardiology Department, Interventional Cardiology Section, Hospital La Princesa, IIS-IP, CIBER-CV, Universidad Autónoma de Madrid, 28006 Madrid, Spain; falf@hotmail.com
* Correspondence: lopez-minguez@hotmail.com

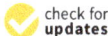

Received: 13 June 2020; Accepted: 13 July 2020; Published: 19 July 2020

Abstract: Introduction and objective: Major bleeding events in patients undergoing left atrial appendage closure (LAAC) range from 2.2 to 10.3 per 100 patient-years in different series. This study aimed to clarify the bleeding predictive factors that could influence these differences. **Methods:** LAAC was performed in 598 patients from the Iberian Registry II (1093 patient-years; median, 75.4 years). We conducted a multivariate analysis to identify predictive risk factors for major bleeding events. The occurrence of thromboembolic and bleeding events was compared to rates expected from CHA2DS2-VASc (congestive heart failure, hypertension, age, diabetes, stroke history, vascular disease, sex) and HAS-BLED (hypertension, abnormal renal and liver function, stroke, bleeding, labile INR, elderly, drugs or alcohol) scores. **Results:** Cox regression analysis revealed that age ≥75 years (HR: 2.5; 95% CI: 1.3 to 4.8; $p = 0.004$) and a history of gastrointestinal bleeding (GIB) (HR: 2.1; 95% CI: 1.1 to 3.9; $p = 0.020$) were two factors independently associated with major bleeding during follow-up. Patients aged <75 or ≥75 years had median CHA2DS2-VASc scores of 4 (IQR: 2) and 5

(IQR: 2), respectively ($p < 0.001$) and HAS-BLED scores were 3 (IQR: 1) and 3 (IQR: 1) for each group ($p = 0.007$). Events presented as follow-up adjusted rates according to age groups were stroke (1.2% vs. 2.9%; HR: 2.4, $p = 0.12$) and major bleeding (3.7 vs. 9.0 per 100 patient-years; HR: 2.4, $p = 0.002$). Expected major bleedings according to HAS-BLED scores were 6.2% vs. 6.6%, respectively. In patients with GIB history, major bleeding events were 6.1% patient-years (HAS-BLED score was 3.8 ± 1.1) compared to 2.7% patients-year in patients with no previous GIB history (HAS-BLED score was 3.4 ± 1.2; $p = 0.029$). **Conclusions:** In this high-risk population, GIB history and age ≥75 years are the main predictors of major bleeding events after LAAC, especially during the first year. Age seems to have a greater influence on major bleeding events than on thromboembolic risk in these patients.

Keywords: atrial fibrillation; bleeding risk; age; left atrial appendage closure

1. Introduction

Left atrial appendage closure (LAAC) is a therapeutic option for patients with a high bleeding risk even in the absence of anticoagulant (AC) treatment after LAAC, and its use has been supported by the increasing body of evidence obtained from several studies and registries [1].

Comparison of results from the series of patients who underwent LAAC may show variations in the percentage of events during follow-up. In spite of some consistency in the relative reduction of stroke (60–80% of CHA2DS2-VASc (congestive heart failure, hypertension, age, diabetes, stroke history, vascular disease, sex) scores), there was a higher variability in bleeding events among the series from the first year of follow-up, with major bleeding events ranging from 2.2% to 10% per year [2–4].

We searched for variables that might be independent predictors for major bleeding events at follow-up. We based our analysis on the Iberian Registry II [5].

2. Methods

Patients and Procedures

Five hundred and ninety-eight patients from the Iberian Registry II referred for LAAC were recruited from 13 hospitals across the Iberian Peninsula (10 from Spain and 3 from Portugal) between 2 March 2009 and 18 December 2015 [5]. These were the set of patients prospectively included in the Iberian Registry I who are continuing long-term follow-up, plus additional patients successively included up to the end of the date set for end of recruitment. Inclusion criteria were one or more of the following conditions: serious hemorrhage during anticoagulant therapy, prior disease or clinical event that contraindicated oral anticoagulants (OACs) or repeated failure to adequately control INR, and hematologist indication to suspend anticoagulation therapy. Exclusion criteria were malignancy, life expectancy less than one year and refusal to provide informed consent for this study.

LAAC indication was as follows: stroke under OAC therapy 6.2%, previous bleeding 73.7%, high risk of bleeding 14.2% and other (poorly controlled INR, patient decision, etc.) 5.9%. Before LAAC, 74.8% and 25.2% of the patients were under OAC and antiplatelet therapy respectively.

The devices used were the Amplatzer® Cardiac Plug (ACP) and its subsequent version, the Amulet® (both from St. Jude Medical; Minneapolis, MN, USA), and the Watchman® (Boston Scientific; Boston, MA, USA).

Thromboembolic and bleeding events were compared with those expected from CHA2DS2-VASc (congestive heart failure, hypertension, age, diabetes, stroke history, vascular disease, sex) and HAS-BLED (hypertension, abnormal renal and liver function, stroke, bleeding, labile INR, elderly, drugs or alcohol) scores in the overall sample [6,7]. Major bleeding events were defined according to VARC-2 classification [8].

The observed incidence of events (number of events during the follow-up period divided by the number of patients per year of follow-up) was calculated per patient and year of follow-up (number of patients at the beginning of the follow-up period multiplied by the mean time of follow-up of those patients expressed in years). The expected incidence of events in the sample was calculated as the mean of the individual risk of each patient. Each patient was assigned an individual risk according to a score of bleeding and ictus risk depending on his or her CHADS2 and HAS-BLED score, as indicated in the work by Friberg and colleagues in the Swedish Atrial Fibrillation cohort study.

All subjects gave their informed consent for inclusion before they participated in the study. The study was conducted in accordance with the Declaration of Helsinki, and the protocol was approved by the Ethics Committee of Hospital Universitario de Badajoz (Project identification 5517).

3. Statistical Analysis

Quantitative variables are expressed as mean (±standard deviation (SD)) or median (interquartile range (IQR)). Categorical variables are expressed as absolute frequency and percentage. Categorical variables were compared using the χ^2 test or Fisher's exact test, and quantitative variables using the Student t-test or Wilcoxon test. Comparisons between rates of observed and expected events were evaluated using binomial tests. Event-free survival analysis was performed using the Kaplan–Meier method and Cox regression. Multivariate analysis (Cox regression) was performed to identify which variables might be independent predictors for bleeding events. Proportional-hazard assumption for Cox Regression was checked by use of Cox proportional hazards regression test with time-dependent covariates. All analyses were carried out using the SPSS statistical package, version 19.0.

All patients gave their consent authorizing the intervention and subsequent follow-up. The study protocol was approved by the hospital ethics committee and conforms to the ethical guidelines of the 1975 Declaration of Helsinki. More details of patients, work methods, variable definitions and statistical analyses were previously reported [5].

4. Results

In the Iberian Registry II, during a mean follow-up of 22.9 months, the observed events for stroke and major bleeding events according to CHA2DS2-VASc and HAS-BLED scores in the total population were 1.6% (vs. expected 8.5%) and 3.9% (vs. expected 6.4%), with a relative risk reduction (RRR) of 81% for stroke and 39% for major bleeding events. In patients monitored for more than 24 months (683 patient-years), stroke and bleeding frequencies were 1.5% and 2.6%, with RRRs of 82% and 59%, respectively.

In the univariate analysis, the variables that were associated with a higher rate of "major bleeding events" at follow-up were: age ≥ 75 years (HR: 2.8; 95% CI: 1.5–5.2; $p = 0.002$), gastrointestinal bleeding (GIB) history (HR: 2.3; 95% CI95: 1.2–4.3; $p = 0.007$) and the antecedent of hypertension (HR: 0.5; 95% CI: 0.3–1; $p = 0.047$). Multivariate analysis (Cox regression analysis) showed that the variables associated with "major bleeding events" during follow-up were only age ≥ 75 years (HR: 2.5; 95% CI: 1.3 to 4.8; $p = 0.004$) and GIB history (HR: 2.1; 95% CI: 1.1 to 3.9; $p = 0.020$).

In patients with previous bleeding, these occurred in 82.1% and 17.9% of patients under OAC and antiplatelet therapy, respectively. GIB accounted for 55% of previous major bleeding events and 82% of major bleeding events during follow-up. Most of GIB (28 of 35) took place during the first 12 months (25 of them in the first 6 months).

Patients were then divided into two different populations according to their age: <75 or ≥ 75years (326 vs. 272 patients). Table 1 shows the main clinical variables between the two groups. The percentage of patients aged ≥75 years with a previous history of bleeding was 81.3%. In general, the percentage of patients with a history of intracranial hemorrhage (ICH) was lower (23.9% and 29.1% in older and younger groups; $p = 0.14$) compared to the percentage with a history of GIB or major bleeding events, which was even significantly higher in patients ≥ 75 years (GIB: 48.5% vs. 32.5%; $p < 0.001$; major bleeding: 53.3% vs. 39.9%; $p = 0.001$). There was also a higher percentage of patients with anemia and renal failure in the elderly group (Table 1). There were no significant differences with regard to the implant used in the procedure or in complications. Table 2 shows the following events presented as follow-up adjusted rates according to age group (<75 or ≥75 years): deaths, 3.9% vs. 11.8% (HR: 3; $p < 0.001$); stroke, 1.2% vs. 2.9% (HR: 2.4; $p = 0.12$); ICH, 1.2% vs. 0.2% (HR: 0.2; $p = 0.09$); GIB, 1.5% vs. 6.9% (OR: 4.6; $p < 0.001$) and major bleeding, 3.7 vs. 9.0 (HR: 2.4; $p = 0.002$) per 100 patient-years (corresponding to patients <75 vs. ≥75 years, respectively). A significant decrease in bleeding events occurred after 1 year of follow-up in both groups (0.5 and 2.9 per 100 patient-years for GIB ($p = 0.045$), and 0.4, and 1.9 per 100 patient-years ($p = 0.018$) for major bleeding, in younger and older patients, although patients aged ≥75 years continued to have more bleeding events) (Figure 1 A,B). Figure 2 shows that survival rate with no GIB was significantly higher in patients aged <75 years compared to the elderly group.

Table 1. Clinical variables in the populations aged <75 and ≥75 years.

	<75 (n = 326)	≥75 (n = 272)	p-Value
Age	67.3 ± 5.8	80.3 ± 3.5	<0.001
Female	112 (34.4%)	116 (42.6%)	0.038
Hypertension	255 (78.2%)	213 (78.3%)	0.979
Diabetes	106 (32.5%)	98 (36.0%)	0.367
Permanent AF	149 (45.7%)	159 (58.5%)	0.002
Previous stroke	111 (34.0%)	77 (28.3%)	0.132
Previous bleeding	170 (52.1%)	221 (81.3%)	<0.001
Previous ICH	95 (29.1%)	65 (23.9%)	0.149
Previous GI bleeding	106 (32.5%)	132 (48.5%)	<0.001
Previous major bleeding	130 (39.9%)	145 (53.3%)	0.001
CHA_2DS_2-VASc *	4 [2]	5 [2]	<0.001
HAS-BLED *	3 [1]	3 [1]	0.007
Anemia	63 (19.3%)	102 (37.5%)	<0.001
Renal failure	42 (12.9%)	85 (31.3%)	<0.001

AF: atrial fibrillation; GI: gastrointestinal; ICH: intracranial hemorrhage. * Median (IQR).

Table 2. Adjusted event rates per 100 patient-years.

	<75 (n = 326)	≥75 (n = 272)	HR (<75 vs. ≥75)	p-Value
Death	3.9	11.8	3.0	<0.001
Stroke	1.2	2.9	2.4	0.120
ICH	1.2	0.2	0.2	0.099
GI bleeding	1.5	6.9	4.6	<0.001
Major bleeding	3.7	9.0	2.4	0.002

GI: gastrointestinal; ICH: intracranial hemorrhage.

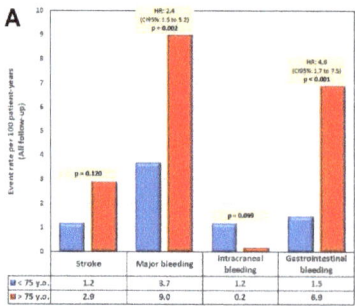
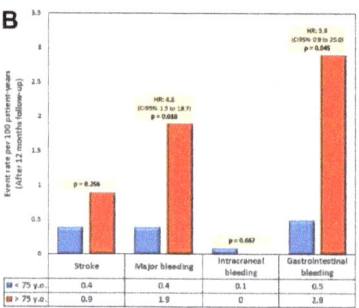

Figure 1. (A) Rate of events in patient-years according to age < or ≥75 years. (B) Rate of events in patients who completed the first year with no events. HR: hazard ratio; CI: confidence interval.

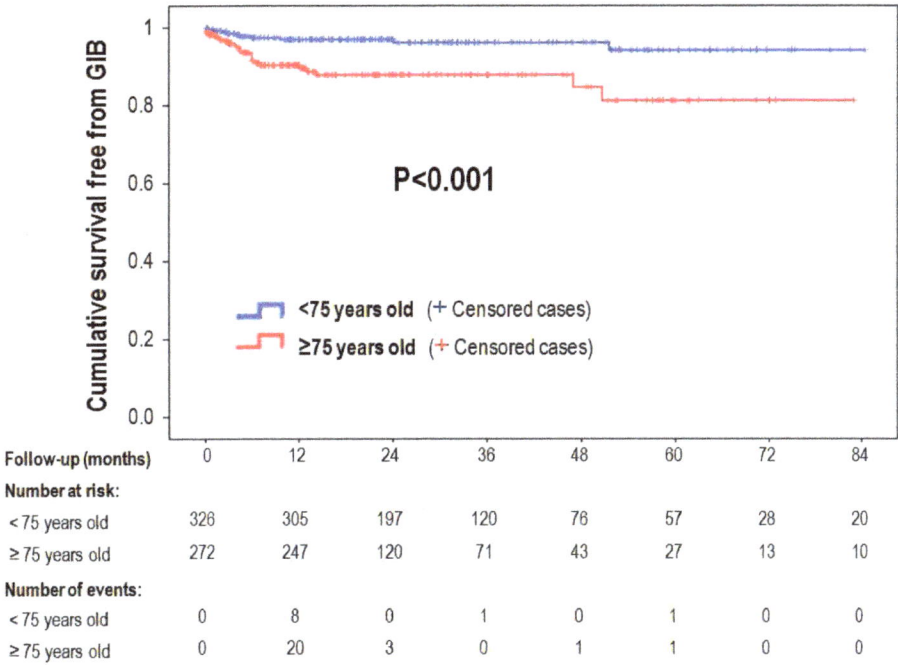

Figure 2. Cumulative survival free from gastrointestinal bleeding (GIB) is significantly higher in patients <75 years compared to patients ≥75 years.

Table 3 shows the rate of events per patient-year in patients aged ≥75 years compared to the rate expected by the risk scores. There were only small differences in stroke and ICH per patient-year between patients aged ≥75 or <75 years. In contrast, there was an increase in major bleeding events in patients aged ≥75 years, which did not occur for the group aged <75 years, in whom bleeding reduction was 40.3%. Most GIB events occurred in the first 6 months of follow-up in both groups. The two variables that were independently associated with the event "gastrointestinal bleeding" after multivariate analysis (Cox regression) were: age ≥75 years (HR: 3.0; 95% CI: 1.4 to 6,3; $p = 0.004$) and gastrointestinal bleeding (GIB) history (HR: 4.3; 95% CI: 2.0 to 9.4; $p < 0.001$).

Table 3. Overall event outcomes in patients aged <75 and ≥75 years.

	Expected events (×100 patient-years) in ≥75 years	Observed events (×100 patient-years) in ≥75 years	Expected events (×100 patient-years) in <75 years	Observed events (×100 patient-years) in <75 years
Ischemic stroke	7.2 CHADs-VASc score	2.9 Reduction, 59.7% $p \leq 0.001$	5.1 CHADs-VASc score	1.2 Reduction, 76.5% $p \leq 0.001$
ICH	1.0 HAS-BLED score	0.3 Reduction, 70.8% $p = 0.220$	0.9 HAS-BLED score	1.2 Increase, 33.3% $p = 0.642$
GI bleeding		6.9		1.5
Major bleeding	6.6 HAS-BLED score (Friberg Registry)	9.0 Increase, 26.7% $p < 0.001$	6.2 HAS-BLED score (Friberg Registry)	3.7 Reduction, 40.3%) $p = 0.007$

GI: gastrointestinal; HT: hypertension; ICH: intracranial hemorrhage.

Table 4 compares treatments at discharge between both age groups of patients, showing no significant differences. Table 5 divides patients in two groups based on new GIB or no new GIB events during follow-up and compares the main variables between the two subpopulations. We found significant differences in GIB history (74.3% vs. 37.7%, $p < 0.001$), HAS-BLED scores (3.8 ± 1.1 vs. 3.4 ± 1.2, $p = 0.029$), ICH (11.4% vs. 27.7%, $p = 0.035$) and death (25.7% vs. 12.6%, $p = 0.027$). Although patients with GIB history showed a higher death rate, multivariate analysis results showed that only age (HR: 1.08; 95% CI: 1.05 to 1.13; $p < 0.001$) and previous stroke (HR: 3.22; 95% CI: 1.64 to 6.34; $p = 0.001$) were predictive factors for death during follow-up.

Table 4. Treatment at discharge according to age group.

	<75 (n = 326)	≥75 (n = 272)	p-Value
AAS	208 (63.8%)	166 (61.0%)	0.485
Clopidogrel	207 (63.5%)	164 (60.3%)	0.422
AAS + Clopidogrel	185 (56.7%)	138 (50.7%)	0.142
Anticoagulants (acenocumarol or LMWH)	45 (13.8%)	40 (14.7%)	0.753
NOAC	9 (2.8%)	9 (3.3%)	0.696

AAS: acetylsalicylic acid; LMWH: low molecular weight heparin; NOAC: non-vitamin K antagonist oral anticoagulant.

Table 5. Comparison of the main variables in patients presenting GIB events or no GIB events during follow-up.

	GIB (n = 35)	No GIB (n = 563)	p-Value
Age	77.0 ± 8.2	74.0 ± 8.0	0.029
Female	15 (42.9%)	213 (37.8%)	0.553
Hypertension	23 (65.7%)	445 (79.0%)	0.064
Diabetes	14 (40.0%)	190 (33.7%)	0.449
Permanent AF	19 (54.3%)	289 (51.3%)	0.734
Previous stroke	7 (20.0%)	181 (32.1%)	0.133
Previous bleeding	26 (74.3%)	365 (64.8%)	0.254
Previous ICH	4 (11.4%)	156 (27.7%)	0.035
Previous GI bleeding	26 (74.3%)	212 (37.7%)	<0.001
Previous major bleeding	16 (45.7%)	259 (56.0%)	0.973
CHA$_2$DS$_2$-VASc *	5 [1]	4 [2]	0.390
HAS-BLED *	4 [2]	3 [1]	0.016
Anemia	13 (37.1%)	152 (27.0%)	0.269
Renal failure	10 (28.6%)	117 (20.8%)	0.766
AAS at discharge	23 (65.7%)	352 (62.3%)	0.689
Clopidogrel at discharge	21 (60.0%)	350 (62.2%)	0.798
AAS + Clopidogrel at discharge	19 (54.3%)	304 (54.0%)	0.973
Acenocumarol at discharge	1 (2.9%)	28 (5.0%)	0.572
LMWH at discharge	2 (5.7%)	54 (9.6%)	0.445
NOAC	1 (2.9%)	17 (3.0%)	0.956
Death in follow-up	9 (25.7%)	71 (12.6%)	0.027

AAS: acetylsalicylic acid; AF: atrial fibrillation; GI: gastrointestinal; ICH: intracranial hemorrhage; LMWH: low molecular weight heparin; NOAC: non-vitamin K antagonist oral anticoagulant. * Median (IQR).

Table 6 presents the main variables of LAAC patients with contraindications for OAC treatment, collected from different registries (data from > 500 patients).

Table 6. Mean variables of patients with contraindication for OAC treatment reported in different registries.

Registry	EWOLUTION Registry	Multicenter Amplatzer	Amulet Registry	Ii Iberian Registry	Italian Registry
Population (n)	n = 1025	n = 1047	n = 1088	n = 598	n = 613
Mean age	73.4 ± 8.9	75 ± 8	74 ± 8	75.4 ± 8.6	75.1 ± 8.0
Follow up (months)	12	13	12	22.9	20
CHA$_2$DS$_2$-VASc score (mean ± SD)	4.5 ± 1.6	4.5 ± 1.6	4.5 ± 1.6	4.4 ± 1.5	4.2 ± 1.5

Table 6. Cont.

Registry	EWOLUTION Registry	Multicenter Amplatzer	Amulet Registry	Ii Iberian Registry	Italian Registry
Population (n)	n = 1025	n = 1047	n = 1088	n = 598	n = 613
HAS-BLED score (mean ± SD)	2.3 ± 1.2	3.1 ± 1.2	3.3 ± 1.1	3.4 ± 1.2	3.2 ± 1.1
Rate of events per 100 patient-years					
Deaths	9.8%	4.3%	8.4%	7%	7.4%
History of Stroke	30.5%	39%	28%	39%	36.3%
History of major Bleeding	31%	47.7%	72%	46%	41.6%
Observed vs. Expected					
Stroke	1.1% vs. 7.2% (CHA_2DS_2-VASc) RRR, 83%	1.8% vs. 5.62% (CHA_2DS_2-VASc) RRR, 59%	2.9 vs. 6.7% (CHA_2DS_2-VASc) RRR, 57%	1.6% vs. 8.5% (CHA_2DS_2-VASc) RRR, 81%	2.9% vs. 8.6% (CHA_2DS_2-VASc) RRR, 66%
Major bleeding	2.7% vs. 5% (HAS-BLED) RRR, 46%	2.1% vs. 5.34% (HAS-BLED) RRR, 46%	7.1% vs. 10.3%	3.9% vs. 6.4% (HAS-BLED) RRR, 39%	4.5% vs. 6.3% (HAS-BLED) RRR, 29%

OAC: Oral anticoagulants; RRR: relative risk reduction; SD: standard deviation.

5. Discussion

Our study shows that during follow-up, both age and major GIB history are the main predictors of major bleeding events and therefore both variables should be taken into account when making comparisons between bleeding percentages in the different series of patients. It is also important that results are interpreted according to the follow-up time, as bleeding rates are higher during the first year [9].

5.1. The Importance of GIB, Major Bleeding History and Follow-up Time

Only around 16%-17% of patients included in randomized trials of both non-vitamin K antagonist oral anticoagulant (NOAC) and LAAC with warfarin therapies have a previous history of bleeding [10]; conversely, in LAAC registries, major bleeding events range from 31% in the EWOLUTION Registry to 72% in the Amulet Registry, with the remainder having conditions associated with a high bleeding risk, such as severe anemia [2,5,11–13].

We show in Table 2 that GIBs represent a higher percentage of severe bleedings in older patients (≥75 years).

In the Amulet and II Iberian Registries, where we find higher HAS-BLED scores and higher percentages of patients with major bleeding history, major bleeding during follow-up rises to 10.3% and 5.4%, respectively, during the first year, in contrast to the results of the Multicentre and EWOLUTION studies, that range from 2.1% to 2.7% [2,9,11,12].

However, in the Iberian Registry II, bleeding events were reduced to 3.9% after two years of follow-up and to 2.6% after more than two years, which corresponded to a relative reduction of more than 21% (39% after two years and 58.7% after more than two years) [5].

Bleeding events, especially GIB, were higher during the first 6 months post-procedure, which is the time window when a higher percentage of patients were receiving dual antithrombotic treatment (therapy changed from two antiplatelet agents to only one after the first 3–6 months). It is interesting to note that bleeding reduction is less dramatic in patients with major bleeding history. The EWOLUTION study reported that after 2 years, patients with HAS-BLED scores <3 showed relative reductions of 50% (1.8% vs. expected 3.6%) compared to relative reductions of 41% in patients with HAS-BLED scores >3 (4.2% vs. expected 7.1%), and these figures were even lower in patients with a major bleeding history (30%) [14]. In our study, in patients with GIB history, major bleeding events were 6.1 per 100 patient-years (HAS-BLED score 3.8 ± 1.1), compared to 2.7 per 100 patient-years in patients with no previous GIB history (HAS-BLED score 3.4 ± 1.2; $p = 0.029$).

5.2. The Importance of Age

Age is a risk factor in the prediction of both stroke and bleeding as a whole [7]. Elderly patients receiving treatment with OAC present a high bleeding risk that ranges from 9% to 13%, and for that reason they are not well represented in NOAC randomized trials [15,16]. It is still debated whether age has more influence on major bleedings than on thromboembolic events, as several studies support opposite claims in this respect [17–19]. Thus, it was observed that even in patients who were able to take OAC in the ENGAGE AF-TIMI 48 study, age had a greater influence on major bleeding than on thromboembolic risk [17].

It is crucial to clarify if age has more impact on major bleeding risk or on thromboembolic events in NVAF patients undergoing left atrial appendage closure (LAAC) and with a history of frequent bleeding events. In our study, patients ≥75 years had higher HAS-BLED scores (3.5 ± 1.1) than patients <75 years (3.3 ± 1.2; $p = 0.004$), and bleeding events were 9 per 100 patient-years (26.7% increase) versus 3.7 per 100 patient-years in the younger group (40.3% decrease).

The question as to whether age is the main factor or a secondary factor responsible for the accumulation in the percentage of patients with bleeding history was clarified by the multivariate analysis, which showed that age and bleeding history were independent predictors of subsequent bleeding events, especially a history of GIB.

There are no specific studies on the importance of age in bleeding events in LAAC patients, although there are two published LAAC series from the Multicentre and EWOLUTION registries [4,20].

The study published by Freixa and colleagues, based on the Multicentre Registry with the AMPLATZER Cardiac Plug, compared two populations of patients under or over 75 years old [4] and found no differences in major bleeding events (1.7% vs. 2.6%; $p = 0.54$) during a mean follow-up of 16.8 months. In addition, in the series of Freixa and collaborators, the percentage of patients <75 or ≥75 years with a previous history of major bleeding was similar between the two groups (48.4% vs. 47.7%; $p = 0.83$), whereas in our study, the percentage was significantly different between the two groups and even higher in patients ≥75 years (39.9% vs. 53.3%; $p = 0.001$) [4,5].

Cruz-González and colleagues published a sub-analysis of the EWOLUTION Registry of patients undergoing LAAC, comparing patients <85 and ≥85 years old. Although the differences between younger and older patients were not statistically significant (due to a limited sample size), after a follow-up of 24 months the group aged >85 years presented higher rates of major or severe non-procedural bleeding events than the younger group (5.1 per 100 patient-years vs. 2.6 per 100 patient-years, or 7.5 vs. 4.3 respectively, if procedural severe bleedings were included) [20].

5.3. Post-Implantation Treatment is an Important Variable

Most of the patients included in our study underwent dual antiplatelet treatment (DAPT) for 3 months, and after that, treatment was reduced to only one antiplatelet agent (APT), which is the usual procedure in current studies. It is clear that post-interventional treatment is an important variable to take into account, but in all studies, with the exception of randomized series, patients present a high percentage of bleeding events of different natures and origins. This makes it difficult to standardize treatment guidelines, and doctors must make decisions based on the specific risk associated with each patient [14]. The analysis of this variable can be confusing as data from the Amulet Registry showed that patients that were not taking antiplatelet agents developed more bleeding events than the group that was medicated, reflecting the current trend to treat patients with lower bleeding risk instead of patients with a very high bleeding risk [2]. The EWOLUTION study showed that patients treated with DAPT presented more major bleeding events after 105 days than those who discontinued this treatment (3.5% vs. 1.1%) [14].

Our study has the limitations of any registry since it is not a randomized trial. However, patients cannot be randomized for ethical reasons. Nevertheless, our data reflect a very exhaustive collection of events in a highly complex population, and their comparison with expected outcomes according to the risk scores has been widely validated. Despite the difficulty of reaching a consensus regarding appropriate post-interventional antiplatelet treatment (generally DAPT for 3 months), our analyses took into consideration the duration of antiplatelet treatment when comparing patients with or without bleeds.

6. Conclusions

In our Iberian Registry II, 46% of patients referred for LAAC had previous major bleedings, mostly of gastrointestinal origin. A history of severe GIB is an independent predictor of new severe bleeding events during follow-up. The percentage of patients aged ≥75 years may also significantly influence the incidence of major bleeding events beyond that expected using the HAS-BLED score, especially due to the high frequency of GIB, as age appears to have greater influence on major bleeding than on thromboembolic risk in these patients. Despite this, after the first year, bleeding events fell significantly, although they continued to be higher than in the group aged <75 years, in whom fewer bleeding complications were observed than expected from the HAS-BLED score. Efficacy in thromboembolic events remains very high, regardless of age, even from the first year.

6.1. What is Known about the Topic?

- LAAC is an effective therapeutic option for atrial fibrillation patients with a contraindication for the use of anticoagulants.
- However, these patients present a high bleeding risk even in the absence of antiplatelet treatment.
- Age influences the emergence of complications during follow-up of LAAC patients.

6.2. What does this Study add?

- This study shows that age has a greater influence on the occurrence of major bleedings than on thromboembolic events.
- Our analysis also shows that GIB history is the main predictive factor of major bleeding events during the first year of follow-up after LAAC.
- Differences in the rates of major bleeding events reported in different series of LAAC patients may be due to the number of patients ≥ 75 years and the percentage of patients with GIB history included in those series.

Author Contributions: J.R.L.-M.: conceptualization, methodology, validation, investigation, writing—original draft preparation, writing—review and editing, visualization, supervision, J.M.N.-A.: methodology, validation, data curation, supervision, project administration, E.I.D.O., L.S., R.R.-S., D.A.-A., M.C., H.G.-G., J.A.F.-D., X.F., I.C.-G., R.M., A.Í.-R., F.A.-M.: methodology, validation, investigation, writing—review and editing, visualization, supervision. All authors have read and agreed to the published version of the manuscript.

Funding: This research received no external funding.

Acknowledgments: Reyes González-Fernández, Ginés Martínez-Cáceres, Roman Arnold, Ignacio J. Amat-Santos, Javier Goicolea Ruigómez, Rocio Gonzalez-Ferreiro, Javier Rodríguez Collado, Guillermo Galeote García, Rodrigo Estevez Loureiro, Guillermo Bastos Fernández, Antonio de Miguel Castro, and Fernando Rivero Crespo: have contributed as collaborators of Iberian Registry II in: methodology and investigation.

Conflicts of Interest: J.R. López-Mínguez, D. Arzamendi-Aizpurua, Ignacio Cruz and Xavi Freixa are proctors of Abbot for LAA closure with Amplatzer Cardiac Plug/Amulet; E. Infante De Oliveira, Ignacio Cruz-González and R. RuizSalmerón are proctors of Boston Scientific with Watchman device. Other authors declare no conflict of interest.

Abbreviations

LAAC	left atrial appendage closure
GIB	gastrointestinal bleeding
OAC	oral anticoagulants
NOAC	new oral anticoagulants
NVAF	non-valvular atrial fibrillation

References

1. Sharma, D.; Reddy, V.Y.; Sandri, M.; Schulz, P.; Majunke, N.; Hala, P.; Wiebe, J.; Mraz, T.; Miller, M.A.; Neuzil, P.; et al. Left Atrial Appendage Closure in Patients With Contraindications to Oral Anticoagulation. *J. Am. Coll. Cardiol.* **2016**, *67*, 2190–2192. [CrossRef] [PubMed]
2. Landmesser, U.; Tondo, C.; Camm, J.; Diener, H.C.; Paul, V.; Schmidt, B.; Settergren, M.; Teiger, E.; Nielsen-Kudsk, J.E.; Hildick-Smith, D. Left atrial appendage occlusion with the AMPLATZER Amulet device: One-year follow-up from the prospective global Amulet observational registry. *EuroIntervention* **2018**, *14*, e590–e597. [CrossRef] [PubMed]
3. Phillips, K.P.; Santoso, T.; Sanders, P.; Alison, J.; Chan, J.L.K.; Pak, H.N.; Chandavimol, M.; Stein, K.M.; Gordon, N.; Razali, O.B. Left atrial appendage closure with WATCHMAN in Asian patients: 2 year outcomes from the WASP registry. *Int. J. Cardiol Heart Vasc.* **2019**, *23*, 100358. [CrossRef] [PubMed]
4. Freixa, X.; Gafoor, S.; Regueiro, A.; Cruz-Gonzalez, I.; Shakir, S.; Omran, H.; Berti, S.; Santoro, G.; Kefer, J.; Landmesser, U.; et al. Comparison of Efficacy and Safety of Left Atrial Appendage Occlusion in Patients Aged <75 to >/= 75 Years. *Am. J. Cardiol.* **2016**, *117*, 84–90. [CrossRef] [PubMed]
5. Lopez-Minguez, J.R.; Nogales-Asensio, J.M.; Infante De Oliveira, E.; De Gama Ribeiro, V.; Ruiz-Salmeron, R.; Arzamendi-Aizpurua, D.; Costa, M.; Gutierrez-Garcia, H.; Fernandez-Diaz, J.A.; Martin-Yuste, V.; et al. Long-term Event Reduction After Left Atrial Appendage Closure. Results of the Iberian Registry II. *Rev. Esp. Cardiol.* **2019**, *72*, 449–455. [CrossRef] [PubMed]
6. Friberg, L.; Rosenqvist, M.; Lip, G.Y. Evaluation of risk stratification schemes for ischaemic stroke and bleeding in 182 678 patients with atrial fibrillation: The Swedish Atrial Fibrillation cohort study. *Eur. Heart J.* **2012**, *33*, 1500–1510. [CrossRef] [PubMed]
7. Lip, G.Y.; Frison, L.; Halperin, J.L.; Lane, D.A. Comparative validation of a novel risk score for predicting bleeding risk in anticoagulated patients with atrial fibrillation: The HAS-BLED (Hypertension, Abnormal Renal/Liver Function, Stroke, Bleeding History or Predisposition, Labile INR, Elderly, Drugs/Alcohol Concomitantly) score. *J. Am. Coll. Cardiol.* **2011**, *57*, 173–180. [CrossRef] [PubMed]
8. Kappetein, A.P.; Head, S.J.; Genereux, P.; Piazza, N.; van Mieghem, N.M.; Blackstone, E.H.; Brott, T.G.; Cohen, D.J.; Cutlip, D.E.; van Es, G.A.; et al. Updated standardized endpoint definitions for transcatheter aortic valve implantation: The Valve Academic Research Consortium-2 consensus document. *EuroIntervention* **2012**, *8*, 782–795. [CrossRef] [PubMed]
9. Lopez Minguez, J.R.; Asensio, J.M.; Gragera, J.E.; Costa, M.; Gonzalez, I.C.; de Carlos, F.G.; Diaz, J.A.; Martin Yuste, V.; Gonzalez, R.M.; Dominguez-Franco, A.; et al. Two-year clinical outcome from the Iberian registry patients after left atrial appendage closure. *Heart* **2015**, *101*, 877–883. [CrossRef] [PubMed]
10. Ruff, C.T.; Giugliano, R.P.; Braunwald, E.; Hoffman, E.B.; Deenadayalu, N.; Ezekowitz, M.D.; Camm, A.J.; Weitz, J.I.; Lewis, B.S.; Parkhomenko, A.; et al. Comparison of the efficacy and safety of new oral anticoagulants with warfarin in patients with atrial fibrillation: A meta-analysis of randomised trials. *Lancet* **2014**, *383*, 955–962. [CrossRef]
11. Boersma, L.V.; Ince, H.; Kische, S.; Pokushalov, E.; Schmitz, T.; Schmidt, B.; Gori, T.; Meincke, F.; Protopopov, A.V.; Betts, T.; et al. Efficacy and safety of left atrial appendage closure with WATCHMAN in patients with or without contraindication to oral anticoagulation: 1-Year follow-up outcome data of the EWOLUTION trial. *Heart Rhythm* **2017**, *14*, 1302–1308. [CrossRef] [PubMed]
12. Tzikas, A.; Shakir, S.; Gafoor, S.; Omran, H.; Berti, S.; Santoro, G.; Kefer, J.; Landmesser, U.; Nielsen-Kudsk, J.E.; Cruz-Gonzalez, I.; et al. Left atrial appendage occlusion for stroke prevention in atrial fibrillation: Multicentre experience with the AMPLATZER Cardiac Plug. *EuroIntervention* **2016**, *11*, 1170–1179. [CrossRef] [PubMed]
13. Berti, S.; Santoro, G.; Brscic, E.; Montorfano, M.; Vignali, L.; Danna, P.; Tondo, C.; D'Amico, G.; Stabile, A.; Sacca, S.; et al. Left atrial appendage closure using AMPLATZER devices: A large, multicenter, Italian registry. *Int. J. Cardiol.* **2017**, *248*, 103–107. [CrossRef] [PubMed]
14. Boersma, L.V.; Ince, H.; Kische, S.; Pokushalov, E.; Schmitz, T.; Schmidt, B.; Gori, T.; Meincke, F.; Protopopov, A.V.; Betts, T.; et al. Evaluating Real-World Clinical Outcomes in Atrial Fibrillation Patients Receiving the WATCHMAN Left Atrial Appendage Closure Technology. *Circ. Arrhythm Electrophysiol.* **2019**, *12*, e006841. [CrossRef] [PubMed]

15. Hylek, E.M.; Evans-Molina, C.; Shea, C.; Henault, L.E.; Regan, S. Major hemorrhage and tolerability of warfarin in the first year of therapy among elderly patients with atrial fibrillation. *Circulation* **2007**, *115*, 2689–2696. [CrossRef] [PubMed]
16. Kwon, C.H.; Kim, M.; Kim, J.; Nam, G.B.; Choi, K.J.; Kim, Y.H. Real-world comparison of non-vitamin K antagonist oral anticoagulants and warfarin in Asian octogenarian patients with atrial fibrillation. *J. Geriatr. Cardiol.* **2016**, *13*, 566–572. [CrossRef] [PubMed]
17. Kato, E.T.; Giugliano, R.P.; Ruff, C.T.; Koretsune, Y.; Yamashita, T.; Kiss, R.G.; Nordio, F.; Murphy, S.A.; Kimura, T.; Jin, J.; et al. Efficacy and Safety of Edoxaban in Elderly Patients With Atrial Fibrillation in the ENGAGE AF-TIMI 48 Trial. *J. Am. Heart Assoc.* **2016**, *5*, e003432. [CrossRef] [PubMed]
18. Lauw, M.N.; Eikelboom, J.W.; Coppens, M.; Wallentin, L.; Yusuf, S.; Ezekowitz, M.; Oldgren, J.; Nakamya, J.; Wang, J.; Connolly, S.J. Effects of dabigatran according to age in atrial fibrillation. *Heart* **2017**, *103*, 1015–1023. [CrossRef] [PubMed]
19. Patti, G.; Lucerna, M.; Pecen, L.; Siller-Matula, J.M.; Cavallari, I.; Kirchhof, P.; De Caterina, R. Thromboembolic Risk, Bleeding Outcomes and Effect of Different Antithrombotic Strategies in Very Elderly Patients With Atrial Fibrillation: A Sub-Analysis From the PREFER in AF (PREvention oF Thromboembolic Events-European Registry in Atrial Fibrillation). *J. Am. Heart Assoc.* **2017**, *6*. [CrossRef] [PubMed]
20. Cruz-Gonzalez, I.; Ince, H.; Kische, S.; Schmitz, T.; Schmidt, B.; Gori, T.; Foley, D.; De Potter, T.; Tschishow, W.; Vireca, E.; et al. Left atrial appendage occlusion in patients older than 85 years. Safety and efficacy in the EWOLUTION registry. *Rev. Esp. Cardiol.* **2019**. [CrossRef] [PubMed]

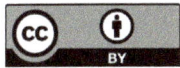

© 2020 by the authors. Licensee MDPI, Basel, Switzerland. This article is an open access article distributed under the terms and conditions of the Creative Commons Attribution (CC BY) license (http://creativecommons.org/licenses/by/4.0/).

MDPI
St. Alban-Anlage 66
4052 Basel
Switzerland
Tel. +41 61 683 77 34
Fax +41 61 302 89 18
www.mdpi.com

Journal of Clinical Medicine Editorial Office
E-mail: jcm@mdpi.com
www.mdpi.com/journal/jcm

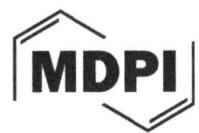

www.ingramcontent.com/pod-product-compliance
Lightning Source LLC
LaVergne TN
LVHW070408100526
838202LV00014B/1414